High Risk Emergencies

Guest Editors

JEFFREY TABAS, MD
TERI REYNOLDS, MD, PhD

EMERGENCY MEDICINE CLINICS OF NORTH AMERICA

www.emed.theclinics.com

Consulting Editor
AMAL MATTU, MD

February 2010 • Volume 28 • Number 1

SAUNDERS an imprint of ELSEVIER, Inc.

W.B. SAUNDERS COMPANY

A Division of Elsevier Inc.

1600 John F. Kennedy Boulevard • Suite 1800 • Philadelphia, Pennsylvania 19103-2899

http://www.theclinics.com

EMERGENCY MEDICINE CLINICS OF NORTH AMERICA Volume 28, Number 1
February 2010 ISSN 0733-8627, ISBN-13: 978-1-4377-1814-0

Editor: Patrick Manley
Developmental Editor: Theresa Collier

Emergency Medicine Clinics of North America (ISSN 0733-8627) is published quarterly by Elsevier Inc., 360 Park Avenue South, New York, NY, 10010-1710. Months of issue are February, May, August, and November. Business and Editorial Offices: 1600 John F. Kennedy Boulevard, Suite 1800, Philadelphia, PA 19103-2899. Customer Service Office: 6277 Sea Harbor Drive, Orlando, FL 32887-4800. Periodicals postage paid at New York, NY, and additional mailing offices. Subscription prices are $127.00 per year (US students), $247.00 per year (US individuals), $414.00 per year (US institutions), $180.00 per year (international students), $354.00 per year (international individuals), $499.00 per year (international institutions), $180.00 per year (Canadian students), $305.00 per year (Canadian individuals), and $499.00 per year (Canadian institutions). International air speed delivery is included in all *Clinics'* subscription prices. All prices are subject to change without notice. **POSTMASTER:** Send address changes to *Emergency Medicine Clinics of North America,* Elsevier Periodicals Customer Service, 11830 Westline Industrial Drive, St. Louis, MO 63146. Customer Service (orders, claims, online, change of address): Elsevier Periodicals Customer Service, 11830 Westline Industrial Drive, St. Louis, MO 63146. Tel: 1-800-654-2452 (U.S. and Canada); 314-453-7041 (outside U.S. and Canada). Fax: 314-453-5170. E-mail: journalscustomerservice-usa@elsevier.com (for print support); journalsonline support-usa@elsevier.com (for online support).

Reprints. For copies of 100 or more of articles in this publication, please contact the Commercial Reprints Department, Elsevier Inc., 360 Park Avenue South, New York, NY 10010-1710. Tel.: 212-633-3812; Fax: 212-462-1935; E-mail: reprints@elsevier.com.

Emergency Medicine Clinics of North America is covered in *MEDLINE/PubMed (Index Medicus), Current Contents/Clinical Medicine, EMBASE/Excerpta Medica, BIOSIS, SciSearch, CINAHL, ISI/BIOMED,* and *Research Alert.*

Printed and bound by CPI Group (UK) Ltd, Croydon, CR0 4YY
Transferred to Digital Print 2011

Contributors

CONSULTING EDITOR

AMAL MATTU, MD, FAAEM, FACEP
Program Director, Emergency Medicine Residency, Associate Professor, Department of Emergency Medicine, University of Maryland School of Medicine, Baltimore, Maryland

GUEST EDITORS

JEFFREY TABAS, MD
Associate Professor of Clinical Emergency Medicine, Director of Outcomes and Innovations for Continuing Medical Education, UCSF School of Medicine; Attending Physician and Director of Performance Improvement San Francisco General Hospital Emergency Department, San Francisco, California

TERI REYNOLDS, MD, PhD
Clinical Fellow in Emergency Ultrasound, Department of Emergency Medicine, UCSF, San Francisco, California

AUTHORS

LARRY J. BARAFF, MD
UCLA Emergency Medicine Center, David Geffen School of Medicine at UCLA, Los Angeles, California

ILENE CLAUDIUS, MD
Department of Emergency Medicine, University of Southern California and Children's Hospital, Los Angeles, California

JAMES D'AGOSTINO, MD
Assistant Professor of Emergency Medicine and Pediatrics, Department of Emergency Medicine, Pediatric Emergency Medicine, Upstate Medical University, Syracuse, New York

MOHAMMAD DIAB, MD
Associate Professor and Chief, Pediatric Orthopaedics, UCSF Department of Orthopaedic Surgery, San Francisco, California

MICHAEL A. GIBBS, MD, FACEP
Chief, Department of Emergency Medicine, Maine Medical Center, Portland, Maine; Professor, Department of Emergency Medicine, Tufts University School of Medicine, Boston, Massachusetts

ERIC D. ISAACS, MD, FACEP, FAAEM
Professor, Department of Emergency Medicine, University of California, San Francisco; Medical Director, Emergency Department, San Francisco General Hospital, San Francisco, California

IAN D. JONES, MD
Associate Professor, Department of Emergency Medicine, Vanderbilt University Medical Center, Oxford House, Nashville, Tennessee; Associate Professor, Department of Biomedical Informatics, Vanderbilt University Medical Center, Oxford House, Nashville, Tennessee; Adult Emergency Department, Vanderbilt University Medical Center, Oxford House, Nashville, Tennessee

SCOTT P. KAISER, MD
Resident, UCSF Department of Orthopaedic Surgery, San Francisco, California

JENNIFER C. LAINE, MD
Resident, UCSF Department of Orthopaedic Surgery, San Francisco, California

WILLIAM B. LENNARZ, MD
Director, Pediatric Emergency Medicine, Legacy Health System, Legacy Emanuel Hospital, Portland, Oregon; Codirector, Legacy Health Pediatric Emergency Medicine Fellowship, Oregon Health Sciences University, Portland, Oregon

DIKU MANDAVIA, MD, FACEP, FRCPC
Clinical Associate Professor in Emergency Medicine, LA County+USC Medical Center; Attending Physician, Cedars-Sinai Medical Center, Los Angeles, California

ROBERT C. MACKERSIE, MD, FACS
Professor of Surgery, University of California, San Francisco; Director, Trauma Services, Department of Surgery, San Francisco General Hospital, San Francisco, California

THOMAS MAILHOT, MD, RDMS
Instructor in Clinical Medicine, Assistant Residency Director, LA County+USC Medical Center, Los Angeles, California

FLAVIA NOBAY, MD
Assistant Professor and Residency Program Director, Department of Emergency Medicine, University of Rochester, Rochester, New York

CHARLOTTE PAGE WILLS, MD
Department of Emergency Medicine, Alameda County Medical Center-Highland Hospital, Oakland, California

PHILLIPS PERERA, MD, RDMS, FACEP
Assistant Clinical Professor of Emergency Medicine, Emergency Ultrasound Director, New York Presbyterian Hospital, Columbia University Medical Center, New York, New York

SUSAN B. PROMES, MD, FACEP
Professor and Vice Chair for Education, Department of Emergency Medicine, University of California San Francisco, San Francisco, California

DAVID RILEY, MD, MS, RDMS
Assistant Clinical Professor of Emergency Medicine, Associate Emergency Ultrasound Director, New York Presbyterian Hospital, Columbia University Medical Center, New York, New York

JENNIFER ROSSI, MD
Resident, Emergency Medicine, Division of Emergency Medicine, Stanford University School of Medicine, Palo Alto, California

CRAIG G. SMOLLIN, MD
Assistant Professor of Emergency Medicine, Department of Emergency Medicine, University of California San Francisco; Assistant Medical Director, California Poison Control System, San Francisco Division; San Francisco General Hospital, Emergency Services, San Francisco, California

COREY M. SLOVIS, MD
Professor of Emergency Medicine and Medicine, Department of Emergency Medicine, Vanderbilt University Medical Center, Oxford House; Medical Director, Metro Nashville Fire Department; Medical Director, Nashville International Airport, Nashville, Tennessee

MATTHEW C. STREHLOW, MD
Assistant Clinical Professor of Emergency Medicine, Assistant Clinical Professor of Surgery, Division of Emergency Medicine, Department of Surgery, Stanford University School of Medicine; Associate Clinical Director, Emergency Department, Stanford University Hospital and Clinics, Stanford, Palo Alto, California

MEGAN C. SWAN, MD
Resident, Emergency Medicine, Division of Emergency Medicine, Stanford University School of Medicine, Palo Alto, California

STUART P. SWADRON, MD, FRCP(C), FAAEM, FACEP
Vice-Chair of Education and Residency Program Director, Department of Emergency Medicine, Los Angeles County/USC Medical Center; Associate Professor, Keck School of Medicine of the University of Southern California, Los Angeles, California

ROBERT J. VISSERS, MD
Director, Emergency Department; and Associate Chief Medical Officer, Legacy Emanuel Hospital; Adjunct Associate Professor, Department of Emergency Medicine, Oregon Health Sciences University, Portland, Oregon

DOUGLAS W. WHITE, MD
Department of Emergency Medicine, Alameda County Medical Center-Highland Hospital, Oakland, California

MEGANN YOUNG, MD
Department of Emergency Medicine, Alameda County Medical Center-Highland Hospital, Oakland, California

Contents

evaluation. MRSA infections are now common and should be considered in all patients with pyoderma, severe pneumonia, and catheter-related sepsis. HSV infection of the CNS should be considered whenever a patient has altered mental status and CSF findings are not diagnostic of bacterial meningitis. Fever rarely represents life-threatening pathology; however, a handful of less common serious causes of pediatric fever exist with the potential for morbidity and mortality.

Pediatric patients often present to the emergency department with orthopedic pathology that can challenge the emergency department physician. This article focuses on key diagnoses that are frequently mismanaged. These diagnoses require specific knowledge to execute appropriate treatment. Pediatric fractures, compartmental syndrome, bone and joint infection, limp and non-accidental trauma are reviewed. Approach to the workup of these patients and treatment algorithms are discussed.

The diagnosis of appendicitis is fraught with potential pitfalls, and despite its prevalence, appendicitis continues to be a condition at high risk for missed and delayed diagnosis. There is no single historical or physical finding or laboratory test that can definitively make the diagnosis. This article discusses the value of presenting signs, symptoms, laboratory testing, and the rational use of various imaging modalities, such as CT scanning and ultrasound. Challenges of special populations, such as children, the elderly, and pregnant patients, are also discussed. Although appendicitis continues to be a source of medical legal risk and misdiagnosis, a clear understanding of the strengths and limitations of all tests in suspected appendicitis can improve the emergency physician's diagnostic accuracy in this high-risk disease.

Pediatric disorders that involve actual or potential airway compromise are among the most challenging cases that emergency department providers face. This article discusses the diagnosis and management of common and uncommon conditions in infants and children who may present with airway obstruction.

Headache is the fifth most common primary complaint of patients presenting to an emergency department (ED) in the United States. The emergency physician (EP) plays a unique role in the management of these patients, one that differs from that of the primary care physician, the neurologist, and other specialists. Diagnostic nomenclature used in the ED is necessarily less specific, as care is more appropriately focused on the relief of symptoms and the identification of life-threatening causes. By seeking a limited number of specific critical features on history and physical examination, the EP can minimize the risk of overlooking one of these dangerous causes of headache. When certain features are present, empirical therapies and diagnostic testing should be initiated in the ED. The most frequently encountered pitfalls in the management of patients with headache in emergency medicine practice, and those with the greatest likelihood to adversely affect patient outcomes, are discussed.

Although most poisonings require only supportive care, the emergency physician must recognize when the use of an antidote is required, and understand the risks and benefits of the treatment rendered. Although the more commonly instituted specific therapy in acute poisoning is the administration of intravenous fluids followed by the administration of oxygen, in certain circumstances prompt administration of a specific antidote may be required, and failure to identify these circumstances may lead to significant morbidity or mortality. This article describes select antidotes, and discusses their indications and potential pitfalls.

This article illustrates the challenges practitioners face evaluating shortness of breath, a common emergency department complaint. Through a series of patient encounters, pitfalls in the evaluation of shortness of breath are reviewed and discussed.

Risk stratification and management of the patient with low-risk chest pain continues to be challenging despite the considerable effort of numerous investigators. Evidence exists that a specific subset of young patients can be defined as low risk in whom further testing may not be necessary. A high index of suspicion of acute coronary syndrome (ACS) and an understanding of the many, subtle, and atypical presentations of ischemic heart disease are required. The initial history, electrocardiogram (ECG), and biomarkers are important, but serial ECGs and biomarkers improve sensitivity in detecting ACS. Unless chest pain is clearly explained, objective testing, such as exercise treadmill testing, nuclear scintigraphy, stress echocardiography, or coronary computed tomography angiogram, should be considered before, or soon after, discharge.

There are few conditions in emergency medicine as potentially challenging and high-risk as the difficult or failed airway. The emergency physician must be able to anticipate the difficult or failed airway, recognize associated physiologic deficits, and plan accordingly. Preparation, pretreatment strategies, and selection of alternative airway devices may mitigate the potential morbidity and management failure associated with the high-risk airway. There are a myriad of airway devices new to emergency medicine, which can increase the chance of successful airway management and rescue. Understanding why the airway is potentially difficult and assessing whether oxygenation can be maintained can guide the clinician's strategy and technique for successful management of the high-risk airway.

The focus of this article is first-trimester bleeding. Vaginal bleeding during the first 3 months of pregnancy is a common event. It is important that the emergency physicians recognize patients with vaginal bleeding who may have an adverse outcome if misdiagnosed or not treated appropriately in the emergency department. Causes of first-trimester vaginal bleeding include implantation bleeding, spontaneous abortions, ectopic pregnancy, and lesions involving the female reproductive system and perineal area infections.

Violent and agitated patients are high risk because they may pose a physical threat to the staff, may harm themselves, and may have dangerous comorbidities and illness that are causing the violence. The emergency physician must quickly control these behaviors, and thoroughly identify and treat their etiology, while simultaneously protecting the patients' rights and reducing the risks of injury to themselves, other patients, and medical staff. This article highlights potentially high-risk situations and describes corresponding mitigation tactics.

THE CLINICS ARE NOW AVAILABLE ONLINE!
Access your subscription at:
www.theclinics.com

GOAL STATEMENT
The goal of *Emergency Medicine Clinics of North America* is to keep practicing physicians up to date with current clinical practice in emergency medicine by providing timely articles reviewing the state of the art in patient care.

ACCREDITATION
The *Emergency Medical Clinics of North America* is planned and implemented in accordance with the Essential Areas and Policies of the Accreditation Council for Continuing Medical Education (ACCME) through the joint sponsorship of the University of Virginia School of Medicine and Elsevier. The University of Virginia School of Medicine is accredited by the ACCME to provide continuing medical education for physicians.

The University of Virginia School of Medicine designates this educational activity for a maximum of 15 *AMA PRA Category 1 Credits*™ for each issue, 60 credits per year. Physicians should only claim credit commensurate with the extent of their participation in the activity.

The American Medical Association has determined that physicians not licensed in the US who participate in this CME activity are eligible for a maximum of 15 *AMA PRA Category 1 Credits*™ for each issue, 60 credits per year.

The Emergency Medicine Clinics of North America CME program is approved by the American College of Emergency Physicians for 60 hours of ACEP Category I Credit per year.

Credit can be earned by reading the text material, taking the CME examination online at http://www.theclinics.com/home/cme, and completing the evaluation. After taking the test, you will be required to review any and all incorrect answers. Following completion of the test and evaluation, your credit will be awarded and you may print your certificate.

FACULTY DISCLOSURE/CONFLICT OF INTEREST
The University of Virginia School of Medicine, as an ACCME accredited provider, endorses and strives to comply with the Accreditation Council for Continuing Medical Education (ACCME) Standards of Commercial Support, Commonwealth of Virginia statutes, University of Virginia policies and procedures, and associated federal and private regulations and guidelines on the need for disclosure and monitoring of proprietary and financial interests that may affect the scientific integrity and balance of content delivered in continuing medical education activities under our auspices.

The University of Virginia School of Medicine requires that all CME activities accredited through this institution be developed independently and be scientifically rigorous, balanced and objective in the presentation/discussion of its content, theories and practices.

All authors/editors participating in an accredited CME activity are expected to disclose to the readers relevant financial relationships with commercial entities occurring within the past 12 months (such as grants or research support, employee, consultant, stock holder, member of speakers bureau, etc.). The University of Virginia School of Medicine will employ appropriate mechanisms to resolve potential conflicts of interest to maintain the standards of fair and balanced education to the reader. Questions about specific strategies can be directed to the Office of Continuing Medical Education, University of Virginia School of Medicine, Charlottesville, Virginia.

The faculty and staff of the University of Virginia Office of Continuing Medical Education have no financial affiliations to disclose.

The authors/editors listed below have identified no professional or financial affiliations for themselves or their spouse/partner:
Larry J. Baraff, MD; Ilene Claudius, MD; James D'Agostino, MD; Mohammad Diab, MD; Michael A. Gibbs, MD, FACEP; Eric D. Isaacs, MD, FACEP, FAAEM; Scott P. Kaiser, MD; Jennifer C. Laine, MD; William B. Lennarz, MD; Robert C. Mackersie, MD, FACS; Thomas Mailhot, MD, RDMS; Patrick Manley (Acquisitions Editor); Amal Mattu, MD, FAAEM, FACEP (Consulting Editor); Flavia Nobay, MD; Charlotte Page Wills, MD; Teri Reynolds, MD, PhD (Guest Editor); David Riley, MD, MS, RDMS; Jennifer Rossi, MD; Corey M. Slovis, MD; Craig Smollin, MD; Matthew C. Strehlow, MD; Stuart Swadron, MD, FRCP(C), FAAEM, FACEP; Megan C. Swan, MD; Jeffrey Tabas, MD (Guest Editor); Robert J. Vissers, MD; Douglas W. White, MD; Bill Woods, MD (Test Author); and Megann Young, MD.

The authors/editors listed below have identified the following professional or financial affiliations for themselves or their spouse/partner:
Ian D. Jones, MD is a patent holder and has stock/ownership in Apogee Informatics Company.
Diku Mandavia, MD, FACEP, FRCPC serves as a consultant for Sonosite, Inc.
Phillips Perera, MD, RDMS FACEP is employed and is a consultant at SonoSite Ultrasound.
Susan B. Promes, MD, FACEP receives royalties as an editor of textbooks for McGraw Hill.

Disclosure of Discussion of Non-FDA Approved Uses for Pharmaceutical Products and/or Medical Devices.
The University of Virginia School of Medicine, as an ACCME provider, requires that all faculty presenters identify and disclose any off-label uses for pharmaceutical and medical device products. The University of Virginia School of Medicine recommends that each physician fully review all the available data on new products or procedures prior to clinical use.

TO ENROLL
To enroll in the Emergency Medicine Clinics of North America Continuing Medical Education program, call customer service at 1-800-654-2452 or visit us online at www.theclinics.com/home/cme. The CME program is available to subscribers for an additional fee of $195.00.

Foreword

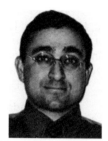

Amal Mattu, MD, FAAEM, FACEP
Consulting Editor

A common teaching in emergency medicine is that the first goal in patient evaluation is to rule out the worst possible condition. Once this goal has been accomplished, whether by history and physical examination alone or with additional testing, one can then proceed to evaluate the patient for the non–life threats and consider discharging the patient for outpatient follow-up. To rule out these high-risk conditions, however, the treating health care provider must first have a sound knowledge of what the life-threats are, the typical and (especially) the atypical presentations of these conditions, and their optimal treatment modalities. The provider must also be aware of the common pitfalls that may occur during the evaluation and treatment process: To avoid a trap, one must first know what a trap looks like.

In this issue of *Emergency Medicine Clinics of North America*, the guest editors, Drs Jeff Tabas and Teri Reynolds, have assembled an outstanding group of authors to address many of the highest-risk medical conditions we face in the specialty of emergency medicine. They specifically focus on the challenges in both diagnosing and treating these conditions. Rather than simply providing a series of diagnosis-related articles, the editors and authors have focused this text on what is most relevant to emergency health care providers: the chief complaint. Most articles address the deadly diseases that present via common chief complaints, such as fever, headache, dyspnea, trauma, chest pain, and vaginal bleeding. Additional articles are added to focus on high-risk patient groups, such as pediatric patients and violent patients. Both pediatric and adult airway disasters are addressed in detail. Two additional articles focus purely on patients in shock. Finally, a separate article is added to address one of the most commonly misdiagnosed high-risk conditions: acute appendicitis.

This issue of *Emergency Medicine Clinics* is an invaluable addition to the library of emergency physicians and other health care providers who diagnose and manage patients in acute care settings. This issue should be considered must-reading for all emergency health care providers, including attending emergency and urgent-care physicians, trainees, and midlevel providers. Knowledge and practice of the concepts

Emerg Med Clin N Am 28 (2010) xiii–xiv
doi:10.1016/j.emc.2009.10.007
0733-8627/09/$ – see front matter © 2010 Elsevier Inc. All rights reserved.

discussed in the following pages are certain to save lives. The guest editors and authors are to be commended for providing this outstanding resource for our specialty.

Amal Mattu, MD, FAAEM, FACEP
Department of Emergency Medicine
University of Maryland School of Medicine
Emergency Medicine Residency
Baltimore, MD, USA

E-mail address:
amattu@smail.umaryland.edu

Preface

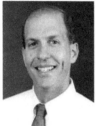 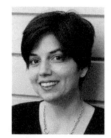

Jeffrey Tabas, MD   Teri Reynolds, MD, PhD
Guest Editors

Every specialty has its high-risk diagnoses, but emergency medicine is its own high-risk diagnosis—doctoring performed emergently and with limited information carries increased risk for provider and patient. Long-term patient relationships in the emergency department are measured in hours and critical decisions made in a fraction of a second. There are sudden sporadic surges in patient volume and acuity, and the majority of care (76%) is delivered during "off hours." Patient-physician communication may be limited by logistics or linguistics, inebriation or intoxication, time constraints or bizarre complaints. In other words, some would argue that emergency medicine and "high-risk" medicine are redundant terms.

At the same time, we are specialists at managing this risk: Emergency medicine offers the opportunity to synthesize history and examination, to make new diagnoses, to intervene quickly and definitively, and, ultimately, to accompany patients through unprecedented moments in their lives. The role of contingency can be overwhelming in a field that has been described as "Anyone, Anything, Anytime,"[1] but we choose it because it offers so many opportunities to do things right.

There will always be, of course, many more ways to do things wrong than there are to do things right, and even doing things right may not be enough: Many lawsuits and judgments have arisen out of cases where everything was done right. In this issue, we address major categories of error and scenarios that consistently challenge clinical reasoning. We also look at the diagnoses responsible for the majority of lawsuits and the majority of dollars awarded in judgments.[2]

We have carefully selected authors who can address and explain these challenges by virtue of their educational leadership and active practice of emergency medicine and related specialties. We may be caught unaware by a common disease because it presents atypically, or miss another because it is rare: "Pitfalls in the Evaluation of Shortness of Breath" addresses both ends of this spectrum. Some environments may challenge our capacities for diagnosis and communication: "Pitfalls in the Evaluation and Resuscitation of the Trauma Patient" examines the culture and chaos of the trauma bay. We address the adult-sized risk that comes with pediatric patients in "Pediatric Emergencies Associated with Fever," "Pediatric Airway Nightmares," and

Emerg Med Clin N Am 28 (2010) xv–xvi
doi:10.1016/j.emc.2009.10.008
0733-8627/09/$ – see front matter © 2010 Elsevier Inc. All rights reserved.

"High-Risk Pediatric Orthopedic Pitfalls," and look at the golden hour of initial intervention in "The High-Risk Airway," "Early Identification of Shock in the Critically Ill," and "The RUSH Examination: Rapid Ultrasound in Shock in the Evaluation of the Critically Ill." We address particular diagnostic and therapeutic challenges with "Toxicology: Pearls and Pitfalls in the Use of Antidotes," "Pitfalls in First-Trimester Bleeding," and "The Violent or Agitated Patient." Finally, we cover the common diagnoses that carry uncommon risk in "Pitfalls in Appendicitis," "Pitfalls in the Management of Headache in the Emergency Department," and "Pitfalls in Evaluating the Low-Risk Chest-Pain Patient."

Turning a clinical eye to risk itself is a means of mitigating its impact on our patients and our practice. In the same way that we learned to integrate multitasking, sign out, diagnostic uncertainty, and the demand for rapid synthesis, so can we manage risk like any other component of our unique practice environment.

Jeffrey Tabas, MD
UCSF School of Medicine, San Francisco, California, USA

Teri Reynolds, MD, PhD
Department of Emergency Medicine
505 Parnassus, Box 0208
UCSF, San Francisco, CA 94143, USA

E-mail addresses:
jeff.tabas@emergency.ucsf.edu (J. Tabas)
teri.reynolds@ucsf.edu (T. Reynolds)

REFERENCES

1. Zink BJ. Anyone, anything, anytime: a history of emergency medicine. 1st edition. Philadelphia: Mosby Elsevier; 2006. xvi, p. 310.
2. Karcz A, Holbrook J, Auerbach BS, et al. Preventability of malpractice claims in emergency medicine: a closed claims study. Ann Emerg Med 1990;19(8):865–73.

Pitfalls in the Evaluation and Resuscitation of the Trauma Patient

Robert C. Mackersie, MD, FACS[a,b,*]

KEYWORDS

• Medical error • Pitfalls • Trauma • Resuscitation

THREATS, VULNERABILITIES, AND ERRORS

Although this article focuses on individual errors, providers are just one component of trauma care. Pitfalls in the management of the trauma patient occur not only as a result of misleading patient presentations but also as a result of inherent vulnerabilities in the system of care.

The care and management of the severely injured multiple trauma patient involves the interaction of various specialists, subspecialists, equipment, and other resources, all within an organized system of care. The infrastructure of this system involves a continuum of response and care from prehospital activation to long-term management. Notification (911 response), prehospital care and transport, the presence of designated and specialized facilities (trauma centers), and an organization that provides oversight are all components of this complex system. The overall structure and function of an ideal trauma system is described in federal documents[1] and by the American College of Surgeons.[2]

The resource-intensive and time-sensitive nature of trauma care creates a complex system with several potential pitfalls and vulnerabilities (**Table 1**). Patient inflow at major trauma centers is unpredictable, with periodic and abrupt surges in volume and acuity. Emergency and trauma physicians are often forced to make time-sensitive decisions with limited information. Opportunities for more extended evaluation, consultation, or even research are rare. The need to function during off-hours, late evenings, and early mornings may add to this effect. The need to provide seamless 24/7 coverage for a wide variety of services may be logistically difficult and

[a] University of California, San Francisco, CA, USA
[b] Department of Surgery, San Francisco General Hospital, 1001 Potrero Avenue, Ward 3A, San Francisco, CA 94110, USA
* Department of Surgery, San Francisco General Hospital, 1001 Potrero Avenue, Ward 3A, San Francisco, CA 94110.
E-mail address: rmackersie@sfghsurg.ucsf.edu

Emerg Med Clin N Am 28 (2010) 1–27
doi:10.1016/j.emc.2009.10.001

Table 1
Errors, pitfalls, and latent failures within a trauma system

Inherent Characteristic of Trauma System	Latent Failure (Vulnerability)	Potential Outcome, Error of Pitfall
Unpredictable and intermittent high patient volume & acuity	Transient staff and resource shortages, system incapacity	Practitioner errors & system "volume saturation" failures
Need for time-sensitive performance of providers and system as a whole	Inadequate response times, untimely communication	Delayed diagnosis & treatment of critical conditions
Long work hours, off-hours, exhausting pace, and high-risk patients	Stress & fatigue, diminished performance	Practitioner technical and/or management errors
Highest risk injuries occurring infrequently in many centers	Insufficient provider experience and/or knowledge base, stress	Practitioner technical and/or management errors
Multisystem injuries with silolike activity of services by specialty	Poor communication & fragmentation of care	Delays in diagnosis or treatment and provider errors
Residency training programs with rotating house staff (learning curve repeated every 1–2 mo)	Insufficient provider experience, inadequate knowledge & training, inadequate supervision	House staff technical and/or management errors
Large service information management demands (many patients, many studies, many details)	Incomplete, untimely, or inaccurate communication of information	Practitioner management errors, delayed diagnosis & treatment
Large potential for clinically occult injuries	Unsuspecting, inexperience, or improperly trained provider	Potentially high incidence of delayed or missed diagnoses
Constantly changing resources: technology, personnel, staffing levels, facilities, organizations, regulations, etc.	Staff and resource shortages, insufficient provider experience and knowledge & training	All of the above

occasionally may require expanding the pool of providers to those with more limited experience, interest, or knowledge. These factors may conspire to degrade the safety and reliability of the overall system of trauma care, creating additional latent hazards.

The goal is to devise a system of care to increase the redundancy of safety-related measures, to improve the resiliency of the system and its providers to errors, and ultimately to improve the outcome. The performance of such a system should be provider-independent, time-of-day-insensitive, and capable of responding to sudden, unexpected increases in volume and acuity.

In a popular model of errors called the "Swiss cheese" model, the environment is constantly producing hazards with the potential to cause adverse events. The safety in this model is created by layers of safeguards or defenses (the slices of cheese). However, each of these safeguards has defects represented by the holes in the slices of Swiss cheese (**Fig. 1**). Most of the time, the layers of defenses are effective at preventing adverse events, but on occasion, the holes in the system line up, creating a confluence of defects resulting in the occurrence of an adverse event.

Human (Provider) Errors

A clinical pitfall is a situation encountered in the course of treating patients that creates a predictable vulnerability to human error. The term "predictable" means that pitfalls are encountered regularly and that the erroneous decision making that occurs in response to the vulnerability may be forecast to some degree.

The study of human error has its roots in cognitive psychology, but it has been a focus for the health care profession only recently.[3,4] As early as the 1970s, Rasmussen and Jensen[5] categorized errors made by skilled electronics repair technicians as skill-based (eg, technical errors), rule-based (eg, deviations from guidelines or established practice patterns), and knowledge-based errors. Helmreich and Foushee[6] further characterized 5 types of errors based on observations conducted in the setting of commercial aviation:

- Task execution errors: typically includes technical slips and psychomotor errors (eg, chipping a tooth during endotracheal intubation), and judgment or perceptual errors causing a technical error (eg, liver injury caused by a chest tube placed much too low).
- Procedural errors: errors involving deviation from existing practice pattern or protocol (eg, failure to obtain a chest radiograph in a stable patient before placing a chest tube).
- Communication errors: communication of incorrect data, failure to communicate important data, delayed communication of critical data, and so on.
- Decision errors: errors in judgment related to patient management caused by the incorrect interpretation of data, insufficient knowledge, or other related factors.
- Intentional noncompliance.

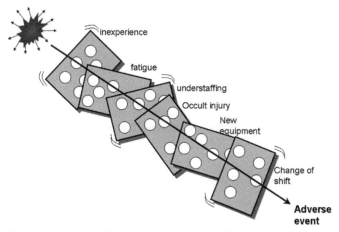

Fig. 1. The "Swiss cheese" model for errors. Hazards and threats spun off in a given environment do not produce adverse events unless defects (failures) in the layers of defenses or safeguards occur in concert with each other. The result of these "holes lining up" is an adverse event. (*Adapted from* Reason J. Human error: models and management. BMJ 2000;320:768–70; with permission.)

Of all the error-based events occurring in the care of trauma patients, missed injuries (or delayed diagnoses) are perhaps the most pervasive and often the most serious. These events typically involve either the improper selection of information (knowledge-based decision errors) or the improper processing of that information (rule-based and procedural errors). Of these decision errors, there are 3 in particular that are regularly made during the diagnostic evaluation of trauma patients.

Diagnostic labeling
Diagnostic labeling involves the use of a premature (and often presumptive) diagnosis as a "label" for a patient. The team of providers then subsequently refer to the patient by this "label" that leads to an assumption by other providers that the diagnosis is definitive, despite the lack of confirmatory data. Labeling may be one of the most tempting and potentially hazardous errors made in the initial assessment of the trauma patient. Even when subsequent diagnostic information conflicts with the labeled diagnosis, changing the label is impeded by "confirmation bias," which is the inherent reluctance to relinquish a current diagnosis despite conflicting clinical information. Diagnostic labeling may also distract from or discourage a more complete diagnostic evaluation and/or intervention. A patient with the label "stab wound to the arm," for example, may be a patient with an obvious upper extremity laceration, whose ruptured spleen is missed. The labeling distracts the clinicians from considering the possibility of both blunt and penetrating injuries.

False-negative prediction
False-negative prediction occurs when an inappropriately high negative predictive value is attributed to a given physical finding, imaging study, or laboratory value. Examples include (1) the abdomen is soft and nontender, so intra-abdominal hemorrhage can be effectively excluded, (2) the heart rate is normal, so the low blood pressure is unlikely to represent hemorrhagic shock, and (3) the computed tomographic (CT) scan is normal, so the patient does not have a serious intra-abdominal injury and the abdominal tenderness must be due to something else (see false attribution in a later section). Most physical findings, laboratory studies, and even imaging studies have insufficient sensitivity to definitively rule out serious injury at initial presentation.

False attribution
False attribution involves erroneously linking a clinical finding to an unrelated cause. False attribution (of signs or symptoms, laboratory or x-ray findings, etc) often involves the cognitive process of selectively using clinical information, and the consequences to a severely injured trauma patient may be devastating. For example, attributing hypotension to a vasovagal response or to a malfunctioning automated blood pressure machine when the actual cause is hemorrhage, or attributing a tender abdomen to an abdominal wall contusion when the actual cause is peritonitis from a perforated viscus can be fatal for the patient.

Approach to the Management of the Trauma Patient
The practice of providing trauma care to victims of critical injury is inherently a rapidly changing, dynamic process. Providers must often make critical decisions in the setting of limited diagnostic information and variable resources, and then they must continually revise these judgments without letting prior decisions limit the perception of a patient's evolving condition. The classical dictum "assume nothing, trust no one" in some respects characterizes a general approach to critically injured patients. Several general principles may also be applicable:

- *Patients should generally be managed according to the worst "reasonable case" scenario*. This is particularly true with respect to diagnostic evaluation and patient monitoring. A more liberal approach to diagnostic studies, including imaging and even invasive procedures when indicated, is often consistent with the goal of minimizing overall risks to the patient.
- *Listen carefully, but remain a bit skeptical about the history of injury*. Injury scenes are often chaotic and the information available to the prehospital crew is incomplete. Falls are not always falls, assaults may involve both blunt and penetrating mechanisms, and patients "found down," particularly in urban environments, may have sustained a wide variety of injuries.
- *Look carefully at the patient*. Subtle findings are often overlooked on rapid physical examination and can make critical differences in some situations: ice pick wounds to the heart with entry at the areolar margin of the nipple, stab wounds to the neck obscured by the cervical collar, the gunshot wound to the tympanic canal that is labeled as a blunt assault with hemotympanum, and the patient "found down" who was actually run over, sustaining massive pelvic fractures, are examples of situations where the clinical history may be misleading.
- *Constantly reassess, never assume "stability."* Trauma patients can deteriorate physiologically in seconds and there is often a tendency to disbelieve this deterioration, wishing the patient to do well. This tendency can lead to complacency in the setting of a critical and rapidly changing condition.
- *Trauma is a team sport; be cooperative and maintain collegiality*. Save interpersonal disputes and confrontation until after the patient has been cared for. Use institutional mechanisms, as needed, for conflict resolution. It is the patient who suffers when there is a team conflict.
- *Maintain the "clock speed"* for diagnosis and management. Be aware of the specific time sensitivities for various injuries (eg, limb ischemia) and prioritize accordingly.
- *Never become married to the initial diagnosis*. This error consists of both diagnostic labeling and cognitive processing in which a provider makes the data fit the diagnosis rather than vice versa (see earlier section).
- Look for risk-reduction strategies in diagnostic monitoring and management.

TEAM DYNAMICS DURING TRAUMA RESUSCITATIONS

The initial evaluation and management of the trauma patient involves a multidisciplinary group of providers and ancillary personnel. The size of the resuscitation team varies from center to center according to the acuity of the patient, with larger teams in academic level I trauma centers. In some situations, members of the resuscitation team might be unfamiliar with the other providers. In teaching environments with rotating resident and attending staff, there is a constantly changing resuscitation team and a wide variation in levels of skill and experience, creating myriad opportunities for knowledge and communication errors. Errors in the resuscitation room (or operating room [OR]) may result more commonly from failure in team dynamics or from the manner in which team members interact than from individual medical errors (**Box 1**).

The management of high risk, high acuity, trauma patients requires frequent monitoring of a large number of rapidly changing physiologic and laboratory parameters. As clinical threats develop, the situational awareness and responsiveness on the part of the resuscitation or operative team becomes a critical determinant of successful management. The use of OR simulation has been used by Gaba and others for the

---

Box 1
Examples of potential problems (failures) in team dynamics during trauma resuscitations

Errors in communication

  Incomplete report by paramedic crew (missing critical information)

  Changes in patient's physiologic status not communicated

  Clinical findings not made clear to the resuscitation team by the team leader

  Overall management plan not clearly outlined by the team leader

  Unavailability of instruments or resuscitation equipment not communicated by the nursing staff

  Failure to notify appropriate consultants

Errors in patient management due to a failure to maintain situational awareness

  Incomplete history or physical examination

  Inadequate patient physiologic monitoring (eg, arterial and central venous pressure [CVP] lines)

  Inadequate patient laboratory monitoring (eg, coagulation rates, hematocrit test, base deficit measurement, and arterial blood gas test)

  Failure to recognize shock and/or ongoing blood loss

  Failure to recognize worsening hypothermia, acidosis, or coagulopathy

  Failure to maintain adequate supply of blood and blood products during massive transfusion

Errors in staffing or workload distribution

  Inexperienced and/or poorly oriented staff (eg, medical students participating in major resuscitations)

  Staffing availability not commensurate with patient volume and acuity

  Insufficiently experienced or trained house staff or an attending staff conducting a difficult procedure

  Surgical or anesthesiology staff distracted or pulled away because of other trauma patients

  Lack of adequate supervision of house staff by attending staff

Conflict resolution issues

  Unresolved hostility due to perceived inadequate performance by other team members

  Disagreement regarding scope of responsibility and team leadership

  Disagreement regarding overall management plans or conduct of a procedure

---

purpose of improving team dynamics and skills in the OR environment.[7–12] Derived from the approach taken by commercial aviation in crew resource management, a program termed Anesthesia Crisis Resource Management (ACRM) can be used to record, analyze, and ultimately improve individual and team interactions in the OR.[13,14] A similar approach has been applied to trauma resuscitations.[15–17]

Clinical medicine clearly has much to learn from studies of team dynamics. Optimal behavior in the setting of major resuscitations and critical operative procedures has not been defined for medical teams, but several specific behavioral markers have been identified in the study of commercial aviation that are seen to help mitigate threats and errors. Some of these behavioral markers, adapted to a medical context, are shown in **Table 2**. Many of these may have applicability both in the OR and in the resuscitation room.[18]

Resuscitation Team Organization and Function

In addition to the behavioral markers outlined in **Table 2**, several other pitfalls in resuscitation team dynamics have been identified:

- Failure to identify the team leader and to establish the roles of team members.
- Changing roles in the midst of a resuscitation, often when a more senior team member usurps the role of team leader. In the absence of clear communication and continuity of purpose, this may lead to redundant or conflicting instructions and general confusion.
- Failure of team members to be assertive in 2 areas: (1) making the team aware of changes in a patient's condition or critical diagnostic findings and (2) making the team leader aware of incipient errors in communication or patient management.
- Failure of the team leader to communicate not only specific instructions but also the overall plan and direction for the resuscitation.
- Failure to maintain situational awareness. This may be related to other problems:
- ○ Failure of the team leader to encourage and be receptive to input from other team members.
- ○ Failure to establish appropriate monitoring and frequently reassess the patient.
- ○ Failure to identify situational threats including risky behaviors, questionable or incorrect decisions by inexperienced personnel, and so on.
- Failure to identify the high-risk patient and institute risk-reduction measures. There is a tendency to standardize treatment and monitoring for a given condition, as opposed to using preventative risk-reduction strategies tailored to a given patient.
- Failure of adequate supervision: teaching programs rely on supervision of less experienced personnel by more experienced personnel. Task execution, procedural, and decision-based errors may be the result of insufficient supervision.
- Crowd control: everyone wants to get into the act, and volunteers, students, and patients' families are often interested in participating. However, the roles of persons not directly administering care must be limited in the context of critical initial resuscitation.

In lieu of trauma simulations, trauma resuscitation videotaping has been used for many years to improve resuscitations.[19–21] The use of these techniques has been limited somewhat by concerns about confidentiality, but properly structured programs for trauma videotaping are consistent with Joint Commission and HIPAA (Health Insurance Portability and Accountability Act of 1996) requirements.

SPECIFIC PITFALLS: RESUSCITATION AND INITIAL EVALUATION
Airway Issues

Airway management remains the top priority in any major trauma resuscitation, and errors in airway management can lead to catastrophic outcomes. Airway management begins in the prehospital arena and is carried through to extubation and even intensive care unit (ICU) discharge. Common problems include the following

- Unrecognized prehospital esophageal intubations: esophageal intubations continue to occur at reported rates ranging from 0.5% to more than 6%.[22] They often occur in the setting of difficult airways, pediatric patients, and/or severely injured patients. The large number of prehospital providers relative to

Table 2
Behavioral markers for team function in medical environments

Briefing	The required briefing was interactive and operationally thorough	Concise, not rushed, and met standard of practice Bottom lines were established
Plans stated	Operational plans and decisions were communicated and acknowledged	Shared understanding about plans—"everybody on the same page"
Workload assignment	Roles and responsibilities were defined for normal and nonnormal situations	Workload assignments were communicated and acknowledged
Contingency management	Team members developed effective strategies to manage threats to safety	Threats and their consequences were anticipated Used all available resources to manage threats
Monitor/Cross-check	Team members actively monitored and cross-checked patient status and team status	Patient and team status were verified
Workload management	Operational tasks were prioritized and properly managed to handle primary patient care responsibilities	Avoided task fixation Did not allow work overload
Vigilance	Team members remained alert of the environment and status of the patient	Team members maintained "situational awareness"
Automation management	Information and other technologies were properly managed to balance workload requirements	Equipment setup was briefed to other members Effective recovery techniques from equipment anomalies
Evaluation of plans	Existing plans were reviewed and modified when necessary	Team decisions and actions were openly analyzed to make sure the existing plan was the best plan
Inquiry	Team members were asked questions to investigate and/or clarify current plans of action	Team members were not afraid to express a lack of knowledge "nothing taken for granted" attitude
Assertiveness	Team members stated critical information and/or solutions with appropriate persistence	Team members spoke up without hesitation
Communication environment	Environment for open communication was established and maintained	Good cross talk—flow of information was fluid, clear, and direct
Leadership	Team leader/surgeon showed leadership and coordinated resus/operative deck activities	In command, decisive, and encouraged team participation

Adapted from Helmreich RL, Musson DM, Sexton JB. Human factors and safety in surgery. In: Manuel BM, Nora PF, editors. Surgical patient safety: essential information for surgeons in today's environment. 1st edition. Chicago (IL): American College of Surgeons; 2004; with permission.

the ongoing experience in endotracheal tube placement creates the latent failure in this setting and may be offset by a program of frequent simulation drills in airway management skills and/or one-on-one airway management instruction in the OR by anesthesiologists. In addition, the increasing use of continuous infrared capnography among prehospital providers has improved performance.[23] Other endotracheal tube misplacements, including supraglottic and right main stem placements, occur regularly but the effect on the patient is typically less. The lesson is to assume that a prehospital endotracheal tube is misplaced until its location is confirmed.

- The airway "flail." Obese patients with short necks, direct airway or neck injuries, aberrant anatomy, and potential C-spine injury create technical challenges. Failures in this setting include those similar to the general resuscitation: failure to identify threats and plan strategically and poor communication. It is imperative in these situations that the provider who is charged with the responsibility for airway management works closely with the surgeon in the event that a surgical airway is required. Techniques for rescue ventilation should ideally be part of a protocol and may include the use of Combitubes (Tyco Healthcare Group, Mansfield, MA, USA), laryngeal mask airways, or video laryngoscopy.[24–26] In addition, the use of potentially difficult airways as "teaching opportunities" must be carefully considered. Although it is crucial to train new providers in difficult intubations, unstable patients with little reserve should be intubated by the most experienced provider available, and the need for a backup and rescue airway approach should be anticipated for every intubation.
- The best surgical airway: with the increased use of percutaneous dilatational tracheostomy in the ICU and improvement in equipment, the percutaneous cricothyroidotomy, using the Seldinger approach, has become increasingly popular. The comfort levels for these techniques appear to be based on a provider's background and training: many surgeons remain most comfortable with surgical cricothyroidotomy while anesthesiologists and emergency physicians are often more comfortable with the percutaneous approach. Cadaveric studies are somewhat variable but may suggest that in nonsurgical hands, the percutaneous approach has some advantages.[27,28] As a general rule however, the provider's level of experience should dictate the technical approach.

In selecting the airway device to be used, it should be kept in mind that tracheostomy tubes may be more difficult to place in the heat of battle than in the controlled OR setting. Hypoxia and/or cricothyroid damage has been associated with attempts to pass larger or more rigid tracheostomy tubes in the emergency situation, and dependence on these tubes creates a latent failure. The use of a size 6 (or relatively small) cuffed endotracheal tube offers a flexible, easily inserted alternative to a rigid tracheostomy tube and can provide a more than adequate airway for temporary ventilation in critical situations.

Failure to Recognize Hemorrhagic Shock

As simple as it sounds, this is one of the more common lethal pitfalls encountered during the initial resuscitation. Although every provider in the trauma bay has an appreciation for the importance and critical nature of hemorrhagic shock, an early presentation of normotension may create the illusion of hemodynamic stability, ignoring the fact that a life-threatening 30% to 35% circulating blood volume loss may occur before the onset of hypotension and that a normal blood pressure is likely to be abnormal in the setting of acute pain and stress. The advanced trauma life support course classifies patients into the following categories[28]

- Normal age-specific blood pressure
- Responders: patients who respond to initial volume resuscitation and maintain an age-specific normal blood pressure thereafter
- Transient responders: patients who initially respond to volume resuscitation but suffer recurrent hypotension despite ongoing fluid or blood administration
- Nonresponders: patients who fail to normalize their blood pressure despite fluid or blood administration

Errors most commonly occur when there is some element of compensated shock. The patient with substantial ongoing hemorrhage and ongoing resuscitation may show an alternating pattern of normotension and hypotension. Providers may be lulled into believing that response to volume resuscitation with elevation of blood pressure, albeit transient, represents the cessation of hemorrhage or at least the cessation of shock. The so-called "saw-toothed" pattern of alternating normo and hypotension often reflects transient response to ongoing or intermittent fluid resuscitation (**Fig. 2**). The error is the assumption that each fluid bolus returns the patient to a state of normal physiology when, in fact, the overall shock state and acidosis is worsening. Patient tolerance of this situation depends on the age and the rate of ongoing blood loss. Eventually, the ability to compensate is overwhelmed, and the progressive ischemia and acidosis compromises myocardial performance, further decreasing cardiac output to the point of irreversible organ damage.

The failure to recognize hemorrhagic shock may also occur in the setting of a patient who is awake with relatively normal mental status. The error involves the misinterpretation of normal mental status as a sign of stability and may be a particular risk in the young adult patient who is awake and alert in the setting of profoundly decompensated shock and low systolic blood pressure. An otherwise healthy patient with an intact mechanism of cerebral autoregulation may have the capacity to maintain near

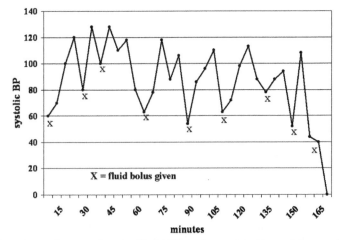

Fig. 2. Intermittent hypotension in the setting of ongoing hemorrhage and recurrent volume resuscitation. Despite the intermittent return of normal systolic BP, the patient remains in a prolonged shock state, which if not definitively corrected results in the patient's demise.

normal cerebral perfusion without major alterations in mental status until they "crash." Even when combative behavior is present, it may be mislabeled as a result of head injury or exogenous substance use rather than a sign of a severe shock state.

Other errors in recognizing a shock state may be made in the very young and very old. The elderly patient with a blood pressure of 120/70 mm Hg (who is normally hypertensive with a pressure of 180/100 mm Hg) may be in a decompensated shock state. Similarly a hypotensive child may be erroneously regarded as having an age-appropriate blood pressure. Other physical findings of a shock state may be overlooked, and the diagnosis is delayed until there is more profound decompensation.

Over- and Under-resuscitation

Most shock seen in the trauma setting is related to hypovolemia or inadequate cardiac preload. In patients with more severe injuries, the shock state and corresponding volume requirements may be extreme and variable, with resuscitation guided by little more than simple clinical monitors (eg, blood pressure, urine output, arterial base deficit). In this setting there is a high potential for either under or overresuscitation. The recognized downsides of underresuscitation include persistent acidosis, coagulopathy, prolonged shock state, and an increased potential risk of acute respiratory distress syndrome (ARDS) and multiple organ failure with increased mortality. The recognized downsides of overresuscitation include pulmonary edema and extensive tissue edema involving the abdominal wall, retroperitoneum, and viscera resulting in secondary abdominal compartment syndrome and the inability to primarily close the abdomen. Massive volume resuscitation may also promote the development of extremity compartment syndrome, even in patients with minor extremity injuries, and may also exacerbate intracranial pressure in the setting of traumatic brain injury.[29,30] Increases in chest wall, airway, and pulmonary edema may result in delayed ventilatory weaning and prolonged ICU stays. Even a minor degree of overresuscitation in the patient with severe pulmonary contusion may exacerbate lung edema and precipitate ARDS.

Theoretically, an optimal level of resuscitation exists for each trauma patient, varying over time and with individual physiology. Defining this optimum "on the fly" is problematic and has been the source of multiple investigations over the years. Shoemaker and colleagues[31] originally formulated a goal-directed approach to resuscitation with the directed augmentation of cardiac index and oxygen delivery. This approach is based on observations that patients with subnormal cardiac indices after shock or sepsis tend to do poorly compared with patients with higher cardiac indices. Several meta-analyses have tried to sort out conflicting reports and have suggested that goal-directed therapy may be of benefit in certain patient populations, such as preoperative and high-risk elective surgery patients.[32–34] In the trauma population, the benefit of goal-directed therapy remains unclear. In one recent prospective study, Velmahos and colleagues[34] failed to find significant overall improvements in mortality, organ failure, complications, or days in the ICU using a goal-directed approach to resuscitation, and concluded that cardiac index, oxygen delivery, and consumption responses were markers of physiologic reserve than valid resuscitation targets.

Although interventions that are designed to drive cardiac output and oxygen delivery to supranormal goals have not been shown to have efficacy in the trauma population, sufficient monitoring to detect deficient physiologic responses, particularly related to inadequate preload or inadequate cardiac reserve, is clearly important. Fluid resuscitation may be guided by the use of appropriate preload monitoring including central venous catheter lines, bedside ultrasonography, or pulmonary artery (PA) catheters. Latent failures in this setting include the lack of training and familiarity with advanced monitoring techniques, lack of knowledge regarding interpretation of the monitoring results, and inappropriate decision making associated with their use.

Failure to Properly Assess the Abdomen and Pelvis

Because abdominal injuries may be severe without manifesting overt clinical signs or symptoms, the abdominal examination is notoriously unreliable in the trauma patient. Mostly, diagnostic adjuncts such as CT, focused abdominal sonography for trauma (FAST), or even diagnostic peritoneal lavage (DPL) offer a means to accurate diagnoses. Despite this, the failure to appropriately evaluate the abdomen has been identified as the most common error in trauma management.[35,36] The most serious errors occur when the potential for major abdominal injury is overlooked altogether.

Strategies to avoid missed abdominal injuries or delayed diagnoses include obtaining an accurate history, maintaining a high index of suspicion, and the liberal use of imaging studies. In the patient without evidence of shock or who responds well to fluid resuscitation, CT scanning offers high sensitivity and specificity and is usually the appropriate diagnostic modality. In the patient with decompensated shock who fails to respond or responds only transiently to fluid resuscitation and is not stable enough for CT, other modalities such as FAST or DPL should be considered. Occasionally, in a patient with shock in the absence of other sources of hemorrhage, laparotomy is the best diagnostic and therapeutic approach.

Serious and potentially fatal errors may occur when the hemodynamic profile of the patient is not matched to the diagnostic modality. Most radiology departments are poorly equipped to run major trauma resuscitations, and preventable deaths have occurred as the result of attempts to complete abdominal CT scanning in patients with decompensated shock. Resuscitation is far from optimal in a CT suite with limited space, lighting, and equipment. The use of FAST for blunt abdominal trauma is well described and has utility as a screening examination for subsequent CT scanning and as a triage instrument for the OR. Extending the use of FAST for penetrating trauma creates a potential pitfall because of its inability to detect small amounts of intra-abdominal fluid associated with hollow viscus injuries. In experienced hands, FAST can detect about 200 mL of fluid in the peritoneal cavity. Subtle hollow viscus injury with little spillage is missed by this technique alone, although these injuries may also remain occult on early CT scan. The reported sensitivity of FAST for intraperitoneal injury varies widely between studies. A meta-analysis of 62 studies found an overall pooled sensitivity of 78.9% and specificity of 99.2%. Inclusion of only highest quality studies yielded a slightly lower sensitivity of 66.0%.[37] Inaccurate examinations can have serious consequences, and factors influencing inaccuracy include improper technique, operator experience, and inappropriate use in stable patients.

DPL is known to be highly sensitive (>97%) for detecting intra-abdominal injury but has low specificity, particularly in blunt trauma where most cases with hemoperitoneum resulting from minor solid organ injuries (eg, liver and spleen) can be managed without operative intervention. The sensitivity for DPL in the setting of penetrating trauma may be improved by adjusting the red blood cell (RBC) count threshold. The risk-reduction trade-offs are an increased sensitivity with lower thresholds (<10,000–15,000 cells/mm^3) and a somewhat higher nontherapeutic laparotomy rate versus a higher incidence of missed injuries or delayed diagnoses associated with higher RBC thresholds (>25,000 cells/mm^3).[38]

FAST and DPL have been used in the setting of hemodynamically normal patients but their utility in this setting, when CT scanning is available, has been questioned and may lead to delays in definitive diagnosis. A literature review conducted by Griffin and Pullinger[39] found little data to support the use of FAST examination to reduce the use of CT scanning in stable patients. Some investigators have suggested that the use of DPL as a "screening" examination along with complimentary CT scanning is more cost-effective and may lead to a low nontherapeutic laparotomy rate.[35,40] If CT scan is not readily available, for example, in a mass casualty situation this may be a viable strategy.

There has been a growing trend toward more liberal use of CT scanning, given its high negative predictive power. As CT equipment continues to improve, with 64, 128, and even 256 slice scanners, the acquisition speed has decreased dramatically allowing "pan-scans" to be performed more routinely for many trauma patients. Although this approach has been condemned by some for its imprecise "shotgun" aspects, for its potential to increase cost and complications with workup of nonspecific findings, and for a significant increase in radiation exposure, recent reports suggest that "pan-scans" may reduce diagnostic errors and delays. In a recent German study, Huber-Wagner and colleagues[41] reported a 25% relative reduction in mortality associated with whole-body CT scanning in a cohort of more severely injured trauma patients with an injury severity score greater than or equal to 16. The utility of "pan-scans" for less severely injured patients, however, remains to be determined, as does the long-term effect of radiation exposure.

Slow or Incomplete Response to the "Bad" Pelvic Fracture

Hemorrhage is the most frequent cause of death associated with pelvic fractures, and management of these patients is a high-risk endeavor that requires a high degree of multidisciplinary coordination. Massive pelvic fracture hemorrhage is often associated with the dreaded "physiologic vortex" of coagulopathy, hypothermia, and acidosis. In addition, many pelvic fracture victims are elderly with limited physiologic reserve and with a relatively poor ability to tamponade hemorrhage within the pelvic bowl.

Methods for hemorrhage control include direct operative control (rarely needed outside of major vascular injury), indirect operative control through the use of packing, pelvic external fixation, and arteriography and embolization for arterial hemorrhage. Patients often do not tolerate delays or strategic management errors, and the use of these modalities must be timely and must be in the proper sequence to maximize survival.

The early detection of hemorrhage amenable to angio/embolization is possible through the use of CT scanning of the abdomen and pelvis, showing evidence of active arterial extravasation from the pelvic vessels. Recognition of pelvic extravasation has been shown to be a reliable predictor of arterial pelvic bleeding and the need for angiographic embolization.[42,43] CT has largely replaced the old strategy of performing arteriography/embolization for only those patients receiving large volume transfusions.

Given the multidisciplinary, multimodality needs of the patient with major pelvic fracture, the most frequent errors often are organizational, and the most accessible opportunities for improvement exist in crafting a scripted, protocolized approach to management. Recent reports suggest significant outcomes benefit to the use of practice management guidelines.[44,45] Protocols are tailored to prevent known risks and should include the following elements

- *Pelvic binders for external compression.* These act to reduce the displacement of the fracture fragments and improve compliance characteristics of the pelvic bowl for subsequent embolization.[46]
- *Massive transfusion protocol (MTP)* using packed red blood cells (PRBCs), fresh frozen plasma, and platelet packs in the ratio of 1:1:1 for patients receiving more than 10 units of PRBCs in the first 6 hours.[47]

- *Early anesthesiology involvement.* From a monitoring and resuscitation standpoint, these cases are similar to major operative cases and should be run accordingly.
- Hypothermia precautions and the use of active warming devices (eg, Bair Hugger [Arizant Inc, Eden Prairie, MN, USA]).
- Preload and arterial monitoring. Central venous lines and arterial lines should be used liberally.
- Procoagluants (rFVIIa [recombinant activated factor VII] and prothrombin complex concentrates for patients on warfarin [Coumadin]). Although proper execution of an MTP helps prevent coagulopathy, patients may benefit from the administration of additional factors.

Cardiac Tamponade

Cardiac tamponade is caused mainly by penetrating chest trauma and often responds well to small volume infusion, leading to the erroneous conclusion that mild hypovolemia is the underlying cause of the hypotension. During fluid resuscitation of cardiac tamponade, a modest fluid bolus of only 300 to 500 mL may increase atrial filling and, by increasing central venous pressure (CVP), restore end-diastolic volumes and systolic blood pressure. This is because of the very steep curve that defines the relationship between preload and blood pressure over a narrow range (**Fig. 3**). The rapid, but temporary, restoration of end-diastolic ventricular volume and resultant improvement in blood pressure may lead to the incorrect assumption that the shock state of the patient is due primarily to hemorrhage.

Failure to look for distended neck veins or the failure to perform a FAST examination early in the resuscitation may compound cardiac tamponade. Chest radiographs are normal under most circumstances because the pericardium does not distend acutely, despite increased cardiac filling pressures.

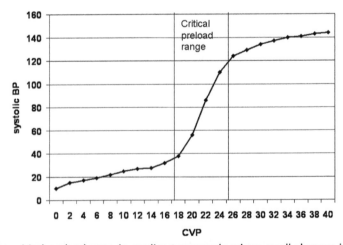

Fig. 3. The critical preload zone in cardiac tamponade where small changes in preload, reflected by CVP, may result in large changes in systolic (BP). As tamponade progresses, the curve flattens and is shifted to the right. The curve provides a snapshot in time that might be seen in early tamponade. Over time, the entire curve becomes rightward shifted and ultimately begins to show a decreased blood pressure at any given CVP.

There is a substantial threat of sudden hemodynamic decompensation, as illustrated in **Fig. 3**, until the tamponade is decompressed. In the same way that patients with tamponade respond to small increases in preload, they may also decompensate, even to the point of cardiac arrest, with equally small decreases in preload. This physiologically precarious situation creates a potential trap: on induction and intubation, positive pressure ventilation increases intrathoracic pressure and preload is suddenly decreased. If the resuscitation team is not ready (with the patient prepared and draped before induction) to perform immediate pericardial decompression, the results may be disastrous. Cardiac tamponade is essentially a compartment syndrome of the heart and progressive myocardial ischemia occurs. Even short delays in pericardial decompression may compromise chances for survival.

Physiologic Traps in Special Populations

Avoiding pitfalls in the pediatric trauma population is largely dependent on being properly prepared with age- or size-specific equipment and resources. An effective system of preparedness may involve, for example, the use of color-coded resuscitation drawers based on the size of the child and the Broselow Pediatric Emergency Tape (Armstrong Medical Industries, Inc, Lincolnshire, IL, USA). Knowledge of age-specific vital signs may prevent misguided assumptions about hypotensive infants having "normal-for-age" blood pressures. Special attention needs to be given to the room temperature, because small children are particularly susceptible to hypothermia. Incorporating pediatric service providers into the trauma team is important, particularly for very young patients.

The elderly trauma patient is intolerant of management missteps and warrants even greater attention to detail. Medications such as β-blockers and calcium channel blockers can blunt the normal tachycardic response associated with many traumatic events and can mask early signs of shock. In addition, physiologic derangements of the normal chronotropic response, and pacemakers, may also lead to erroneous assumptions about the (normal) state of a patient's hemodynamics. In general, a normal heart rate is a poor indicator of the absence of a shock state and may be particularly misleading in an elderly patient.

The elderly patient is highly susceptible to noncavitary hemorrhage, because of the relative loss of connective tissue integrity and the loss of the normal ability to tamponade soft tissue hemorrhage. The presence of fragile blood vessels contributes to the potential for occult bleeding within subcutaneous, retroperitoneal, or intramuscular spaces. A list of specific considerations in the elderly population appears in **Table 3**.

The management of trauma in pregnancy has some unique pitfalls. Every female trauma patient who may be of childbearing age should have a urine pregnancy test sent as part of the initial resuscitation. Providers should also consider performing a preliminary ultrasound evaluation of the uterus for obvious findings of pregnancy during the FAST scan to minimize the delays that may occur while waiting for urine test results. Failure to recognize pregnancy early leads to serious delays in diagnosis and avoidable radiation exposure. Obstetrics consultation should be sought for all pregnant patients.

Many pitfalls and errors in the setting of managing the pregnant patient result from inexperience. Risk reduction is directed at the early diagnosis of fetal hypoxia from placental injuries and also diagnosing direct fetal injury. The key steps to initial evaluation should involve an assessment of abnormal fetal heart rate or rhythm, the presence of contractions, any vaginal bleeding, ruptured amniotic membranes, or a distended perineum. Continuous cardiotocographic fetal monitoring should be performed for virtually all pregnant trauma patients who may have viable pregnancies

Table 3
Potential pitfalls in the management of the elderly patient

What The Injured Elderly Would Tell You (if they could)	Related Physiology and Rationale
"I can go from normotensive to hypotensive in a heartbeat."	Profound, life-threatening hypovolemia may occur in the setting of normal blood pressure. Physiologic reserve is minimal, and hemodynamic decompensation can occur quickly
"I respond poorly to too much or too little fluid."	The therapeutic window for cardiac preload is narrow, and inadequate preload monitoring may lead to errors in volume resuscitation
"My subdural hematoma hasn't expanded enough yet to really affect my level of consciousness."	Cortical atrophy, common in the elderly, may act to delay the clinical manifestations of serious intracranial hemorrhage. This hemorrhage may be clinically occult
"Trauma is not really my major problem."	Stroke, myocardial infarction, and seizures may result from falls or motor vehicle crashes and delayed diagnosis of the principal underlying problem
"I only look like I have adequate ventilatory reserve."	Ventilatory failure & respiratory arrest may occur suddenly in conjunction with chest or abdominal injuries despite a benign outward clinical appearance
"I get demand ischemia if I have too much pain or my hematocrit drops below 29."	Myocardial (demand) ischemia may result from severe or prolonged pain or from transfusion thresholds that have not been appropriately liberalized in the setting of coronary artery disease
"I can't stand even a little shock or hypoxia.... and neither can my myocardium."	Even minor perturbations in perfusion, oxygenation, or vasoconstriction may lead to major cardiac complications

"My connective tissue just ain't what it used to be..."	Decrease in connective tissue integrity with less "tamponade effect" for hemorrhage into soft tissues. Blood loss into soft tissue spaces, including subcutaneous loss, may be excessive and is often overlooked
"The sensitivity of my abdominal examination is better than flipping a coin....but not much."	Clinical manifestations of serious abdominal injury in elderly patients are often minimal. Reliance on the abdominal examination often leads to missed abdominal injuries
"My bones are brittle...my hip bone, my shin bone, and my aortic bone!"	BAI may occur in the elderly in the absence of conventional signs or symptoms. A low threshold for CT imaging should exist
"A little medication goes a long way with me...."	Failure to adjust medication dosage, particularly sedative-hypnotics and analgesics, may result in serious complications
"I just haven't been eating so well lately"	Chronic malnutrition is common and often undiagnosed
"My injuries weren't accidental"	Elder abuse is common and often unreported and undiagnosed
"Major trauma? Heck, I wouldn't even tolerate a brisk haircut..."	Underestimating and undermanaging comorbidities (eg, chronic obstructive pulmonary disease, coronary artery disease, smoking, ethyl alcohol [ETOH] consumption) may result in preventable morbidity/mortality

(more than 24 weeks gestation). Providers should keep in mind that reported dates may be unreliable and that a patient whose uterine fundus is at or above the umbilicus on abdominal examination should be considered viable until evaluated by ultrasound for dates. An assessment of fetomaternal hemorrhage using the Kleihauer-Betke test may provide an indicator of placental injury and guide treatment to avoid sensitization in Rh-negative gravidas.

It is occasionally forgotten that the management of the term pregnant patient involves the balanced management of 2 considerations. Too much emphasis on fetal management may result in maternal complications ("treat the mother to treat the fetus"). Conversely, in situations where cesarean section delivery is necessary (>26 week gestation), the potential for direct injury to the fetus-now-newborn may be overlooked in the setting of major maternal injuries.

Pitfalls in the Performance of Procedures

Most major trauma resuscitations involve the performance of invasive procedures. It is wise to remember the old dictum that "there is no such thing as a small procedure." Risks of resuscitation procedures exist for both high- and low-volume centers, but for different reasons. The risks for high-volume centers (mostly academic level I centers) are related to the relative inexperience of the trainees in teaching programs. The risks for low-volume centers (community or rural level III–IV centers) may be related to the lack of ongoing experience by the providers staffing those centers. Most technical mishaps occur in patients with higher risk (elderly, obese, and uncooperative) and in higher risk settings (critical injury and need for multiple simultaneous interventions). In teaching programs, watchful senior supervision is essential. At lower volume centers, surgical and emergency medicine providers may improve and/or maintain their procedural skills through coursework, such as ATLS or simulation skills training, using models specifically adapted to individual procedures.[48]

Infectious complications may be increased by inability to ensure aseptic techniques in the emergent setting. In addition, providers may assume that a small incision size or a percutaneous procedure is somehow associated with less procedural or infectious risk when the opposite may be true. Examples include empyema with lung entrapment after chest tube placement requiring thoracotomy or decortication and prolonged hospitalization, septic thrombophlebitis from intravenous or cut down lines, and arterial injuries sustained during central line placement with subsequent hemorrhage or pseudoaneurysm requiring operative repair (**Table 4**). Strict adherence to aseptic techniques and assurance that providers who perform these procedures are technically proficient and well supervised helps avoid many of these procedural pitfalls.

Missed Injuries

Avoidance of missed injuries depends on an understanding of injury patterns, a thorough primary evaluation, and a systematic follow-up examination and review of imaging studies. The reported incidence of missed injuries (or delayed diagnoses) in trauma patients varies from 2% to 3% to more than 60%.[49–51] Most of these are low-effect "misses" that have limited clinical sequelae and many are more accurately termed "delayed presentations." These include minor fractures (eg, patella or metatarsal fractures, chip fractures of the pelvis) that are diagnosed later in a patient's hospital course. Conditions that blunt the normal response to pain, including neurologic injury, sedation, drugs, and even major distracting injuries, may diminish the accuracy of the physical examination as a primary means of detection. The increasing use of whole-body CT radiography has provided a means of counteracting these effects.[40]There is a general recognition that primary and secondary surveys for traumatic injuries, despite being carefully conducted, still result in missed injuries. In teaching programs, radiologic misreads may occur in the setting of less experienced physicians providing preliminary radiologic interpretations and there continue to be diagnostic pitfalls with respect to certain types of injuries (**Table 5**).

Measures to reduce the incidence of missed injury in a system of trauma care must balance the resources required to achieve a near-100% capture rate for significant diagnoses and the effect of complications resulting from diagnostic delays. A protocol-driven process involving a follow-up, complete and detailed head-to-toe physical examination, and systematic review of all diagnostic studies has been termed a "tertiary survey." This process has been shown to significantly reduce the incidence of missed injuries[52,53] and may be performed by advance practice nurses (eg, nurse practitioners) or mid-level providers (eg, physician assistants). The tertiary survey process seems to be cost-effective and demonstrates the viability of a "systems" approach to error reduction in a heavily provider-dependent arena.

Technical improvement in speed and resolution of diagnostic imaging and increased use has served to decrease the overall incidence of some types of missed injuries. The overuse of imaging, particularly CT, may create problems with false-positive results. Some examples include splenic clefts mistaken for major splenic injury, standing wave artifact masquerading as blunt aortic injury (BAI), or volume averaging artifacts creating the impression of a ruptured diaphragm.[54–56] The obvious pitfall is predicating decisions entirely on a radiographic image.

Despite improved imaging and increased sensitivity of missed injuries, a few troublesome areas continue to exist.

Missed blunt intestinal injuries

Despite improvements in CT imaging, missed and delayed diagnoses of blunt intestinal injuries (BIIs) continue to occur. The miss rate for this injury has been reported to be around 10% based on the initial CT scan, with an associated mortality as high as 40%.[57] The radiographic hallmarks of BII may be subtle and include (1) unexplained free intraperitoneal fluid, (2) bowel wall thickening, (3) mesenteric stranding, and (4) extravasation of intraluminal contrast. Associated clinical findings include seat belt contusions, Chance fractures, and abdominal pain. The major pitfall resulting in missed injury and preventable morbidity and mortality is the tendency to disregard subtle CT findings in a higher-risk clinical setting. Most errors of this nature may be avoided by undertaking further diagnostic investigations in any patient at risk, including serial abdominal examinations, repeat CT scanning, DPL, laparoscopy, or even exploratory laparotomy.

Missed blunt pancreatic injuries

The pancreas, despite being well protected in the midretroperitoneum, is still susceptible to blunt fracture caused by anterior abdominal impact, typically near its point of contact with the anterior spinal column. CT findings may be subtle or even nonexistent initially, consisting of nothing more than local edema or some irregularities in pancreatic perfusion. In most cases, short delays in the diagnosis of isolated blunt pancreatic injuries, in the absence of major hemorrhage, are reasonably well tolerated, allowing repeated CT imaging or even ERCP (endoscopic retrograde cholangiopancreatography) in highly suspicious cases. The threshold for repeat imaging should be low, and most injuries involving the main pancreatic duct should be evident before proceeding to the OR.

Table 4
Technical pitfalls and complications in trauma resuscitation procedures

Procedure	Threat, Pitfall, Error, or Complication
Chest tubes	
Misplacement	Inexperienced personnel, poor supervision, incision size too small, failure to confirm chest entry by palpation, excessive force, & other psychomotor errors
Infection/Empyema	Poor antiseptic preparation, inadequate patient draping, inadequate analgesia or local anesthesia, chest tube manipulation, use of same incision for chest tube replacement
Lung, liver, and spleen injury	Failure to establish landmarks. Failure to palpate pleural space before tube placement, inexperience, and lack of competence
Intercostal injury	Failure to incise or dissect above the rib and excessive force
Pain	Failure to administer appropriate analgesia and local anesthesia. Poor understanding of anatomic structures
Occlusion	Misplacement (kinking) of chest tube. Failure to use appropriate tube size, failure to "milk" tubes with high blood volume output
Groin lines & CVP lines	
Venous injury	Back wall perforations related to inadequate skin incision size (loss of sensitivity to increased use of force)
Arterial injury	Failure to palpate artery, failure to assess back bleeding, inappropriate puncture location (typically too low), poor understanding of anatomic relationships
False passage	Failure to assess bleed-back, excessive force, inadequate skin incision size
Infection	Poor or lack of antiseptic preparation, poor aseptic technique
Insertion of sub-clavian or internal jugular centra line	Pneumothorax due to improper patient positioning (Trendelenburg), improper puncture site or direction, application of excessive force
DPL	
Bowel, bladder injury	Failure to distinguish between bowel and peritoneum (open procedures), use of DPL at old laparotomy site (adhesions), failure to decompress stomach or bladder, excessive force

False passage	Fascial incision site too small (increased sliding resistance), failure to elevate fascia on trochar insertion (semiopen procedures)
Infection	Poor or lack of antiseptic preparation, poor aseptic technique, occult bowel injury
Needle thoracostomy	
Ineffective	Needle/catheter too small. Failure to dislodge fat plug, improper location, catheter or needle too short for location
Injury to vessels, heart	Inappropriate location of puncture site, failure to establish proper landmarks
Unresolved pneumo	Failure to place chest tube after needle thoracostomy
Resus thoracotomy	
Poor exposure	Failure to extend incision or create "trap door" by dividing medial costal cartilage. Inadequate retractors
Injury to phrenic nerve	Inappropriate pericardiotomy incision (anteroposterior vs superior-inferior)
Injury to heart	Technical error in pericardiotomy with epicardial laceration. Digital injury to atria during manual cardiac compression
Injury to lung hilum	Failure to take down inferior pulmonary ligament, clamp injury to pulmonary vessels during cross-clamping
Needle sticks & blood/fluids exposure (providers)	Failure to take appropriate body-substance isolation precautions (masks, hats, eye protection, gloves, gowns). Failure to handle and dispose off "sharps" properly, inexperienced or inadequately trained personnel, failure of crowd control, cramped resuscitation space

Table 5
Potential missed injuries (selected) and approaches to error reduction

Missed Injury Type	Presentation or Common Factors Associated With Delay/Miss	Error Reduction Strategies
Traumatic brain injury	False attribution (drugs, ETOH consumption, seizures). Errors in CT interpretation	Routine CT scans based on threshold GCS/neurologic examination
Axial spine injuries	Reliance on physical examination, false attribution of subtle signs and symptoms	Protocol-driven radiograph series for obtunded patients, CT for primary cervical spine evaluation in higher risk patients
Carotid, vertebral dissections	Unexplained decreases in LOC	Protocols for duplex scans/ magnetic resonance imaging in selected c-spine injuries
BAI	Initial false-negative chest radiograph	Guidelines for chest CT based on age, mechanism, etc
BII	Initial false-negative CT, false-negative prediction based on CT. Errors in CT interpretation missing subtle signs	DPL or repeat CT scan for suspicious or equivocal studies. DPL or repeat CT scan for associated seat belt signs or Chance fractures
Blunt cardiac injury	Nonspecific signs/ symptoms, failure to obtain ECG	Protocol-driven ECG assessment. TEE/TTE for hemodynamic manifestations
Pancreatic injury	Initial false negative CT. Errors in CT interpretation, false negative DPL	Mandatory follow-up CT examination for equivocal studies
Pelvic fractures	Obtunded patient, false negative prediction based on physical examination	Protocol-driven radiograph series for obtunded patients
Tibial plateau fracture	Obtunded patient, false negative prediction based on examination	Protocol-driven radiograph series for obtunded patients
Extremity vascular injury	False negative prediction based on pulse examination	ABI screening for all proximity injuries

Abbreviations: ABI, ankle/brachial index; BAI, blunt aortic injury; BII, blunt intestinal injury; ECG, electrocardiogrphy; GCS, Glasgow Coma Scale; LOC, level of consciousness; TEE, transesophageal echocardiography; TTE, transthoracic echocardiogram.

Missed cervical spine injuries

Missed cervical spine injuries with resultant neurologic damage have historically been one of the most treacherous areas in terms of impact to the patient and medicolegal cost. Horror stories of occult injuries are well documented in the literature, but most occur in the setting of inadequate diagnostic imaging. In some centers, the high-impact potential for misses in these areas has resulted in an almost defensive over-diagnosis with increasing reliance on CT and magnetic resonance imaging. Although appropriate in many circumstances, the widespread application of these imaging techniques to most at-risk patients raises questions about proper resource use.

The most common pitfalls in these areas are the over-reliance on the physical examination for purposes of cervical spine clearance in a lower risk setting. Most centers now have protocols in place for clearance of the cervical spine in the patient who is awake. These same protocols avoid clinical clearance in the setting of interfering effects such as drugs or alcohol, altered mental status, distracting injuries, neurologic findings on clinical examination, or other concomitant axial spine injuries. Stiell and colleagues[58] demonstrated that a rule-based approach to cervical spine diagnosis can be effectively implemented and can result in a minimal number of diagnostic errors. This rule-based approach was validated in the prehospital arena.[59]

Missed blunt cerebrovascular injuries
Carotid and vertebral dissections can result in devastating neurologic sequelae and likely occur with greater regularity than was originally suspected. Faster CT imaging has made screening arteriograms more accessible, and recent literature suggests that a protocolized approach for screening for blunt cerebrovascular injuries may be warranted.[60] Despite improvements in early diagnosis, not all reports show concomitant improvements in patient outcomes.[61]

Missed BAIs
Historically, clinicians have relied on plain, upright anteroposterior chest radiograph as a screening modality for detection of BAIs. Increasingly, it has been recognized that occult injuries may occur without the typical findings on plain radiographs, particularly in the elderly population, and the increasingly liberal use of CT has decreased the problem of missed BAIs. The classic chest radiograph indications of BAI include mediastinal widening, depression of the left main-stem bronchus, obliteration of the PA window, apical capping, and deviation of a nasogastric tube, but they may also include evidence of associated chest injuries, including pleural effusion, rib fractures, scapular fractures, clavicular fractures, and so on. Elderly patients with "eggshell" aortas may sustain potentially lethal injuries in the absence of any imaging findings whatsoever. Therefore, the presence of chest or torso trauma, chest pain, or concerning mechanism of injury in this patient group may provide adequate indication for dynamic CT of the chest.

SUMMARY

It has been said that 2 types of diagnostic errors occur: one is where the diagnosis is not known and the other is where the diagnosis is not considered ("the ones you don't know about and the ones you don't think about"). This may be true of pitfalls in general. These traps occur more frequently when they are not learned or not considered. Patients benefit from providers being acutely aware of their own fallibility, from providers recognizing the latent threats and errors inherent in any complex system of care, and from providers developing strategies that allow them to recognize and respond to inevitable errors. The recognition and avoidance of attribution, labeling, and specific management errors; the development of systems of high-fidelity communication; and an appreciation for the capacity of human biology to confound even the most carefully laid diagnostic and therapeutic plans can lead to a safer environment and improved care.

REFERENCES

1. Health Resources and Services Administration. Model trauma system planning and evaluation. Merrifield (VA): U.S. Department of Health & Human Services; 2006.
2. Regional Trauma Systems. Optimal elements, integration, and assessment. American College of Surgeons: Chicago (IL); 2007. Available at: http://www. facs.org/trauma/consultationguide-prq.pdf.
3. Reason J. Human error. 1st edition. Cambridge (UK): Cambridge University Press; 1990.
4. Kohn LT, Corrigan JM, Donaldson MS, editors. To err is human: building a safer health system. 1st edition. Washington, DC: National Academies Press; 2000.
5. Rasmussen J, Jensen A. Mental procedures in real-life tasks: a case study of electronic troubleshooting. Ergonomics 1974;17:293–307.
6. Helmreich RL, Foushee HC. Why crew resource management? Empirical and theoretical bases of human factors training in aviation. In: Wiener E, Kanki B, Helmreich R, editors. Cockpit resource management. San Diego (CA): Academic Press; 1993. p. 3–45.
7. Mackersie RC, Rhodes M. Patient safety and trauma care. In: Manuel BM, Nora PF, editors. Surgical patient safety: essential information for surgeons in today's environment. 1st edition. Chicago (IL): American College of Surgeons; 2004. p. 61–77.
8. Lester H, Tritter JQ. Medical error: a discussion of the medical construction of error and suggestions for reforms of medical education to decrease error. Med Educ 2001;35:855–61.
9. Sox HC Jr, Woloshin S. How many deaths are due to medical error? Getting the number right. Eff Clin Pract 2000;3(6):277–83.
10. Ioannidis J, Lau J. Evidence on interventions to reduce medical errors. An overview and recommendations for future research. J Gen Intern Med 2001;16: 325–34.
11. Gaba DM. Research techniques in human performance using realistic simulation. In: Henson L, Lee A, Basford A, editors. Simulators in anesthesiology education. New York: Plenum Publishing Corporation; 1998. p. 93–102.
12. Lee SK, Pardo M, Gaba D, et al. Trauma assessment training with a patient simulator: a prospective, randomized study. J Trauma 2003;55(4):651–7.
13. Howard SK, Gaba DM, Fish KJ, et al. Anesthesia crisis resource management training: teaching anesthesiologists to handle critical incidents. Aviat Space Environ Med 1992;63(9):763–70.
14. Holzman RS, Cooper JB, Gaba DM, et al. Anesthesia crisis resource management: real-life simulation training in operating room crises. J Clin Anesth 1995; 7(8):675–87.
15. Knudson MM, Khaw L, Bullard MK, et al. Trauma training in simulation: translating skills from SIM time to real time. J Trauma 2008;64(2):255–63 [discussion: 263–4].
16. Holcomb JB, Dumire RD, Crommett JW, et al. Evaluation of trauma team performance using an advanced human patient simulator for resuscitation training. J Trauma 2002;52:1078–85.
17. Helmreich RL, Schaefer HG. Team performance in the operating room. In: Bogner MS, editor. Human error in medicine. Hillside (NJ): Erlbaum & Associates; 1994.
18. Carthey J, deLeval MR, Wright DJ, et al. Behavioural makers of surgical success. Safety Sci 2003;41:409–25.

19. Hoyt DB, Shackford SR, Fridland PH, et al. Video recording trauma resuscitations: an effective teaching technique. J Trauma 1988;28(4):435–40.
20. Michaelson M, Levi L. Videotaping in the admitting area: a most useful tool for quality improvement of the trauma care. Eur J Emerg Med 1997;4(2):94–6.
21. Oakley E, Stocker S, Staubli G, et al. Using video recording to identify management errors in pediatric trauma resuscitation. Pediatrics 2006;117(3):658–64.
22. Jemmett ME, Kendal KM, Fourre MW, et al. Unrecognized misplacement of endotracheal tubes in a mixed urban to rural emergency medical services setting. Acad Emerg Med 2003;10(9):961–5.
23. Bair AE, Smith D, Lichty L. Intubation confirmation techniques associated with unrecognized non-tracheal intubations by pre-hospital providers. J Emerg Med 2005;28(4):403–7.
24. Dorges V, Wenzel V, Knacke P, et al. Comparison of different airway management strategies to ventilate apneic, nonpreoxygenated patients. Crit Care Med 2003; 31(3):800–4.
25. Davis DP, Valentine C, Ochs M, et al. The Combitube as a salvage airway device for paramedic rapid sequence intubation. Ann Emerg Med 2003; 42(5):697–704.
26. Rabitsch W, Schellongowski P, Staudinger T, et al. Comparison of a conventional tracheal airway with the Combitube in an urban emergency medical services system run by physicians. Resuscitation 2003;57(1):27–32.
27. Schaumann N, Lorenz V, Schellongowski P, et al. Evaluation of Seldinger technique emergency cricothyroidotomy versus standard surgical cricothyroidotomy in 200 cadavers 2005;102(1):7–11.
28. American College of Surgeons, Committee on Trauma. Advanced trauma life support. 7th edition. Chicago (IL): American College of Surgeons; 2004.
29. Scalea TM, Bochicchio GV, Habashi N, et al. Increased intra-abdominal, intrathoracic, and intracranial pressure after severe brain injury: multiple compartment syndrome. J Trauma 2007;62(3):647–56.
30. Tremblay LN, Feliciano DV, Rozycki GS. Secondary extremity compartment syndrome. J Trauma 2002;53(5):833–7.
31. Shoemaker WC, Appel P, Bland R. Use of physiologic monitoring to predict outcome and to assist in clinical decisions in critically ill postoperative patients. Am J Surg 1983;146(1):43–50.
32. Poeze M, Greve JW, Ramsay G. Meta-analysis of hemodynamic optimization: relationship to methodological quality. Crit Care 2005;9(6):R771–9.
33. Kern JW, Shoemaker WC. Meta-analysis of hemodynamic optimization in high-risk patients. Crit Care Med 2002;30(8):1686–92.
34. Velmahos GC, Demetriades D, Shoemaker WC, et al. Endpoints of resuscitation of critically injured patients: normal or supranormal? A prospective randomized trial. Ann Surg 2000;232(3):409–18.
35. Gonzalez RP, Ickler J, Gachassin P. Complementary roles of diagnostic peritoneal lavage and computed tomography in the evaluation of blunt abdominal trauma. J Trauma 2001;51(6):1128–34 [discussion: 1134–6].
36. Davis JW, Hoyt DB, McArdle S, et al. An analysis of errors causing morbidity and mortality in a trauma system: a guide for quality improvement. J Trauma 1992; 32(5):660–6.
37. Stengel D, Bauwens K, Rademacher G, et al. Association between compliance with methodological standards of diagnostic research and reported test accuracy: meta-analysis of focused assessment of US for trauma. Radiology 2005; 236(1):102–11.

38. Alyono D, Morrow CE, Perry JF Jr. Reappraisal of diagnostic peritoneal lavage criteria for operation in penetrating and blunt trauma. Surgery 1982;92(4):751–7.
39. Griffin XL, Pullinger R. Are diagnostic peritoneal lavage or focused abdominal sonography for trauma safe screening investigations for hemodynamically stable patients after blunt abdominal trauma? A review of the literature. J Trauma 2007; 62(3):779–84.
40. Mele TS, Stewart K, Marokus B, et al. Evaluation of a diagnostic protocol using screening diagnostic peritoneal lavage with selective use of abdominal computed tomography in blunt abdominal trauma. J Trauma 1999;46(5):847–52.
41. Huber-Wagner S, Lefering R, Qvick LM, et al. Effect of whole-body CT during trauma resuscitation on survival: a retrospective, multicentre study. Lancet 2009;373(9673):1455–61.
42. Stephen DJ, Kreder HJ, Day AC, et al. Early detection of arterial bleeding in acute pelvic trauma. J Trauma 1999;47(4):638–42.
43. Pereira SJ, O'Brien DP, Luchette FA, et al. Dynamic helical computed tomography scan accurately detects hemorrhage in patients with pelvic fracture. Surgery 2000;128(4):678–85.
44. Biffl WL, Smith WR, Moore EE, et al. Evolution of a multidisciplinary clinical pathway for the management of unstable patients with pelvic fractures. Ann Surg 2001;233(6):843–50.
45. Balogh Z, Caldwell E, Heetveld M, et al. Institutional practice guidelines on management of pelvic fracture-related hemodynamic instability: do they make a difference? J Trauma 2005;58(4):778–82.
46. Krieg JC, Mohr M, Ellis TJ, et al. Emergent stabilization of pelvic ring injuries by controlled circumferential compression: a clinical trial. J Trauma 2005;59(3): 659–64.
47. Zink KA, Sambasivan CN, Holcomb JB, et al. A high ratio of plasma and platelets to packed red blood cells in the first 6 hours of massive transfusion improves outcomes in a large multicenter study. Am J Surg 2009;197(5): 565–70.
48. Cherry RA, Williams J, George J, et al. The effectiveness of a human patient simulator in the ATLS shock skills station. J Surg Res 2007;139(2):229–35.
49. Houshian S, Larsen MS, Holm C. Missed injuries in a level I trauma center. J Trauma 2002;52(4):715–9.
50. Janjua KJ, Sugrue M, Deane SA. Prospective evaluation of early missed injuries and the role of tertiary trauma survey. J Trauma 1998;44(6):1000–6 [discussion: 1006–7].
51. Buduhan G, McRitchie DI. Missed injuries in patients with multiple trauma. J Trauma 2000;49(4):600–5.
52. Enderson BL, Reath DB, Meadors J, et al. The tertiary trauma survey: a prospective study of missed injury. J Trauma 1990;30(6):666–9.
53. Biffl WL, Harrington DT, Cioffi WG. Implementation of a tertiary trauma survey decreases missed injuries. J Trauma 2003;54(1):38–43.
54. Koenig TR, West OC. Diagnosing acute traumatic aortic injury with computed tomography angiography: signs and potential pitfalls. Curr Probl Diagn Radiol 2004;33(3):97–105.
55. Brennan TV, Lipshutz GS, Posselt AM, et al. Congenital cleft spleen with CT scan appearance of high-grade splenic laceration after blunt abdominal trauma. J Emerg Med 2003;25(2):139–42.
56. Lynch RM, Neary P, Jackson T, et al. Traumatic pseudorupture of the diaphragm. Accid Emerg Nurs 2004;12(1):58–9.

57. Miller PR, Croce MA, Bee TK, et al. Associated injuries in blunt solid organ trauma: implications for missed injury in nonoperative management. J Trauma 2002;53(2):238–42 [discussion: 242–4].
58. Stiell IG, Clement CM, McKnight RD, et al. The Canadian C-spine rule versus the NEXUS low-risk criteria in patients with trauma. N Engl J Med 2003;349(26): 2510–8.
59. Vaillancourt C, Stiell IG, Beaudoin T, et al. The out-of-hospital validation of the Canadian C-Spine rule by paramedics. Ann Emerg Med 2009;54(5):672–3.
60. Schneidereit NP, Simons R, Nicolaou S, et al. Utility of screening for blunt vascular neck injuries with computed tomographic angiography. J Trauma 2006;60(1): 209–15.
61. Mayberry JC, Brown CV, Mullins RJ, et al. Blunt carotid artery injury: the futility of aggressive screening and diagnosis. Arch Surg 2004;139(6):609–12.

The RUSH Exam: Rapid Ultrasound in SHock in the Evaluation of the Critically Ill

Phillips Perera, MD, RDMS, FACEP[a],*, Thomas Mailhot, MD, RDMS[b],
David Riley, MD, MS, RDMS[a], Diku Mandavia, MD, FACEP, FRCPC[b,c]

KEYWORDS

- Rapid ultrasound in shock examination • RUSH exam
- Shock • Ultrasound

Care of the patient with shock can be one of the most challenging issues in emergency medicine. Even the most seasoned clinician, standing at the bedside of the patient in extremis, can be unclear about the cause of shock and the optimal initial therapeutic approach. Traditional physical examination techniques can be misleading given the complex physiology of shock.[1] Patients in shock have high mortality rates, and these rates are correlated to the amount and duration of hypotension. Therefore, diagnosis and initial care must be accurate and prompt to optimize patient outcomes.[2] Failure to make the correct diagnosis and act appropriately can lead to potentially disastrous outcomes and high-risk situations.

Ultrasound technology has been rapidly integrated into Emergency Department care in the last decade. More practicing emergency physicians (EPs) are now trained in bedside point of care or goal-directed ultrasound, and this training is now included in all United States Accreditation Council for Graduate Medical Education Emergency Medicine residency programs.[3,4] Furthermore, the American College of Emergency Physicians (ACEP) has formally endorsed and embraced bedside ultrasound by the EP for multiple applications.[5] This technology is ideal in the care of the critical patient in shock, and the most recent ACEP guidelines further delineate a new category of

[a] New York Presbyterian Hospital, Columbia University Medical Center, Division of Emergency Medicine, 622 West 168th Street, PH1-137, New York, NY 10032, USA
[b] LA County+USC Medical Center, Department of Emergency Medicine, General Hospital, 1200 State Street, Room 1011, Los Angeles, California 90033, USA
[c] Cedars-Sinai Medical Center, Department of Emergency Medicine, General Hospital, 1200 State Street, Room 1011, Los Angeles, California 90033, USA
* Corresponding author.
E-mail address: pperera1@mac.com (P. Perera).

Emerg Med Clin N Am 28 (2010) 29–56
doi:10.1016/j.emc.2009.09.010
0733-8627/09/$ – see front matter © 2010 Elsevier Inc. All rights reserved.

"resuscitative" ultrasound. Studies have demonstrated that initial integration of bedside ultrasound into the evaluation of the patient with shock results in a more accurate initial diagnosis with an improved patient care plan.[1,6,7] Instead of relying on older techniques, like listening for changes in sound coming from the patient's body suggestive of specific pathology, bedside ultrasound now allows direct visualization of pathology or abnormal physiological states. Thus, bedside ultrasound has become an essential component in the evaluation of the hypotensive patient.

CLASSIFICATIONS OF SHOCK

Many authorities categorize shock into 4 classic subtypes.[8] The first is hypovolemic shock. This condition is commonly encountered in the patient who is hemorrhaging from trauma, or from a nontraumatic source of brisk bleeding such as from the gastrointestinal (GI) tract or a rupturing aortic aneurysm. Hypovolemic shock may also result from nonhemorrhagic conditions with extensive loss of body fluids, such as GI fluid loss from vomiting and diarrhea. The second subtype of shock is distributive shock. The classic example of this class of shock is sepsis, in which the vascular system is vasodilated to the point that the core vascular blood volume is insufficient to maintain end organ perfusion. Other examples of distributive shock include neurogenic shock, caused by a spinal cord injury, and anaphylactic shock, a severe form of allergic response. The third major form of shock is cardiogenic shock, resulting from pump failure and the inability of the heart to propel the needed oxygenated blood forward to vital organs. Cardiogenic shock can be seen in patients with advanced cardiomyopathy, myocardial infarction, or acute valvular failure. The last type of shock is obstructive shock. This type is most commonly caused by cardiac tamponade, tension pneumothorax, or large pulmonary embolus. Many patients with obstructive shock will need an acute intervention such as pericardiocentesis, tube thoracostomy or anticoagulation, or thrombolysis.

   At the bedside of a critical patient, it is often difficult to assess clinically which classification of shock best fits the patient's current clinical status. Physical findings often overlap between the subtypes. For example, patients with tamponade, cardiogenic shock and sepsis (when myocardial depression compounds this form of distributive shock) may all present with distended neck veins and respiratory distress. Because of this diagnostic challenge, practitioners used to perform Swan-Ganz catheterization in hypotensive patients, providing immediate intravascular hemodynamic data. Although the data obtained from these catheters was detailed and often helpful at the bedside, large studies demonstrated no improvement in mortality in the patients who received such prolonged invasive monitoring.[9] Swan-Ganz catheterization has thus declined in use, and the stage has now been set for development of a noninvasive hemodynamic assessment using point of care ultrasound.

SHOCK ULTRASOUND PROTOCOL: THE RUSH EXAM

Given the advantages of early integration of bedside ultrasound into the diagnostic workup of the patient in shock, this article outlines an easily learned and quickly performed 3-step shock ultrasound protocol. The authors term this new ultrasound protocol the RUSH exam (Rapid Ultrasound in SHock). This protocol involves a 3-part bedside physiologic assessment simplified as:

   Step 1: The pump
   Step 2: The tank
   Step 3: The pipes

This examination is performed using standard ultrasound equipment present in many emergency departments today. The authors recommend a phased-array transducer (3.5–5 MHz) to allow adequate thoracoabdominal intercostal scanning, and a linear array transducer (7.5–10 MHz) for the required venous examinations and for the evaluation of pneumothorax.

The first, and most crucial, step in evaluation of the patient in shock is determination of cardiac status, termed for simplicity "the pump" (Table 1). Clinicians caring for the patient in shock begin with a limited echocardiogram. The echo examination is focused on looking for 3 main findings. First, the pericardial sac can be visualized to determine if the patient has a pericardial effusion that may be compressing the heart, leading to a mechanical cause of obstructive shock. Second, the left ventricle can be analyzed for global contractility. Determination of the size and contractility status of the left ventricle will allow for those patients with a cardiogenic cause of shock to be rapidly identified.[10,11] The third goal-directed examination of the heart focuses on determining the relative size of the left ventricle to the right ventricle. A heart that has an increased size of the right ventricle relative to the left ventricle may be a sign of acute right ventricular strain from a massive pulmonary embolus in the hypotensive patient.[12,13]

The second part of the RUSH shock ultrasound protocol focuses on the determination of effective intravascular volume status, which will be referred to as "the tank." Placement of the probe in the subxiphoid position, along both the long and short axis of the inferior vena cava (IVC), will allow correct determination of the size of the vessel. Looking at the respiratory dynamics of the IVC will provide an assessment of the patient's volume status to answer the clinical question, "how full is the

Table 1			
Rapid Ultrasound in SHock (RUSH) protocol: ultrasonographic findings seen with classic shock states			
RUSH Evaluation	**Hypovolemic Shock**	**Cardiogenic Shock**	**Obstructive Shock**	**Distributive Shock**
Pump	Hypercontractile heart Small chamber size	Hypocontractile heart Dilated heart	Hypercontractile heart Pericardial effusion Cardiac tamponade RV strain Cardiac thrombus	Hypercontractile heart (early sepsis) Hypocontractile heart (late sepsis)
Tank	Flat IVC Flat jugular veins Peritoneal fluid (fluid loss) Pleural fluid (fluid loss)	Distended IVC Distended jugular veins Lung rockets (pulmonary edema) Pleural fluid Peritoneal fluid (ascites)	Distended IVC Distended jugular veins Absent lung sliding (pneumothorax)	Normal or small IVC (early sepsis) Peritoneal fluid (sepsis source) Pleural fluid (sepsis source)
Pipes	Abdominal aneurysm Aortic dissection	Normal	DVT	Normal

Abbreviations: DVT, deep venous thrombosis; IVC, inferior vena cava; RV, right ventricle.

tank?"[14,15] The clinician can also place a transducer on the internal jugular veins to view their size and changes in diameter with breathing to further assess volume.[16] Also included in evaluation of the tank is an assessment of the lung, pleural cavity, and abdominal cavities for pathology that could signal a compromised vascular volume. Integration of lung ultrasound techniques can quickly allow the clinician to identify a pneumothorax, which in the hypotensive patient may represent a tension pneumothorax requiring immediate decompression. Tension pneumothorax presumably limits venous return into the heart due to increased pressure within the chest cavity.[17,18] The lung can also be examined for ultrasonic B lines, a potential sign of volume overload and pulmonary edema. The clinician can further examine the thoracic cavity for a pleural effusion. Last, the clinician can perform a FAST exam (Focused Assessment with Sonography in Trauma examination), to look for fluid in the abdomen, indicating a source for "loss of fluid from the tank."

The third and final part of the shock ultrasound protocol is evaluation of the large arteries and veins of the body, referred to as "the pipes." Clinicians should answer the clinical question "are the pipes ruptured or obstructed" by first evaluating the arterial side of the vascular system to specifically examine the abdominal and thoracic aorta for an aneurysm or dissection. Next the clinician should turn to evaluation of the venous side of the vascular system. The femoral and popliteal veins can be examined with a high frequency linear array transducer for compressibility. Lack of full venous compression with direct pressure is highly suggestive of a deep venous thrombosis (DVT).[19,20] Presence of a venous thrombus in the hypotensive patient may signal a large pulmonary thromboembolus.

RUSH Protocol: Step 1—Evaluation of the Pump

Focused echocardiography is a skill that is readily learned by the EP. A smaller footprint phased-array transducer is ideal for this examination as it permits the intercostal scanning required of the heart. Imaging of the heart usually involves 4 views. The traditional views of the heart for bedside echocardiography are the parasternal long- and short-axis views, the subxiphoid view, and the apical 4-chamber view (**Fig. 1**). The parasternal views are taken with the probe positioned just left of the sternum at intercostal space 3 or 4. The subxiphoid 4-chamber view is obtained with the probe aimed up toward the left shoulder from a position just below the subxiphoid tip of the sternum (**Fig. 2**). The apical 4-chamber view of the heart is best evaluated by turning the patient into a left lateral decubitus position and placing the probe just below the nipple line at the point of maximal impulse of the heart. It is important for the EP to know all 4 views

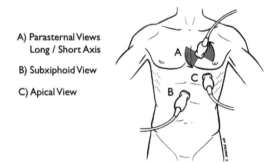

A) Parasternal Views
   Long / Short Axis

B) Subxiphoid View

C) Apical View

Fig. 1. Rapid Ultrasound in SHock (RUSH) step 1. Evaluation of the pump.

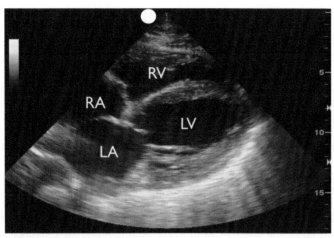

Fig. 2. Subxiphoid view: cardiomyopathy with enlarged heart. LA, left atrium; LV, left ventricle; RA, right atrium; RV, right ventricle.

of the heart, as some views may not be well seen in individual patients, and an alternative view may be needed to answer the clinical question at hand.

"Effusion around the pump": evaluation of the pericardium

The first priority is to search for the presence of a pericardial effusion, which may be a cause of the patient's hemodynamic instability. The heart should be imaged in the planes described here, with close attention to the presence of fluid, usually appearing as a dark or anechoic area, within the pericardial space (**Fig. 3**). Small effusions may be seen as a thin stripe inside the pericardial space, whereas larger effusions tend to wrap circumferentially around the heart.[21,22] Isolated small anterior anechoic areas on the parasternal long-axis view often represent a pericardial fat pad, as free flowing pericardial effusions will tend to layer posteriorly and inferiorly with gravity. Fresh fluid

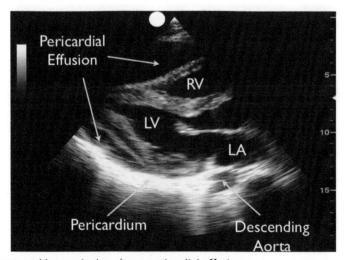

Fig. 3. Parasternal long-axis view: large pericardial effusion.

or blood tends to have a darker or anechoic appearance, whereas clotted blood or exudates may have a lighter or more echogenic look.

Pericardial effusions can result in hemodynamic instability, due to increased pressure within the sac leading to compression of the heart. Because the pericardium is a relatively thick and fibrous structure, acute pericardial effusions may result in cardiac tamponade despite only small amounts of fluid. In contrast, chronic effusions can grow to a large volume without hemodynamic instability.[23] Once a pericardial effusion is identified, the next step is to evaluate the heart for signs of tamponade. Thinking of the heart as a dual chamber in-line pump, the left side of the heart is under considerably more pressure, due to the high systemic pressures against which it must pump. The right side of the heart is under relatively less pressure, due to the lower pressure within the pulmonary vascular circuit. Thus, most echocardiographers define tamponade as compression of the right side of the heart (**Fig. 4**). High pressure within the pericardial sac keeps the chamber from fully expanding during the relaxation phase of the cardiac cycle and thus is best recognized during diastole. As either chamber may be affected by the effusion, both the right atrium and right ventricle should be closely inspected for diastolic collapse. Diastolic collapse of the right atrium or right ventricle appears as a spectrum from a subtle inward serpentine deflection of the outer wall to complete compression of a chamber.[24] Whereas most pericardial effusions are free flowing in the pericardial sac, occasionally effusions may be loculated. This phenomenon is more commonly seen in patients following heart surgery, in whom a clot can form in only one area of the sac.[25] In these cases, effusions can preferentially form posteriorly, and in tamponade, the left side of the heart may be compressed before the right side of the heart. The IVC can also be evaluated for additional confirmatory signs of tamponade.[26] IVC plethora will be recognized by distention of the IVC without normal respiratory changes. (see later discussion on IVC in the section "Evaluation of the tank").

Previous published studies have demonstrated that EPs, with a limited amount of training, can correctly and accurately identify the presence of a pericardial effusion.[27] Studies examining the incidence of pericardial effusions in Emergency Department or

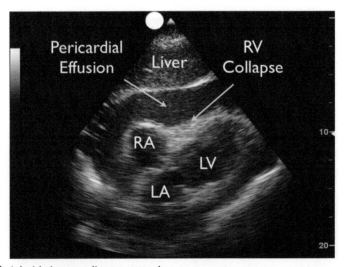

Fig. 4. Subxiphoid view: cardiac tamponade.

Intensive Care patients suffering acute shortness of breath, respiratory failure, or shock have found effusions in as many as 13% of these patients.[21] Another study looked specifically at patients arriving at the Emergency Department in near-cardiac arrest states, and found a relatively large number of these cases had pericardial effusions.[28] Thus, symptomatic pericardial effusions may be a cause of hemodynamic instability in a significant number of acute patients, and EPs can quickly and accurately diagnose this condition using bedside ultrasound.

As a general principle, it is easier for an EP to diagnose a pericardial effusion than to evaluate for the specific signs of tamponade.[29] It is thus safer to assume tamponade physiology in the hypotensive patient if a significant pericardial effusion is identified. Under ideal circumstances, the EP can obtain a formal echocardiogram in conjunction with Cardiology to specifically examine for cardiac tamponade. In the rare cases where there is not enough time for consultation and the patient is unstable, a pericardiocentesis under echo guidance by the EP may be life-saving. In these cases, employing bedside echocardiography also allows the EP to determine the optimal needle insertion site for pericardiocentesis. Of note, most EPs have classically been taught the subxiphoid approach for pericardiocentesis. However, a large review from the Mayo Clinic looked at 1127 pericardiocentesis procedures, and found that the optimal placement of the needle was where the distance to the effusion was the least and the effusion size was maximal.[30] The apical position at the point of maximal impulse on the left lateral chest wall was chosen in 80% of these procedures, based on these variables. The subxiphoid approach was only chosen in 20% of these procedures, as the investigators recognized the large distance the needle had to travel through the liver to enter the pericardial sac. EPs should therefore anatomically map out the effusion before a pericardiocentesis procedure to plan the most direct and safest route. If the apical approach is selected, the patient should optimally be rolled into a left lateral decubitus position to bring the heart closer to the chest wall, and after local anesthesia, a pericardiocentesis drainage catheter should be introduced over the rib and into the pericardial sac. To maximize success and to avoid complications, the transducer should be placed in a sterile sleeve adjacent to the needle, and the procedure performed under real-time ultrasound guidance.

"Squeeze of the pump": determination of global left ventricular function
The next step in the RUSH protocol is to evaluate the heart for contractility of the left ventricle. This assessment will give a determination of "how strong the pump is." The examination focuses on evaluating motion of the left ventricular endocardial walls, as judged by a visual calculation of the percentage change from diastole to systole. Whereas in the past echocardiographers used radionuclide imaging to determine ejection fraction, published studies have demonstrated that visual determination of contractility is roughly equivalent.[31] A ventricle that has good contractility will be observed to have a large percentage change from the 2 cycles, with the walls almost coming together and touching during systole. As an example, a vigorously contracting ventricle will almost completely obliterate the ventricular cavity during systole. In comparison, a poorly contracting heart will have a small percentage change in the movement of the walls between diastole and systole. In these hearts, the walls will be observed to move little during the cardiac cycle, and the heart may also be dilated in size, especially if a long-standing cardiomyopathy with severe systolic dysfunction is present. Motion of anterior leaflet of the mitral valve can also be used to assess contractility. In a normal contractile state, the anterior leaflet will vigorously touch the wall of the septum during ventricular filling when examined using the parasternal long-axis view.

The parasternal long-axis view of the heart is an excellent starting view to assess ventricular contractility. Moving the probe into the parasternal short-axis orientation will give confirmatory data on the strength of contractions. In this view, a left ventricle with good contraction will appear as a muscular ring that squeezes down concentrically during systole. Whereas cardiologists often use the parasternal short-axis view to evaluate for segmental wall motion abnormalities, this is a more subjective measurement, and determinations may differ among different clinicians. For that reason, it is better for the EP to initially concentrate on the overall contractility of the ventricle, rather than to evaluate for segmental wall motion deficits. An easy system of grading is to judge the strength of contractions as good, with the walls of the ventricle contracting well during systole; poor, with the endocardial walls changing little in position from diastole to systole; and intermediate, with the walls moving with a percentage change in between the previous 2 categories. If the parasternal views are inadequate for these determinations, moving the patient into the left lateral decubitus position and examining from the apical view often gives crucial data on left ventricular contractility. The subxiphoid view can be used for this determination, but the left ventricle is farther away from the probe in this view.

Published studies confirm that EPs can perform this examination and get an estimate of left ventricular contractility that compares well with that measured by a cardiologist.[32] Because a large proportion of shock patients (up to 60% in one study) will have a cardiac cause for their hypotension, this part of the examination can be very high yield.[10] Immediate identification of cardiogenic shock by the EP can lead to more rapid transfer of the patient to the cardiac catheterization suite for revascularization, especially in suspected cases of cardiac ischemia.[33,34] Other types of shock can be evaluated by knowing the strength of the left ventricle during systole. Strong ventricular contractility (often termed hyperdynamic, because of the strength of contractions of the left ventricle in addition to a rapid heart rate) is often seen in early sepsis and in hypovolemic shock.[35] In severe hypovolemic conditions, the heart is often small in size with complete obliteration of the ventricular cavity during systole. Bedside echocardiography also allows for repeated evaluation of the patient's heart, looking for changes in contractility over time, especially when if a patient's status deteriorates. For example, later in the course of sepsis there may be a decrease in contractility of the left ventricle due to myocardial depression.[36]

Knowing the strength of left ventricular contractility will give the EP a better idea of how much fluid "the pump" or heart of the patient can handle, before manifesting signs and symptoms of fluid overload. This knowledge will serve as a critical guide for the clinician to determine the amount of fluid that can be safely given to a patient. As an example, in a heart with poor contractility, the threshold for initiation of vasopressor agents for hemodynamic support should be lower. In contrast, sepsis patients have been shown to benefit with aggressive early goal-directed therapy, starting with large amounts of fluids before use of vasopressor medications.[37] Because many Emergency Departments do not currently use the invasive catheter needed to optimally monitor the hemodynamic goals outlined for treatment of sepsis patients, bedside ultrasound gives the clinician a noninvasive means to identify and follow a best management strategy.

In cardiac arrest, the clinician should specifically examine for the presence or absence of cardiac contractions. If contractions are seen, the clinician should look for the coordinated movements of the mitral and aortic valves. In this scenario, the absence of coordinated opening of mitral and aortic valves will require chest compressions to maintain cardiac output. Furthermore, if after prolonged advanced cardiac life support resuscitation the bedside echocardiogram shows cardiac standstill, it is unlikely that the adult patient will have return of spontaneous circulation.[38,39]

"Strain of the pump": assessment of right ventricular strain

In the normal heart, the left ventricle is larger than the right ventricle. This aspect is predominantly a cause of the muscular hypertrophy that takes place in the myocardium of the left ventricle after birth, with the closure of the ductus arteriosus. The left ventricle is under considerably more stress than the right ventricle, to meet the demands of the higher systemic pressure, and hypertrophy is a normal compensatory mechanism. On bedside echocardiography, the normal ratio of the left to right ventricle is 1:0.6.[40] The optimal cardiac views for determining this ratio of size between the 2 ventricles are the parasternal long and short-axis views and the apical 4-chamber view. The subxiphoid view can be used, but care must be taken to fan through the entire right ventricle, as it is easy to underestimate the true right ventricular size in this view.

Any condition that causes pressure to suddenly increase within the pulmonary vascular circuit will result in acute dilation of the right heart in an effort to maintain forward flow into the pulmonary artery. The classic cause of acute right heart strain is a large central pulmonary embolus. Due to the sudden obstruction of the pulmonary outflow tract by a large pulmonary embolus, the right ventricle will attempt to compensate with acute dilation. This process can be seen on bedside echocardiography by a right ventricular chamber that is as large, or larger, than the left ventricle (**Fig. 5**).[41] In addition, deflection of the interventricular septum from right to left toward the left ventricle may signal higher pressures within the pulmonary artery.[42] In rare cases, intracardiac thrombus may be seen floating free within the heart (**Fig. 6**).[43] In comparison, a condition that causes a more gradual increase in pulmonary artery pressure over time, such as smaller and recurrent pulmonary emboli, cor pulmonale with predominant right heart strain, or primary pulmonary artery hypertension, will cause both dilation and thickening or hypertrophy of the right ventricular wall.[44] These mechanisms can allow the right ventricle to compensate over time and to adapt to pumping

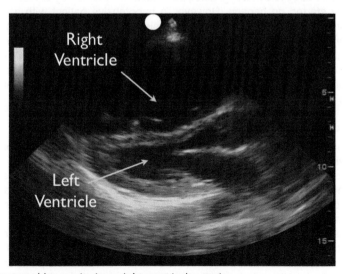

Fig. 5. Parasternal long-axis view: right ventricular strain.

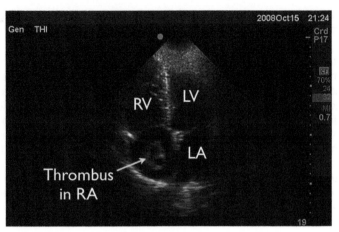

Fig. 6. Apical view: floating thrombus in right atrium.

blood against the higher pressures in the pulmonary vascular circuit. Acute right heart strain thus differs from chronic right heart strain in that although both conditions cause dilation of the chamber, the ventricle will not have the time to hypertrophy if the time course is sudden.

Previous published studies have looked at the sensitivity of the finding of right heart dilation in helping the clinician to diagnose a pulmonary embolus. The results show that the sensitivity is moderate, but the specificity and positive predictive value of this finding are high in the correct clinical scenario, especially if hypotension is present.[12,13,45–47] The finding of acute right heart strain due to a pulmonary embolus correlates with a poorer prognosis.[12,48,49] This finding, in the setting of suspected pulmonary embolus, suggests the need for immediate evaluation and treatment of thromboembolism.[50] The EP should also proceed directly to evaluation of the leg veins for a DVT (covered in detail later under "Evaluation of the pipes").

The literature suggests that in general, patients with a pulmonary embolus should be immediately started on heparin. However, a hypotensive patient with a pulmonary embolus should be considered for thrombolysis.[51,52] Bedsides, ultrasound gives the treating clinician the clinical confidence to proceed in this more aggressive fashion. Clinical status permitting, a chest computed tomography (CT) scan using a dedicated pulmonary embolus protocol should be obtained. If the patient is not stable enough for CT, an emergent echocardiogram in conjunction with Cardiology or bilateral duplex ultrasound of the legs should be considered.

RUSH Protocol Step 2: Evaluation of the Tank

"Fullness of the tank": evaluation of the inferior cava and jugular veins for size and collapse with inspiration

The next step for the clinician using the RUSH protocol in the hypotensive patient is to evaluate the effective intravascular volume as well as to look for areas where the intravascular volume might be compromised (**Fig. 7**). An estimate of the intravascular volume can be determined noninvasively by looking initially at the IVC.[14,15] The ultrasound transducer should be positioned in the epigastric area in a long-axis configuration along the IVC as it runs from the abdomen into the heart. A good way of obtaining this image is to first examine the heart in the subxiphoid 4-chamber plane and then to move the probe into the subxiphoid 2-chamber plane, with the probe marker oriented

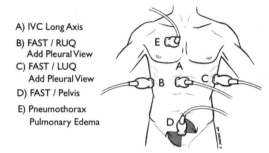

A) IVC Long Axis
B) FAST / RUQ
   Add Pleural View
C) FAST / LUQ
   Add Pleural View
D) FAST / Pelvis
E) Pneumothorax
   Pulmonary Edema

Fig. 7. RUSH step 2. Evaluation of the tank. IVC exam, inferior vena cava; FAST views (Focused Sonography in Trauma), right upper quadrant, left upper quadrant and suprapubic; lung exam, pneumothorax and pulmonary edema.

anteriorly. The aorta will often come quickly into view from this plane as a thicker walled and deeper structure. Moving the probe to the patient's right will bring the IVC into view, running longitudinally adjacent to the aorta. The IVC should be examined at the junction of the right atrium and the cava and followed 2 to 3 cm caudally along the vessel. Moving the probe into short axis to further evaluate the IVC is complementary as it will display the structure as an oval and allow confirmation of size by avoiding underestimation of the structure with the cylinder effect. As the patient breathes, the IVC will have a normal pattern of collapse during inspiration, due to the negative pressure generated in the chest, causing increased flow from the abdominal to the thoracic cavity (**Fig. 8**). This respiratory variation can be further augmented by having the patient sniff or inspire forcefully. M-mode Doppler, positioned on the IVC, can graphically document the dynamic changes in the vessel caliber during the patient's respiratory cycle (**Fig. 9**).

Previous studies have demonstrated a correlation between the size and percentage change of the IVC with respiratory variation to central venous pressure (CVP) using an indwelling catheter. A smaller caliber IVC (<2 cm diameter) with an inspiratory collapse

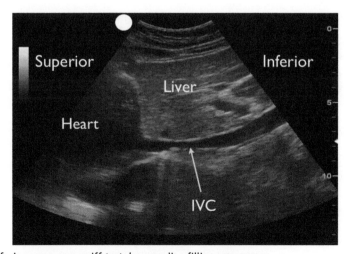

Fig. 8. Inferior vena cava sniff test: low cardiac filling pressures.

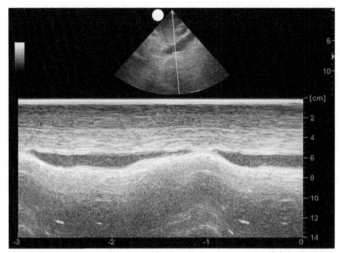

Fig. 9. Inferior vena cava sniff test: M-mode Doppler showing collapsible IVC.

greater than 50% roughly correlates to a CVP of less than 10 cm of water. This phenomenon may be observed in hypovolemic and distributive shock states. A larger sized IVC (>2 cm diameter) that collapses less than 50% with inspiration correlates to a CVP of more than 10 cm of water (**Fig. 10**).[53,54] This phenomenon may be seen in cardiogenic and obstructive shock states. Two caveats to this rule exist. The first is in patients who have received treatment with vasodilators and/or diuretics prior to ultrasound evaluation in whom the IVC may be smaller than prior to treatment, altering the initial physiological state. The second caveat exists in intubated patients receiving positive pressure ventilation, in which the respiratory dynamics of the IVC are reversed. In these patients, the IVC is also less compliant and more distended throughout all respiratory cycles. However, crucial physiologic data can still be

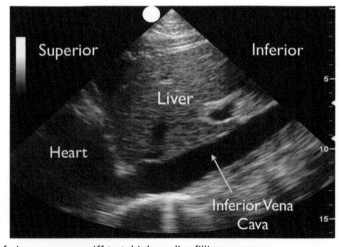

Fig. 10. Inferior vena cava sniff test: high cardiac filling pressures.

obtained in these ventilated patients, as fluid responsiveness has been correlated with an increase in IVC diameter over time.[55]

Evidence suggests that the bedside ultrasound estimate of CVP is most accurate when the IVC is small and inspiratory collapse is high. However, rather than relying on a single measurement of the IVC, it is better to determine the effective vascular volume by following changes in size and respiratory dynamics over time with fluid challenges.[56] Observing a change in IVC size from small, with a high inspiratory collapse, to a larger IVC with little inspiratory collapse, suggests that the CVP is increasing and "the tank" is more full.[57]

The internal jugular veins can also be examined with ultrasound to further evaluate the intravascular volume. As with visual evaluation of the jugular veins, the patient's head is placed at a 30° angle. Using a high-frequency linear array transducer, the internal jugular veins can first be found in the short-axis plane, then evaluated more closely by moving the probe into a long-axis configuration. The location of the superior closing meniscus is determined by the point at which the walls of the vein touch each other. Similar to the IVC, the jugular veins can also be examined during respiratory phases to view inspiratory collapse. Veins that are distended, with a closing meniscus level that is high in the course of the neck, suggest a higher CVP.[16] Coupling this data with the evaluation of the IVC may give a better overall assessment of the effective intravascular volume.

"Leakiness of the tank": FAST exam and pleural fluid assessment

Once a patient's intravascular volume status has been determined, the next step in assessing the tank is to look for "abnormal leakiness of the tank." Leakiness of the tank refers to 1 of 3 things leading to hemodynamic compromise: internal blood loss, fluid extravasation, or other pathologic fluid collections. In traumatic conditions, the clinician must quickly determine whether hemoperitoneum or hemothorax is present, as a result of a "hole in the tank," leading to hypovolemic shock. In nontraumatic conditions, accumulation of excess fluid into the abdominal and chest cavities often signifies "tank overload," with resultant pleural effusions and ascites that may build-up with failure of the heart, kidneys, and/or liver. However, many patients with intrathoracic or intra-abdominal fluid collections are actually intravascularly volume depleted, confusing the clinical picture. Focusing on "tank fullness" by assessment of IVC and jugular veins in conjunction with the aforementioned findings can be very helpful in elucidating these conditions. In infectious states, pneumonia may be accompanied by a complicating parapneumonic pleural effusion, and ascites may lead to spontaneous bacterial peritonitis. Depending on the clinical scenario, small fluid collections within the peritoneal cavity may also represent intra-abdominal abscesses leading to a sepsis picture.

The peritoneal cavity can be readily evaluated with bedside ultrasound for the presence of an abnormal fluid collection in both trauma and nontrauma states. This assessment is accomplished with the FAST exam. This examination consists of an inspection of the potential spaces in the right and left upper abdominal quadrants and in the pelvis. Specific views include the space between the liver and kidney (hepatorenal space or Morison pouch), the area around the spleen (perisplenic space), and the area around and behind the bladder (rectovesicular/rectovaginal space or pouch of Douglas). A dark or anechoic area in any of these 3 potential spaces represents free intraperitoneal fluid (**Fig. 11**). These 3 areas represent the most common places for free fluid to collect, and correspond to the most dependent areas of the peritoneal cavity in the supine patient. Because the FAST exam relies on free fluid settling into these dependent areas, the patient's position should be taken into account while

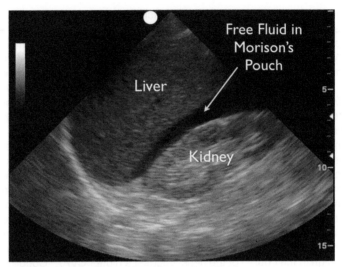

Fig. 11. Right upper quadrant/hepatorenal view: free fluid.

interpreting the examination. Trendelenburg positioning will cause fluid to shift to the upper abdominal regions, whereas an upright position will cause shift of fluid into the pelvis.

The FAST exam has been reported to detect intraperitoneal fluid collections as small as 100 mL, with a range of 250 to 620 mL commonly cited.[58–60] How much fluid can be detected depends on the clinician's experience as well as the location of the free fluid, with the pelvic view best able to detect small quantities of fluid.[60] The overall sensitivity and specificity of the FAST exam have been reported to be approximately 79% and 99%, respectively.[61]

Ultrasound can also assist in evaluating the thoracic cavity for free fluid (pleural effusion or hemothorax) in an examination known as the extended FAST, or E-FAST. This evaluation is easily accomplished by including views of the thoracic cavity with the FAST examination. In both the hepatorenal and perisplenic views, the diaphragms appear as bright or hyperechoic lines immediately above, or cephalad to, the liver and spleen respectively. Aiming the probe above the diaphragm will allow for identification of a thoracic fluid collection. If fluid is found, movement of the probe 1 or 2 intercostal spaces cephalad provides a better view of the thoracic cavity, allowing quantification of the fluid present. In the normal supradiaphragmatic view, there are no dark areas of fluid in the thoracic cavity, and the lung can often be visualized as a moving structure. In the presence of an effusion or hemothorax, the normally visualized lung above the diaphragm is replaced with a dark, or anechoic, space. The lung may also be visualized floating within the pleural fluid (**Fig. 12**). Pleural effusions often exert compression on the lung, causing "hepatization," or an appearance of the lung in the effusion similar to a solid organ, like the liver. The literature supports the use of bedside ultrasound for the detection of pleural effusion and hemothorax. Several studies have found Emergency Department ultrasound to have a sensitivity in excess of 92% and a specificity approaching 100% in the detection of hemothorax.[62–65] Assessing the patient with the head slightly elevated may improve the sensitivity of this examination, as this will cause intrathoracic fluid to accumulate just above the diaphragms.

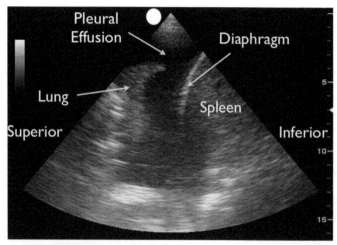

Fig. 12. Left upper quadrant: pleural effusion.

Free fluid in the peritoneal or thoracic cavities in a hypotensive patient in whom a history of trauma is present or suspected should initially be presumed to be blood, leading to a diagnosis of hemorrhagic shock. Although a history of trauma is commonly elicited in such cases, the trauma may be occult or minor, making diagnosis sometimes difficult. One circumstance of occult trauma is a delayed splenic rupture resulting from an enlarged and more fragile spleen, such as in a patient with infectious mononucleosis. Although rare, this entity may occur several days following a minor trauma, and may thus be easily overlooked by both patient and clinician.[66] Leakage of intestinal contents from rupture of a hollow viscus or urine extravasation from intraperitoneal bladder rupture may also demonstrate free intraperitoneal fluid.

Nontraumatic conditions may also lead to hemorrhagic shock, and must remain on the EP's differential diagnosis. Ruptured ectopic pregnancy and hemorrhagic corpus luteum cyst are 2 diagnoses that should not be overlooked in women of childbearing age. In an elderly patient, an abdominal aortic aneurysm may occasionally rupture into the peritoneal cavity and thoracic aneurysms may rupture into the chest cavity. Once the diagnosis of hemorrhagic shock is made, treatment should be directed toward transfusion of blood products and surgical or angiographic intervention.

In the nontrauma patient, ascites and pleural effusions will appear as dark, or anechoic, fluid collections, similar to blood. Parapneumonic inflammation may cause considerable pleural effusions and/or empyema. Differentiating blood from other fluids can be suggested from the history, clinical examination, and chest radiograph. There may occasionally be some signature sonographic findings that help make a diagnosis. In hemorrhagic conditions, blood often has a mixed appearance, with areas of both anechoic fresh blood and more echogenic blood clot present. In an infectious parapneumonic pleural effusion, gas bubbles may be seen within the fluid. In cases of uncertainty, a diagnostic thoracentesis or paracentesis (under ultrasound guidance) will most accurately evaluate the nature of the fluid.[67]

"Tank compromise": pneumothorax

Although the exact mechanism by which tension pneumothorax causes shock is controversial, it has historically been thought to produce obstructive shock.[17,18,68] According to this theory, severely increased intrathoracic pressure produces mediastinal shift, which kinks and compresses the inferior and superior vena cava at their insertion into the right atrium, obstructing venous return to the heart. Regardless of the exact mechanism, detection is critical.

Although chest radiography reveals characteristic findings in tension pneumo-thorax, therapy should not be delayed while awaiting radiographic studies. With bedside ultrasound, the diagnosis of tension pneumothorax can be accomplished within seconds. Pneumothorax detection with ultrasound relies on the fact that free air (pneumothorax) is lighter than normal aerated lung tissue, and thus will accumulate in the nondependent areas of the thoracic cavity. Therefore, in a supine patient a pneu-mothorax will be found anteriorly, while in an upright patient a pneumothorax will be found superiorly at the lung apex.

Multiple studies have shown ultrasound to be more sensitive than supine chest radi-ography for the detection of pneumothorax.[69–74] Sensitivities for these various studies ranged from 86% to 100%, with specificities ranging from 92% to 100%. A study by Zhang and colleagues[71] that focused on trauma victims found the sensitivity of ultra-sound for pneumothorax was 86% versus 27% for chest radiography; furthermore, this same study reported the average time to obtain ultrasound was 2.3 minutes versus 19.9 minutes for chest radiography.

To assess for pneumothorax with ultrasound, the patient should be supine. Position a high-frequency linear array or a phased-array transducer in the mid-clavicular line at approximately the third through fifth intercostal spaces to identify the pleural line. This line appears as an echogenic horizontal line located approximately half a centimeter deep to the ribs. The pleural line consists of both the visceral and parietal pleura closely apposed to one another. In the normal lung, the visceral and parietal pleura can be seen to slide against each other, with a glistening or shimmering appearance, as the patient breathes (**Fig. 13**). The presence of this lung sliding excludes a pneumo-thorax.[75] This lung sliding motion can be graphically depicted by using M-mode Doppler. A normal image will depict "waves on the beach," with no motion of the chest wall anteriorly, represented as linear "waves," and the motion of the lung posteriorly, representing "the beach" (**Fig. 14**). When a pneumothorax is present, air gathers between the parietal and visceral pleura, preventing the ultrasound beam from detect-ing lung sliding. In pneumothorax, the pleural line seen consists only of the parietal layer, seen as a stationary line. M-mode Doppler through the chest will show only repeating horizontal linear lines, demonstrating a lack of lung sliding or absence of the "beach" (see **Fig. 14**). Although the presence of lung sliding is sufficient to rule

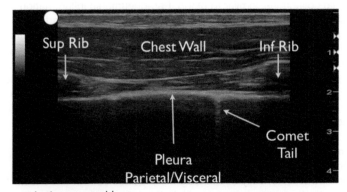

Fig. 13. Long-axis view: normal lung.

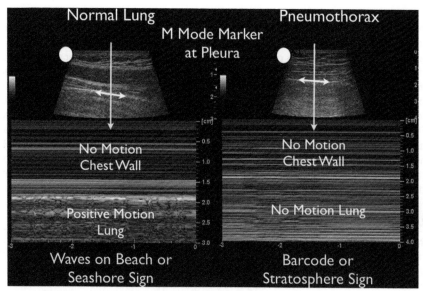

Fig. 14. M-mode: normal lung versus pneumothorax.

out pneumothorax, the absence of lung sliding may be seen in other conditions in addition to pneumothorax, such as a chronic obstructive pulmonary disease bleb, consolidated pneumonia, atelectasis, or mainstem intubation.[76–78] Thus the absence of lung sliding, especially as defined in one intercostal space, is not by itself diagnostic of a pneumothorax. The clinician can examine through several more intercostal spaces, moving the transducer more inferiorly and lateral, to increase the utility of the test. This maneuver may also help identify the lung point, or the area where an incomplete pneumothorax interfaces with the chest wall, as visualized by the presence of lung sliding on one side and the lack of lung sliding on the other.[79]

Another sonographic finding seen in normal lung, but absent in pneumothorax, is the comet tail artifact. Comet tail artifact is a form of reverberation echo that arises from irregularity of the lung surface. This phenomenon appears as a vertical echoic line originating from the pleural line and extending down into the lung tissue. The presence of comet tail artifact rules out a pneumothorax.[80] The combination of a lack of lung sliding and absent comet tail artifacts strongly suggests pneumothorax. In the setting of undifferentiated shock, the EP should strongly consider that a tension pneumothorax may be present, and immediate needle decompression followed by tube thoracostomy should be considered.

"Tank overload": pulmonary edema

Pulmonary edema often accompanies cardiogenic shock, in which weakened cardiac function causes a backup of blood into the pulmonary vasculature, leading to tank overload. Yet the clinical picture can be misleading, as patients in pulmonary edema may present with wheezing, rather than rales, or may have relatively clear lung sounds. The ability to quickly image the lung fields with ultrasound can rapidly lead the EP to the correct diagnosis. Although it is a relatively new concept, ultrasound has been shown to be helpful in the detection of pulmonary edema.[81] The sonographic signs of pulmonary edema correlate well with chest radiography.[82]

To assess for pulmonary edema with ultrasound, the lungs are scanned with the phased-array transducer in the anterolateral chest between the second and fifth rib interspaces. Detection of pulmonary edema with ultrasound relies on seeing a special subtype of comet tail artifact, called B lines (**Fig. 15**). These B lines appear as a series of diffuse, brightly echogenic lines originating from the pleural line and projecting in a fanlike pattern into the thorax (described as "lung rockets"). In contrast to the smaller comet tail artifacts seen in normal lung that fade out within a few centimeters of the pleural line, the B lines of pulmonary edema are better defined and extend to the far field of the ultrasound image. B lines result from thickening of the interlobular septa, as extravascular water accumulates within the pulmonary interstitium.[81,83] The presence of B lines coupled with decreased cardiac contractility and a plethoric IVC on focused sonographic evaluation should prompt the clinician to consider the presence of pulmonary edema and initiate appropriate treatment.

RUSH Protocol: Step 3—Evaluation of the Pipes

"Rupture of the pipes": aortic aneurysm and dissection

The next step in the RUSH exam is to examine the 'Pipes' looking first at arterial side of circulatory system and then at the venous side (**Fig. 16**). Vascular catastrophes, such as ruptured abdominal aortic aneurysms (AAA) and aortic dissections, are life-threatening causes of hypotension. The survival of such patients may often be measured in minutes, and the ability to quickly diagnose these diseases is crucial.

A ruptured AAA is classically depicted as presenting with back pain, hypotension, and a pulsatile abdominal mass. However, fewer than half of cases occur with this triad, and some cases will present with shock as the only finding.[84] A large or rupturing AAA can also mimic a kidney stone, with flank pain and hematuria. Fortunately for the EP, ultrasound can be used to rapidly diagnose both conditions.[85] Numerous studies have shown that EPs can make the diagnosis of AAA using bedside ultrasound, with a high sensitivity and specificity.[86–89] The sensitivity of EP-performed ultrasound for the detection of AAA ranges from 93% to 100%, with specificities approaching 100%.[86–88]

A complete ultrasound examination of the abdominal aorta involves imaging from the epigastrium down to the iliac bifurcation using a phased-array or curvilinear

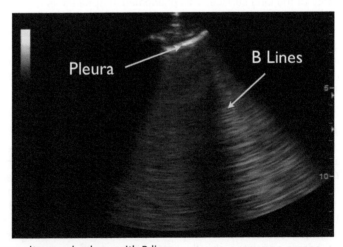

Fig. 15. Lung ultrasound: edema with B lines.

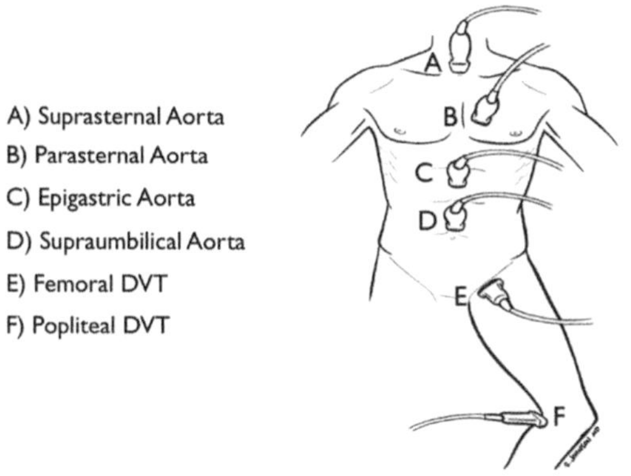

A) Suprasternal Aorta
B) Parasternal Aorta
C) Epigastric Aorta
D) Supraumbilical Aorta
E) Femoral DVT
F) Popliteal DVT

Fig. 16. RUSH step 3. Evaluation of the pipes.

transducer. Aiming the transducer posteriorly in a transverse orientation in the epigastric area, the abdominal aorta can be visualized as a circular vessel seen immediately anterior to the vertebral body and to the left of the paired IVC. Application of steady pressure to the transducer to displace bowel gas, while sliding the probe inferiorly from a position just below the xiphoid process down to the umbilicus, allows for visualization of the entire abdominal aorta. The aorta should also be imaged in the longitudinal orientation for completion. Measurements should be obtained in the short axis, measuring the maximal diameter of the aorta from outer wall to outer wall, and should include any thrombus present in the vessel. A measurement of greater than 3 cm is abnormal and defines an abdominal aortic aneurysm (**Fig. 17**). Smaller aneurysms may be symptomatic, although rupture is more common with aneurysms measuring larger than 5 cm.[90] Studies have also confirmed that the EP can reliably make a correct determination of the size of an AAA.[87,91]

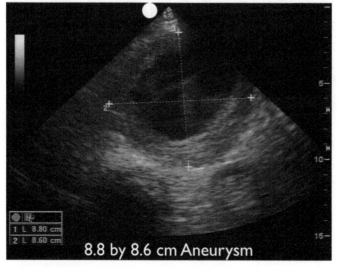

1 L 8.80 cm
2 L 8.60 cm
8.8 by 8.6 cm Aneurysm

Fig. 17. Short-axis view: large abdominal aortic aneurysm.

Identifying the abdominal aorta along its entire course is essential to rule out an aneurysm, paying special attention below the renal arteries where most AAAs are located. Rupture of an abdominal aortic aneurysm typically occurs into the retroperitoneal space, which unfortunately is an area difficult to visualize with ultrasound. In a stable patient, a CT scan with intravenous contrast can be ordered to investigate leakage of an aneurysm. However, a hypotensive patient with sonographic evidence of an AAA should be considered to have acute rupture, and a surgeon should be consulted with plans for immediate transport to the operating room.

Another crucial part of "the pipes" protocol is evaluation for an aortic dissection. The sensitivity of transthoracic echocardiography to detect aortic dissection is poor (approximately 65% according to one study), and is limited compared with CT, MRI, or transesophageal echocardiography.[92] Despite this, EP-performed bedside ultrasound has been used to detect aortic dissections and has helped many patients.[93–95] Sonographic findings suggestive of the diagnosis include the presence of aortic root dilation and an aortic intimal flap. The parasternal long-axis view of the heart permits an evaluation of the proximal aortic root, and a measurement of more than 3.8 cm is considered abnormal. An echogenic intimal flap may be recognized within the dilated root or anywhere along the course of the thoracic or abdominal aorta (**Fig. 18**). The suprasternal view allows imaging of the aortic arch and should be performed in high-suspicion scenarios by placing the phased-array transducer within the suprasternal notch and aiming caudally and anteriorly (**Fig. 19**). Color flow imaging can further delineate 2 lumens with distinct blood flow, confirming the diagnosis. In patients with acute proximal dissection, aortic regurgitation or a pericardial effusion may also be recognized. Abdominal aortic ultrasound may reveal a distal thoracic aortic dissection that extends below the diaphragm, and in the hands of skilled sonographers has been shown to be 98% sensitive.[96]

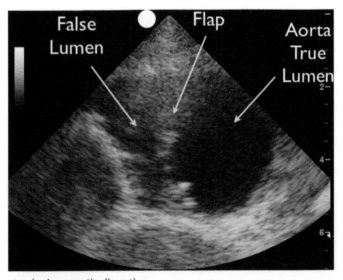

Fig. 18. Short-axis view: aortic dissection.

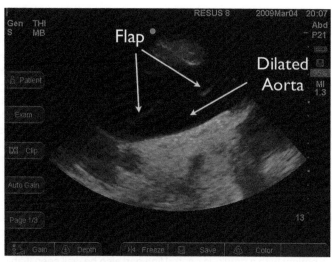

Fig. 19. Suprasternal view: aortic dissection.

"Clogging of the pipes": venous thromboembolism

Bedside ultrasound for DVT In the patient in whom a thromboembolic event is suspected as a cause of shock, the EP should then move to an assessment of the venous side of "the pipes." As the majority of pulmonary emboli originate from lower extremity DVT, the examination is concentrated on a limited compression evaluation of the leg veins. Simple compression ultrasonography, which uses a high frequency linear probe to apply direct pressure to the vein, has a good overall sensitivity for detection of DVT of the leg.[97] An acute blood clot forms a mass in the lumen of the vein, and the pathognomonic finding of DVT will be incomplete compression of the anterior and posterior walls of the vein (**Fig. 20**).[98,99] In contrast, a normal vein will completely collapse with simple compression. Most distal deep venous thromboses can be detected through

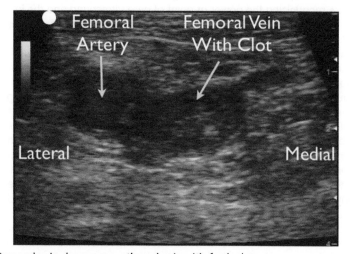

Fig. 20. Femoral vein deep venous thrombosis with fresh clot.

simple compression ultrasonography of the leg using standard B-mode imaging, and more complicated Doppler techniques add little utility to the examination.[100]

Ultrasound may miss some clots that have formed in the calf veins, a difficult area to evaluate with sonography.[101] However, most proximal DVTs can be detected by a limited compression examination of the leg that can be rapidly performed by focusing on 2 major areas.[102,103] The proximal femoral vein just below the inguinal ligament is evaluated first, beginning at the common femoral vein, found below the inguinal ligament. Scanning should continue down the vein through the confluence with the saphenous vein to the bifurcation of the vessel into the deep and superficial femoral veins. The second area of evaluation is the popliteal fossa. The popliteal vein, the continuation of the superficial femoral vein, can be examined from high in the popliteal fossa down to trifurcation into the calf veins. If an upper extremity thrombus is clinically suspected, the same compression techniques can be employed, following the arm veins up to the axillary vein and into the subclavian vein. Although a good initial test, the sensitivity of ultrasound for proximal upper extremity clots is lower than for lower extremity clots, as the subclavian vein cannot be fully compressed behind the clavicle.[104] Although clinically less common, an internal jugular vein thrombosis that may form in a patient with a previous central line can also be well seen with ultrasound.

Previous studies have shown that EPs can perform limited ultrasound compression for lower extremity venous clots with good sensitivity in patients with a high pretest probability for the disease.[105–108] The examination can also be performed rapidly, and can be integrated into the overall RUSH protocol with a minimum of added time.[109]

SUMMARY

Bedside ultrasound technology has evolved to the point that it offers a powerful, yet easy to use tool for the clinician faced with a critical patient. The initial imaging focus of ultrasound as used by Radiologists was on anatomy and pathology. Now with clinicians actively using this technology at the bedside, attention has shifted to the crucial evaluation of *physiology*. The ability to recognize both abnormal pathology and physiology in a critical patient, recognize a distinctive shock state, and arrive at a more precise diagnosis represents a new paradigm in resuscitation care. Clinicians around the world are recognizing the power of point of care ultrasound and the impact it will have on critical care resuscitation in the Emergency Department, as well as in Intensive Care Units.

The individual components of the *Rapid Ultrasound in SHock* protocol have been studied and published prior, but this new protocol represents the first synthesis of these sonographic techniques into a unified 3 step algorithm. The protocol simplifies the ultrasound evaluation into the physiological paradigm of "pump, tank, and pipes," allowing the clinician to easily remember the critical aspects of the exam components. Although described in a sequential 3-step approach, clinicians are expected to alter the components and sequence of sonographic techniques based on the clinical scenario presented. Unlike previous published studies that have examined ultrasound protocols in the hypotensive patient, the described RUSH exam presents the most detailed shock algorithm for use by EPs to date.[110] By focusing on both the anatomy and the physiology of these complex patients, in shock, bedside ultrasound provides the opportunity for improved clinical treatments and patient outcomes.

For educational ultrasound videos covering all RUSH applications, please go to http://www.sound-bytes.tv where a downloadable pocket card on RUSH is also available.

ACKNOWLEDGMENTS

We would like to acknowledge the work of Scott Weingart, MD and Brett Nelson, MD on ultrasound evaluation of the hypotensive patient.

REFERENCES

1. Jones AE, Tayal VS, Sullivan DM, et al. Randomized, controlled trial of immediate versus delayed goal directed ultrasound to identify the cause of nontraumatic hypotension in emergency department patients. Crit Care Med 2004;32: 1703–8.
2. Jones AE, Aborn LS, Kline JA. Severity of emergency department hypotension predicts adverse hospital outcome. Shock 2004;22:410–4.
3. Thomas HA, Beeson MS, Binder LS, et al. The 2005 model of the clinical practice of emergency medicine: the 2007 update. Acad Emerg Med 2008;15(8): 776–9.
4. Heller MB, Mandavia D, Tayal VS. Residency training in emergency ultrasound: fulfilling the mandate. Acad Emerg Med 2002;9:835–9.
5. ACEP emergency ultrasound guidelines. Ann Emerg Med 2009;14:550–70.
6. Pershad J, Myers S, Plouman C, et al. Bedside limited echocardiography by the emergency physician is accurate during evaluation of the critically ill patient. Pediatrics 2004;114:e667–71.
7. Plummer D, Heegaard W, Dries D, et al. Ultrasound in HEMS: its role in differentiating shock states. Air Med J 2003;22:33–6.
8. Kline JA. Shock. In: Rosen P, Marx J, editors. Emergency medicine; concepts and clinical practice. 5th edition. St Louis (MO): Mosby; 2002. p. 33–47.
9. Shah MR, Hasselblad V, Stevenson LW, et al. Impact of the pulmonary artery catheter in critically ill patients: meta-analysis of randomized clinical trials. JAMA 2005;294:1664–70.
10. Joseph M, Disney P. Transthoracic echocardiography to identify or exclude cardiac cause of shock. Chest 2004;126:1592–7.
11. Bealieu Y. Specific skill set and goals of focused echocardiography for critical care physicians. Crit Care Med 2007;35:S144–9.
12. Viellard-Baron A, Page B, Augarde R, et al. Acute cor pulmonale in massive pulmonary embolism: incidence, echocardiography pattern, clinical implications and recovery rate. Intensive Care Med 2001;27:1481–6.
13. Grifoni S, Olivotto I, Cecchini P, et al. Utility of an integrated clinical, echocardiographic and venous ultrasound approach for triage of patients with suspected pulmonary embolism. Am J Cardiol 1998;82:1230–5.
14. Jardin F, Veillard-Baron A. Ultrasonographic examination of the vena cavae. Intensive Care Med 2006;32:203–6.
15. Randazzo MR, Snoey ER, Levitt MA, et al. Accuracy of emergency physician assessment of left ventricular ejection fraction and central venous pressure using echocardiography. Acad Emerg Med 2003;10:973–7.
16. Jang T, Aubin C, Naunheim R, et al. Ultrasonography of the internal jugular vein in patients with dyspnea without jugular venous distention on physical examination. Ann Emerg Med 2004;44:160–8.
17. Connolly JP. Hemodynamic measurements during a tension pneumothorax. Crit Care Med 1993;21:294–6.
18. Carvalho P, Hilderbrandt J, Charan NB. Changes in bronchial and pulmonary arterial blood flow with progressive tension pneumothorax. J Appl Physiol 1996;81:1664–9.

19. Lensing AW, Prandoni P, Brandjes D, et al. Detection of deep vein thrombosis by real time B-mode ultrasonography. N Engl J Med 1989;320:342–5.

20. Birdwell BG, Raskob GE, Whitsett TL, et al. The clinical validity of normal compression ultrasonography in outpatients suspected of having deep venous thrombosis. Ann Intern Med 1998;128:1–7.

21. Blaivas M. Incidence of pericardial effusions in patients presenting to the emergency department with unexplained dyspnea. Acad Emerg Med 2001;8: 1143–6.

22. Shabetai R. Pericardial effusions: haemodynamic spectrum. Heart 2004;90: 255–6.

23. Spodick DH. Acute cardiac tamponade. N Engl J Med 2003;349:684–90.

24. Trojanos CA, Porembka DT. Assessment of left ventricular function and hemodynamics with transesophageal echocardiography. Crit Care Clin 1996;12: 253–72.

25. Russo AM, O'Connor WH, Waxman HL. Atypical presentations and echocardiographic findings in patients with cardiac tamponade occurring early and late after cardiac surgery. Chest 1993;104:71–8.

26. Poelaert J, Schmidt C, Colardyn F. Transesophageal echocardiography in the critically ill patient. Anaesthesia 1998;53:55–68.

27. Mandavia DP, Hoffner RJ, Mahaney K, et al. Bedside echocardiography by emergency physicians. Ann Emerg Med 2001;38:377–82.

28. Tayal VS, Kline JA. Emergency echocardiography to determine pericardial effusions in patients with PEA and near PEA states. Resuscitation 2003;59:315–8.

29. Merce J, Sagrista SJ. Correlation between clinical and Doppler echocardiographic findings in patients with moderate and large pericardial effusions. Am Heart J 1999;138:759–64.

30. Tsang T, Enriquez-Sarano M, Freeman WK. Consecutive 1127 therapeutic echocardiographically guided pericardiocenteses: clinical profile, practice patterns and outcomes spanning 21 years. Mayo Clin Proc 2002;77:429–36.

31. Amico AF, Lichtenberg GS, Reisner SA, et al. Superiority of visual versus computerized echocardiographic estimation of radionuclide left ventricular ejection fraction. Am Heart J 1989;118:1259–65.

32. Moore CL, Rose GA, Tayal VS, et al. Determination of left ventricular function by emergency physician echocardiography of hypotensive patients. Acad Emerg Med 2002;9:186–93.

33. Reynolds HR, Hochman JS. Cardiogenic shock: current concepts and improving outcomes. Circulation 2008;117:686–97.

34. Picard MH, Davidoff R, Sleeper LA. Echocardiographic predictors of survival and response to early revascularization in cardiogenic shock. Circulation 2003;107:279–84.

35. Jones AE, Craddock PA, Tayal VS, et al. Diagnostic accuracy of identification of left ventricular function among emergency department patients with nontraumatic symptomatic undifferentiated hypotension. Shock 2005;24:513–7.

36. Parker M, Shelhamer J, Baruch S, et al. Profound but reversible myocardial depression in patients with septic shock. Ann Intern Med 1984;100:483–90.

37. Rivers E, Nguyen B, Haystad S, et al. Early goal directed therapy in the treatment of severe sepsis and septic shock. N Engl J Med 2001;345:1368–77.

38. Blaivas M, Fox JC. Outcome in cardiac arrest patients found to have cardiac standstill on bedside emergency department echocardiogram. Acad Emerg Med 2001;8:616–21.

39. Salen P, Melniker L, Choolijan C, et al. Does the presence or absence of sono-graphically identified cardiac activity predict resuscitation outcomes of cardiac arrest patients? Am J Emerg Med 2005;23:459–62.
40. Nazeyrollas D, Metz D, Jolly D, et al. Use of transthoracic Doppler echocardiog-raphy combined with clinical and electrographic data to predict acute pulmo-nary embolism. Eur Heart J 1996;17:779–86.
41. Jardin F, Duborg O, Bourdarias JP. Echocardiographic pattern of acute cor pulmonale. Chest 1997;111:209–17.
42. Jardin F, Dubourg O, Gueret P, et al. Quantitative two dimensional echocar-diography in massive pulmonary embolism: emphasis on ventricular interde-pendence and leftward septal displacement. J Am Coll Cardiol 1987;10:1201–6.
43. Madan A, Schwartz C. Echocardiographic visualization of acute pulmonary embolus and thrombolysis in the ED. Am J Emerg Med 2004;22:294–300.
44. Stein J. Opinions regarding the diagnosis and management of venous thrombo-embolic disease. ACCP Consensus Committee on pulmonary embolism. Chest 1996;109:233–7.
45. Jackson RE, Rudoni RR, Hauser AM, et al. Prospective evaluation of two dimen-sional transthoracic echocardiography in emergency department patients with suspected pulmonary embolism. Acad Emerg Med 2000;7:994–8.
46. Rudoni R, Jackson R. Use of two-dimensional echocardiography for the diag-nosis of pulmonary embolus. J Emerg Med 1998;16:5–8.
47. Miniati M, Monti S, Pratali L, et al. Value of transthoracic echocardiography in the diagnosis of pulmonary embolism: results of a prospective study in unselected patients. Am J Med 2001;110(7):528–35.
48. Gifroni S, Olivotto I, Cecchini P, et al. Short term clinical outcome of patients with acute pulmonary embolism, normal blood pressure and echocardiographic right ventricular dysfunction. Circulation 2000;101:2817–22.
49. Becattini C, Agnelli G. Acute pulmonary embolism: risk stratification in the emer-gency department. Intern Emerg Med 2007;2:119–29.
50. Frazee BW, Snoey ER. Diagnostic role of ED ultrasound in deep venous throm-bosis and pulmonary embolism. Am J Emerg Med 1999;17:271–8.
51. Konstantinides S, Geibel A, Heusel G, et al. Heparin plus alteplase compared with heparin alone in patients with submassive pulmonary embolus. N Engl J Med 2002;347:1143–50.
52. Kucher N, Goldhaber SZ. Management of massive pulmonary embolism. Circu-lation 2005;112:e28–32.
53. Kircher B, Himelman R. Noninvasive estimation of right atrial pressure from the inspiratory collapse of the inferior vena cava. Am J Cardiol 1990;66:493–6.
54. Simonson JS, Schiller NB. Sonospirometry: a new method for noninvasive measurement of mean right atrial pressure based on two dimensional echocar-diographic measurements of the inferior vena cava during measured inspiration. J Am Coll Cardiol 1988;11:557–64.
55. Barbier C, Loubieres Y, Schmit C, et al. Respiratory changes in inferior vena cava diameter are helpful in predicting fluid responsiveness in ventilated septic patients. Intensive Care Med 2004;30:1704–46.
56. Lyon M, Blaivas M, Brannam L. Sonographic measurement of the inferior vena cava as a marker of blood loss. Am J Emerg Med 2005;23:45–50.
57. Feissel M, Michard F. The respiratory variation in inferior vena cava diameter as a guide to fluid therapy. Intensive Care Med 2004;30:1834–7.

58. Gracias VH, Frankel HL, Gupta R, et al. Defining the learning curve for the Focused Abdominal Sonogram for Trauma (FAST) examination: implications for credentialing. Am Surg 2001;67:364–8.

59. Branney SW, Wolfe RE, Moore EE, et al. Quantitative sensitivity of ultrasound in detecting free intraperitoneal fluid. J Trauma 1995;39:375–80.

60. Von Kuenssberg Jehle D, Stiller G, Wagner D. Sensitivity in detecting free intraperitoneal fluid with the pelvic views of the FAST exam. Am J Emerg Med 2003; 21:476–8.

61. Stengel D, Bauwens K, Rademacher G, et al. Association between compliance with methodological standards of diagnostic research and reported test accuracy: meta-analysis of focused assessment of US for trauma. Radiology 2005;236: 102–11.

62. Sisley AC, Rozycki GS, Ballard RB, et al. Rapid detection of traumatic effusion using surgeon-performed ultrasonography. J Trauma 1998;44:291–6.

63. Ma OJ, Mateer JR. Trauma ultrasound examination versus chest radiography in the detection of hemothorax. Ann Emerg Med 1997;29:312–5.

64. Brooks A, Davies B, Smethhurst M, et al. Emergency ultrasound in the acute assessment of haemothorax. Emerg Med J 2004;21:44–6.

65. McEwan K, Thompson P. Ultrasound to detect haemothorax after chest injury. Emerg Med J 2007;24:581–2.

66. Gamblin TC, Wall CE Jr, Rover GM, et al. Delayed splenic rupture: case reports and review of the literature. J Trauma 2005;59:1231–4.

67. Blaivas M. Emergency department paracentesis to determine intraperitoneal fluid identity discovered on bedside ultrasound of unstable patients. J Emerg Med 2005;29:461–5.

68. Subotich D, Mandarich D. Accidentally created tension pneumothorax in patient with primary spontaneous pneumothorax—confirmation of the experimental studies, putting into question the classical explanation. Med Hypotheses 2005;64:170–3.

69. Soldati G, Testa A, Sher S, et al. Occult traumatic pneumothorax: diagnostic accuracy of lung ultrasonography in the emergency department. Chest 2008; 133:204–11.

70. Sartori S, Tombesi P, Trevisani L, et al. Accuracy of transthoracic sonography in detection of pneumothorax after sonographically guided lung biopsy: prospective comparison with chest radiography. Am J Roentgenol 2007;188:37–41.

71. Zhang M, Liu ZH, Yang JX, et al. Rapid detection of pneumothorax by ultrasonography in patients with multiple trauma. Crit Care 2006;10:R112.

72. Garofalo G, Busso M, Perotto F, et al. Ultrasound diagnosis of pneumothorax. Radiol Med 2006;11:516–25.

73. Blaivas M, Lyon M, Duggal S. A prospective comparison of supine chest radiography and bedside ultrasound for the diagnosis of traumatic pneumothorax. Acad Emerg Med 2005;12:844–9.

74. Knudtson JL, Dort JM, Helmer SD, et al. Surgeon-performed ultrasound for pneumothorax in the trauma suite. J Trauma 2004;56:527–30.

75. Lichtenstein DA, Menu Y. A bedside ultrasound sign ruling out pneumothorax in the critically ill. Lung sliding. Chest 1995;108:1345–8.

76. Slater A, Goodwin M, Anderson KE, et al. COPD can mimic the appearance of pneumothorax on thoracic ultrasound. Chest 2006;129:545–50.

77. Lichtenstein DA, Meziere GA. Relevance of lung ultrasound in the diagnosis of acute respiratory failure: the BLUE protocol. Chest 2008;134:117–25.

78. Blaivas M, Tsung JW. Point-of-care sonographic detection of left endobronchial main stem intubation and obstruction versus endotracheal intubation. J Ultrasound Med 2008;27:785–9.
79. Lichtenstein D, Meziere G, Biderman P, et al. The "lung point": an ultrasound sign specific to pneumothorax. Intensive Care Med 2000;26:1434–40.
80. Lichtenstein D, Meziere G, Biderman P, et al. The comet-tail artifact: an ultrasound sign ruling out pneumothorax. Intensive Care Med 1999;25:383–8.
81. Lichtenstein D, Meziere G, Biderman P, et al. The comet-tail artifact. An ultrasound sign of alveolar-interstitial syndrome. Am J Respir Crit Care Med 1997; 156:1640–6.
82. Agricola E, Bove T, Oppizzi M, et al. "Ultrasound comet-tail images": a marker of pulmonary edema: a comparative study with wedge pressure and extravascular lung water. Chest 2005;127:1690–5.
83. Soldati G, Copetti R, Sher S. Sonographic interstitial syndrome: the sound of lung water. J Ultrasound Med 2009;28:163–74.
84. Rohrer MJ, Cutler BS, Wheeler HB. Long-term survival and quality of life following ruptured abdominal aneurysm. Arch Surg 1988;123:1213–7.
85. Hendrickson RG, Dean AJ, Costantino TG. A novel use of ultrasound in pulseless electrical activity: the diagnosis of an acute abdominal aortic aneurysm rupture. J Emerg Med 2001;21:141–4.
86. Dent B, Kendall RJ, Boyle AA, et al. Emergency ultrasound of the abdominal aorta by UK emergency physicians: a prospective cohort study. Emerg Med J 2007;24:547–9.
87. Costantino TG, Bruno EC, Handly N, et al. Accuracy of emergency medicine ultrasound in the evaluation of abdominal aortic aneurysm. J Emerg Med 2005;29:455–60.
88. Tayal VS, Graf CD, Gibbs MA. Prospective study of accuracy and outcome of emergency ultrasound for abdominal aortic aneurysm over two years. Acad Emerg Med 2003;10:867–71.
89. Kuhn M, Bonnin RL, Davey MJ, et al. Emergency department ultrasound scanning for abdominal aortic aneurysm: accessible, accurate, and advantageous. Ann Emerg Med 2000;36:219–23.
90. Nevitt MP, Ballard DJ, Hallett JW Jr. Prognosis of abdominal aortic aneurysms. A population-based study. N Engl J Med 1989;321:1009–14.
91. Moore CL, Holliday RS, Hwang JQ, et al. Screening for abdominal aortic aneurysm in asymptomatic at-risk patients using emergency ultrasound. Am J Emerg Med 2008;26:883–7.
92. Kodolitsch Y, Krause N, Spielmann R, et al. Diagnostic potential of combined transthoracic echocardiography and x-ray computed tomography in suspected aortic dissection. Clin Cardiol 1999;22:345–52.
93. Budhram G, Reardon R. Diagnosis of ascending aortic dissection using emergency department bedside echocardiogram. Acad Emerg Med 2008;15:584.
94. Fojtik JP, Costantino TG, Dean AJ. The diagnosis of aortic dissection by emergency medicine ultrasound. J Emerg Med 2007;32:191–6.
95. Blaivas M, Sierzenski PR. Dissection of the proximal thoracic aorta: a new ultrasonographic sign in the subxiphoid view. Am J Emerg Med 2002;20:344–8.
96. Clevert DA, Rupp N, Reiser M, et al. Improved diagnosis of vascular dissection by ultrasound B-flow: a comparison with color-coded Doppler and power Doppler sonography. Eur Radiol 2005;15:342–7.

97. Kearon CK, Julian JA, Math M, et al. Noninvasive diagnosis of deep venous thrombosis. Ann Intern Med 1998;128:663–77.
98. Pezullo JA, Perkins AB, Cronan JJ. Symptomatic deep vein thrombosis: diagnosis with limited compression US. Radiology 1996;198:67–70.
99. Blaivas M. Ultrasound in the detection of venous thromboembolism. Crit Care Med 2007;35(5 suppl):S224–34.
100. Jolly BT, Massarin E, Pigman EC. Color Doppler ultrasound by emergency physicians for the diagnosis of acute deep venous thrombosis. Acad Emerg Med 1997;4:129–32.
101. Eskandari MK, Sugimoto H, Richardson T, et al. Is color flow duplex a good diagnostic test for detection of isolated calf vein thrombosis in high risk patients? Angiology 2000;51:705–10.
102. Poppiti R, Papinocolau G, Perese S. Limited B-mode venous scanning versus complete color flow duplex venous scanning for detection of proximal deep venous thrombosis. J Vasc Surg 1995;22:553–7.
103. Bernardi E, Camporese G, Buller H, et al. Serial 2 point ultrasonography plus d-dimer vs. whole leg color ceded Doppler ultrasonography for diagnosing suspected symptomatic deep vein thrombosis. JAMA 2008;300:1653–9.
104. Baarslag HJ, Van Beek EJ, Koopman MM. Prospective study of color duplex ultrasonography compared with contrast venography in patients suspected of having deep venous thrombosis of the upper extremities. J Intern Med 2002; 136:865–72.
105. Frazee BW, Snoey ER, Levitt A. Emergency department compression ultrasound to diagnose proximal deep vein thrombosis. J Emerg Med 2001;20:107–11.
106. Jang T, Docherty M, Aubin S, et al. Resident performed compression ultrasonography for the detection of proximal deep vein thrombosis: fast and accurate. Acad Emerg Med 2004;11:319–22.
107. Burnside PR, Brown MD, Kline JA. Systematic review of emergency physician-performed ultrasonography for lower-extremity deep vein thrombosis. Acad Emerg Med 2008;15:493–8.
108. Kline JA, O'Malley PM, Tayal VS, et al. Emergency clinician-performed compression ultrasonography for deep venous thrombosis of the lower extremity. Ann Emerg Med 2008;52:437–45.
109. Blaivas M, Lambert MJ, Harwood RA, et al. Lower extremity Doppler for deep venous thrombosis: can emergency physicians be accurate and fast? Acad Emerg Med 2000;7:120–6.
110. Rose JS, Bair AE, Mandavia DP. The UHP ultrasound protocol: a novel ultrasound approach to the empiric evaluation of the undifferentiated hypotensive patient. Am J Emerg Med 2001;19:299–302.

Early Identification of Shock in Critically Ill Patients

Matthew C. Strehlow, MD[a,b,*]

KEYWORDS

• Shock • Hypotension • Lactate • Base deficit • Evaluation

In the eighteenth century the French surgeon Le Dran coined the term *choc* for soldiers suffering from severe traumatic injuries and heavy blood loss. Shock began appearing in the medical literature in the nineteenth century, and in 1872 the venerated trauma surgeon Samuel D. Gross defined shock as "the rude unhinging of the machinery of life."[1] Over the centuries the term shock became synonymous with hypotension.

The misconception that hypotension is necessary to define shock persists, despite evidence and international consensus recommendations to the contrary. More appropriately, shock is defined as a life-threatening condition characterized by inadequate delivery of oxygen and nutrients to vital organs relative to their metabolic demand. Inadequate oxygen delivery typically results from poor tissue perfusion but occasionally, may also be caused by an increase in metabolic demand.[2]

In the setting of persistent inadequate oxygen delivery, cells are unable to produce adenosine triphosphate (ATP) to power vital functions. Cells transition to anaerobic metabolism to continue production of ATP, generating lactic acid, which accumulates in the cell and is transported into the blood. The accumulation of lactic acid in the cell is compounded by an increase in production of its precursor, pyruvate, via the stress response.[3] Increased production of lactate accounts for most elevation in blood levels, but a reduction in lactate metabolism also occurs.[4,5]

Systemically, the stress response is intended to release energy stores and augment perfusion to vital organs. Receptors in large arteries detect a decrease in wall tension, activating a hormonal response via the hypothalamus-pituitary-adrenal axis and a neurogenic response through sympathetic stimulation. The resultant increase in circulating levels of epinephrine, norepinephrine, corticosteroids, renin, and glucagon

The author has no financial interests to disclose.

[a] Division of Emergency Medicine, Department of Surgery, Stanford University School of Medicine, 701 Welch Road, Building C, Palo Alto, CA 94304, USA

[b] Emergency Department, Stanford University Hospital and Clinics, Stanford, 701 Welch Road, Building C, Palo Alto, CA 94304, USA

* Department of Surgery, Division of Emergency Medicine, Stanford University School of Medicine, 701 Welch Road, Building C, Palo Alto, CA 94304.

E-mail address: Strehlow@stanford.edu

Emerg Med Clin N Am 28 (2010) 57–66
doi:10.1016/j.emc.2009.09.006
0733-8627/09/$ – see front matter © 2010 Elsevier Inc. All rights reserved.

elevates the heart rate and produces vasoconstriction of peripheral arteries. As a whole, cardiac output is augmented, blood pressure elevated, and increased glucose and fatty acids are available to cells as energy precursors.

Counteracting these effects is the build-up of toxic metabolites and inflammatory mediators. Endogenous toxic metabolites derived from damaged cells and exogenous toxins can cause cellular dysfunction, myocardial depression, and vasodilation. Inflammatory mediators are released from the up-regulated immune system, leading to further organ dysfunction and microischemia. The corresponding acidemia potentiates cellular and organ dysfunction.

If the imbalance between oxygen delivery and demand persists, compensatory mechanisms fail, blood pressure and cardiac output decrease, and multiple organ dysfunction syndrome (MODS) develops. Once MODS develops, mortality is high and it is challenging to reverse the cycle of cellular death and dysfunction.

Despite the high prevalence and morbidity of shock, the lack of a widely accepted definition and clear diagnostic criteria have limited the development of robust epidemiologic data. Estimates suggest that more than 1.2 million emergency department (ED) visits annually are for patients in shock.[6,7] Mortality for patients in shock varies depending on the cause, but common causes of shock including sepsis, trauma, and cardiac failure have mortality ranging from 20% to 50%.[8-10] ED patients with persistent hypotension incur the highest rate of death, but mortality is also substantial in those with cryptic shock, or shock without overt hypotension. In patients with presumed septic shock without hypotension, for example, mortality ranges from 18% to 27%.[11,12]

EARLY DETECTION OF SHOCK

Early recognition and, correspondingly, early intervention before the onset of multiple organ dysfunction have been demonstrated to decrease morbidity and mortality in critically ill patients. The "golden hour" of trauma care has been a tenant for emergency practitioners for decades and more recently the "golden hour" for medical patients is being hailed as imperative to improving outcomes.[13] Goal-directed therapy, attempted for years in the intensive care unit (ICU) with variable results, when implemented within the first 6 hours of presentation to the ED improved absolute mortality by 16% in the original study by Rivers.[14] Evidence has continued to accumulate and more recently a meta-analysis reported that an early, quantitative resuscitation strategy in patients with severe sepsis and septic shock significantly reduced mortality. In contrast, the same investigators concluded that equivalent strategies initiated later in the patient's course were not effective.[15]

Although most recent research has focused on septic shock, studies of alternate causes of shock have also shown that early intervention is a critical factor in determining outcomes. Sebat and colleagues[16] described a 5-year process of implementing an early recognition and rapid-response strategy for patients with all forms of shock. Mortality was reduced by a factor of 3 (40%–12%). Although results of this magnitude are difficult to replicate, they suggest that reducing time to recognition is a critical aspect of caring for patients in shock. In contrast to the mortality reductions seen with strategies that target early recognition and intervention, care decisions in later stages of shock, such as choice of vasopressor, administration of steroids, and implementation of tight glycemic control, have proven to have minimal if any effects.[17-21]

HISTORY AND PHYSICAL EXAMINATION

Emergency providers are frequently presented with the undifferentiated patient and must be intimately familiar with the elements of history, physical examination, and diagnostic testing that may suggest early shock, before the onset of significant organ dysfunction (**Box 1**).

Vital-sign abnormalities have long been the cornerstone of shock recognition. Traditionally, a patient was deemed to be in shock when tachycardic, tachypneic, and possessing a systolic blood pressure (SBP) less than 90 mm Hg. Current evidence suggests that traditional vital signs are insensitive markers of early hypoperfusion. Advanced trauma life support (ATLS) teaches that decreased blood pressure is a marker of hemorrhage that is already moderate to severe. Despite this, a SBP of less than 90 mm Hg is still used as a screening criterion for the activation of trauma patients. Recent evidence supports ATLS teaching that a SBP less than 90 mm Hg is a late and insensitive finding of hemorrhage and shock.[22–27] Parks and colleagues[26] performed a retrospective evaluation of the National Trauma Database. They evaluated a cohort of trauma patients with a median initial SBP of 90 mm Hg; mortality in these patients was 65% and the base deficit 20. Lipsky and colleagues[28] determined that patients who were hypotensive (<90 mm Hg) in the prehospital setting but normotensive in the ED had a 2-fold increase in mortality and a 3-fold increase in injuries requiring an emergency therapeutic operation when compared with patients normotensive in both settings. Although an SBP of less than 90 mm Hg is a marker of severe disease in trauma patients, higher cut-offs could improve sensitivity for life-threatening injury. Studies in the ED and prehospital setting show an increase in patients' mortality and injuries when blood pressure decreases to less than 110 mm Hg.[22,24] As a result of these studies many trauma experts now argue that blood pressures less than 110 mm Hg should be considered hypotension.

Box. 1
Signs of shock

Early signs[a]

　Tachypnea

　Tachycardia

　Weak or bounding peripheral pulses

　Delayed capillary refill (>2 seconds)

　Pale or cool skin

　Narrowed pulse pressure

　Oliguria

　Lactic acidosis

　Elevated base deficit

Late signs

　Decreased mental status

　Weak or absent central pulses

　Central cyanosis

　Hypotension

　Bradycardia

[a] Early signs of shock are frequently seen in later stages and late signs such as altered mental status may present early depending on the cause and the patient.

In nontrauma patients systemic hypotension is likewise a late finding of critical illness and mortality ranges from 20% to 60% for common causes of hypotensive shock.[29,30] A single episode of hypotension (<100 mm Hg) in the prehospital or ED setting portends an increased risk of death during hospital admission.[31,32] As the frequency or duration of hypotension increases, so does the patient's risk of death. Although concerning when identified, ED hypotension is an insensitive marker of critical illness and in-hospital mortality.[33,34]

Likewise, an elevated heart rate has limited predictive value in trauma and nontrauma patients.[35] Despite ATLS teaching that tachycardia is present after moderate acute blood loss, studies in healthy phlebotomized patients and trauma patients reveal supine heart rate to be an insensitive marker of injury severity and mortality.[25,27,36] Furthermore, tachycardia is frequently absent in patients with significant dehydration and hypovolemia.[25]

Calculation of the shock index—the heart rate divided by the SBP—can improve the detection of critically ill patients compared to HR and BP alone.[34,37] Values falling significantly outside normal (0.5–0.7), those greater than 0.9, indicate impaired cardiac function and correspondingly a reduced cardiac output. Although an elevated shock index heralds an increased risk of critical illness and mortality, its sensitivity remains low and it cannot be used in isolation to evaluate for occult shock.

In addition to vital signs, which focus on the cardiac and respiratory systems, other physical examination findings are helpful in the recognition of tissue hypoperfusion. Altered mental status, poor skin perfusion, and oliguria are markers of decreased end-organ perfusion and have been found to be independent predictors of 30-day mortality in patients with cardiogenic shock.[38]

Lima and colleagues[39] studied poor peripheral skin perfusion, defined as a delayed capillary refill time greater than 4.5 seconds or extremity coolness to the examiner's touch, in recently admitted, critically ill patients in the ICU after resolution of hypotension. Poor peripheral skin perfusion was identified as an independent predictor of worsening organ failure and persistent lactic acidosis. Other studies have determined signs of poor perfusion on extremity skin examination to correlate with global hemodynamic dysfunction, such as decreased cardiac output.[40,41] In children with meningococcal disease, cool extremities and abnormal skin signs have been shown to be an early indicator of disease before the onset of other, more classic findings.[42]

Urine output is a marker of kidney perfusion. In the setting of decreased blood flow, blood redistributes from the renal cortex to the renal medulla, lowering the glomerular filtration rate and urine production. Urine output should be monitored by Foley catheter placement early in the ED course, because an accurate estimation requires at least 30 minutes of collection. During resuscitation, urine production is considered normal if greater than 1 mL/kg/h, reduced if 0.5 to 1 mL/kg/h, or severely reduced if less than 0.5 mL/kg/h.

LABORATORY MARKERS OF HYPOPERFUSION
Lactate

Elevated lactate levels in the setting of critical illness are associated with a worse prognosis for medical and trauma patients. Multiple conditions resulting in inadequate oxygen delivery, disproportionate oxygen demand, and diminished oxygen use may lead to elevated lactate levels (**Box 2**), but most of these conditions are readily apparent or cause only modest, transient elevations in the blood lactate levels. An abnormal lactate level is generally considered greater than 2 mmol/L. A level greater

| **Box. 2** |
| **Causes of an elevated lactate** |

Inadequate oxygen delivery

    Volume depletion or profound dehydration

    Significant blood loss

    Septic shock

    Profound anemia

    Severe hypoxemia

    Prolonged carbon monoxide exposure

    Trauma

Disproportionate oxygen demands

    Hyperthermia

    Shivering

    Seizures

    Strenuous exercise

Inadequate oxygen use

    Systemic inflammatory response syndrome

    Diabetes mellitus

    Total parenternal nutrition

    Human immunodeficiency virus infection

    Drugs such as metformin, salicylate, antiretroviral agents, isoniazid, propofol, cyanide.

than 4 mmol/L is significantly elevated and in most settings is a sign of tissue hypoperfusion.

Several trials have demonstrated the prognostic value of lactate levels.[11,12,43–45] Mikkelsen[12] studied initial ED lactate levels in patients with presumed sepsis and determined that elevations predicted an increased 28-day mortality independent of organ dysfunction and hypotension. A corresponding study by Howell[11] looked at patients with presumed sepsis but who did not qualify as having septic shock; patients with a lactate level greater than 4 mmol/L at the time of admission had a mortality of 26.5%.

Lactate clearance can be used to risk stratify patients and determine their response to therapy.[33,46] One ED study determined that a lactate reduction of greater than 10% at 6 hours was associated with a 3-fold lower mortality and reduced need for vasopressors. It has been recommended that patients with a decline in lactate of less than 50% at 1 hour require additional resuscitation measures.[6]

Lactate levels may be arterial, central venous, or peripherally obtained. Studies document good correlation between samples acquired from different locations.[47,48] Ideally, peripheral venous lactates should be drawn without the use of a tourniquet as prolonged tourniquet times may falsely elevate levels.

Arterial Base Deficit

Arterial base deficit is a calculation of the quantity of base required to raise the pH of blood to the expected level. It is calculated from the partial pressure of carbon dioxide ($Paco_2$), pH, and serum bicarbonate. Base deficit is more sensitive to tissue hypoperfusion than pH or serum bicarbonate levels alone. A normal value is −2 to 2 and a significantly elevated base deficit is greater than 6. Similar to lactate, it has been shown in trauma patients to predict the severity of injury and mortality during initial resuscitation.[26,43,49,50] Because many hospitals can perform bedside arterial blood gas analysis, determination of base deficit is a useful screening tool for trauma patients. Evidence as to its utility in nontrauma patients with shock or later in the course of patients with traumatic injuries is less robust, although base deficit can be used in these circumstances to identify occult hypoperfusion and guide resuscitation when lactate is unavailable.[51–53]

Various other biomarkers of shock and organ dysfunction have been proposed. A recent study by Shapiro and colleagues[54] identified 3 biomarkers (neutrophil gelatinase-associated lipocalin, protein C, interleukin 1) that, when used in conjunction, predicted severe sepsis, septic shock, and death in ED patients. This unique biomarker panel and other biomarkers hold promise but require further study before their widespread clinical implementation.

Noninvasive Monitoring of Regional Tissue Perfusion

Multiple noninvasive techniques to monitor regional tissue perfusion have been developed. The most established of these include sublingual capnometry ($Slco_2$), near-infrared spectroscopy to monitor muscle tissue oxygen saturation (Sto_2), and transcutaneous tissue oxygenation and capnometry ($Ptco_2$, $Ptcco_2$). These techniques are based on the concept that under physiologic stress the body will preferentially shunt blood away from the peripheral and splanchnic tissues to augment perfusion of vital organs, primarily the brain and heart. Therefore, unlike more global markers of tissue hypoperfusion such as lactate and base deficit, these regional markers will demonstrate abnormalities in perfusion and oxygenation earlier in the course of the patient's illness. Furthermore, most can be rapidly obtained and continuously monitored.

Sublingual capnometry is a measurement of the carbon dioxide (CO_2) level in the vascular bed underlying the tongue. It is measured in a manner similar to an oral temperature. $Slco_2$ has been demonstrated to be a sensitive marker of splanchnic perfusion and gut ischemia.[55–57] In the critical-care setting, splanchnic perfusion has long been identified as an early marker of hypoperfusion. Multiple studies in trauma and nontrauma patients have determined $Slco_2$ to be a predictor of injury severity, organ dysfunction, and mortality.[43,49,58,59] Widespread adoption of sublingual capnometry monitoring in the ED has been limited by the requirement for new equipment, difficulties with obtaining accurate, reproducible measurements, and the need for further study.

Muscle Sto_2 uses light absorption to determine the oxygen saturation in the microcirculation in muscle tissue. An external probe is commonly placed on the biceps or thenar eminence. Continuous monitoring can be performed similarly to pulse oximetry. Recently, Cohn and colleagues[50] demonstrated that an Sto_2 less than 75% during the initial resuscitation of trauma patients performed equivalently to an arterial base deficit as a predictor of MODS. This cut-off was found to have a high sensitivity but low specificity for significant injury. Other studies of muscle Sto_2 found similar results in trauma patients, but it has not performed so well in patients with sepsis.[60–62]

Transcutaneous tissue oxygenation and capnometry measurements most often use heated probes placed on the skin to determine peripheral tissue perfusion. Studies have shown $Stco_2$ and $Stcco_2$ to be markers of early hemodynamic compromise and increased mortality.[23,63–65] Tissue trauma resulting from the probes and a lack of established critical values have limited its widespread adoption.

Bedside Ultrasonography

Bedside ultrasonography has become an essential tool in the evaluation of shock patients in the ED. In addition to the focused abdominal sonography in trauma examination, bedside ultrasound can augment the assessment and management of critically ill patients. Although most ED-based ultrasound studies of critically ill have focused on the evaluation of hypotensive patients, a recent study evaluated trauma patients who were normotensive after initial resuscitation. The study found that patients with a smaller interior vena cava diameter were at increased risk for recurrent hypotension.[66] Furthermore, determining the correct etiology of shock in ED patients is challenging, with providers able to accurately diagnose only 25% to 50% of cases.[67,68] Early, protocol-driven bedside ultrasound performed by emergency physicians can improve diagnostic accuracy to 80%.[68] Overall, the literature illustrates that bedside ultrasonography performed by ED providers plays a crucial role in the early recognition and evaluation of patients in shock. See also article by Perera and colleagues elsewhere in this issue.

SUMMARY

Shock is a state of inadequate tissue perfusion and, although hypotension is often present, it is a late finding and not necessary for the diagnosis. Timely recognition and intervention are critical to reducing the morbidity and mortality of shock. Clinical suspicion, thorough physical examination, and laboratory screening using base deficit or lactate can improve early identification of patients suffering from shock.

REFERENCES

1. Cairns CB. Rude unhinging of the machinery of life: metabolic approaches to hemorrhagic shock. Curr Opin Crit Care 2001;7:437.
2. Antonelli M, Levy M, Andrews PJ, et al. Hemodynamic monitoring in shock and implications for management. International Consensus Conference, Paris, France, 27–28 April 2006. Intensive Care Med 2007;33:575.
3. Gore DC, Jahoor F, Hibbert JM, et al. Lactic acidosis during sepsis is related to increased pyruvate production, not deficits in tissue oxygen availability. Ann Surg 1996;224:97.
4. Levraut J, Ciebiera JP, Chave S, et al. Mild hyperlactatemia in stable septic patients is due to impaired lactate clearance rather than overproduction. Am J Respir Crit Care Med 1998;157:1021.
5. Levraut J, Ichai C, Petit I, et al. Low exogenous lactate clearance as an early predictor of mortality in normolactatemic critically ill septic patients. Crit Care Med 2003;31:705.
6. Marx JA, editor. Marx: Rosen's emergency medicine: concepts and clinical practice, vol. 1. 6th edition. Philadelphia: Mosby Elsevier, 2006.
7. Pitts SR, Niska RW, Xu J, et al. National Hospital Ambulatory Medical Care Survey: 2006 emergency department summary. Natl Health Stat Report 2008;7:1–38.
8. Astiz ME, Rackow EC. Septic shock. Lancet 1998;351:1501.
9. Janssens U, Graf J. [Shock–what are the basics?] Internist (Berl) 2004;45:758–66 [in German].
10. Shoemaker WC, Peitzman AB, Bellamy R, et al. Resuscitation from severe hemorrhage. Crit Care Med 1996;24:S12.
11. Howell MD, Donnino M, Clardy P, et al. Occult hypoperfusion and mortality in patients with suspected infection. Intensive Care Med 2007;33:1892.

12. Mikkelsen ME, Miltiades AN, Gaieski DF, et al. Serum lactate is associated with mortality in severe sepsis independent of organ failure and shock. Crit Care Med 2009;37:1670.
13. Shapiro NI, Howell MD, Talmor D, et al. Implementation and outcomes of the Multiple Urgent Sepsis Therapies (MUST) protocol. Crit Care Med 2006;34:1025.
14. Rivers E, Nguyen B, Havstad S, et al. Early goal-directed therapy in the treatment of severe sepsis and septic shock. N Engl J Med 2001;345:1368.
15. Jones AE, Brown MD, Trzeciak S, et al. The effect of a quantitative resuscitation strategy on mortality in patients with sepsis: a meta-analysis. Crit Care Med 2008; 36:2734.
16. Sebat F, Musthafa AA, Johnson D, et al. Effect of a rapid response system for patients in shock on time to treatment and mortality during 5 years. Crit Care Med 2007;35:2568.
17. Abraham WT, Adams KF, Fonarow GC, et al. In-hospital mortality in patients with acute decompensated heart failure requiring intravenous vasoactive medications: an analysis from the Acute Decompensated Heart Failure National Registry (ADHERE). J Am Coll Cardiol 2005;46:57.
18. Annane D, Vignon P, Renault A, et al. Norepinephrine plus dobutamine versus epinephrine alone for management of septic shock: a randomised trial. Lancet 2007;370:676.
19. Cuffe MS, Califf RM, Adams KF Jr, et al. Short-term intravenous milrinone for acute exacerbation of chronic heart failure: a randomized controlled trial. JAMA 2002;287:1541.
20. Finfer S, Chittock DR, Su SY, et al. Intensive versus conventional glucose control in critically ill patients. N Engl J Med 2009;360:1283.
21. Sprung CL, Annane D, Keh D, et al. Hydrocortisone therapy for patients with septic shock. N Engl J Med 2008;358:111.
22. Bruns B, Gentilello L, Elliott A, et al. Prehospital hypotension redefined. J Trauma 2008;65:1217.
23. Chien LC, Lu KJ, Wo CC, et al. Hemodynamic patterns preceding circulatory deterioration and death after trauma. J Trauma 2007;62:928.
24. Eastridge BJ, Salinas J, McManus JG, et al. Hypotension begins at 110 mm Hg: redefining "hypotension" with data. J Trauma 2007;63:291.
25. McGee S, Abernethy WB 3rd, Simel DL. The rational clinical examination. Is this patient hypovolemic? JAMA 1999;281:1022.
26. Parks JK, Elliott AC, Gentilello LM, et al. Systemic hypotension is a late marker of shock after trauma: a validation study of Advanced Trauma Life Support principles in a large national sample. Am J Surg 2006;192:727.
27. American College of Surgeons Committee on Trauma, editor. Advanced trauma life support for doctors. 7th edition. Chicago: American College of Surgeons; 2004.
28. Lipsky AM, Gausche-Hill M, Henneman PL, et al. Prehospital hypotension is a predictor of the need for an emergent, therapeutic operation in trauma patients with normal systolic blood pressure in the emergency department. J Trauma 2006;61:1228.
29. Menon V, White H, LeJemtel T, et al. The clinical profile of patients with suspected cardiogenic shock due to predominant left ventricular failure: a report from the SHOCK Trial Registry. SHould we emergently revascularize Occluded Coronaries in cardiogenic shocK? J Am Coll Cardiol 2000;36:1071.
30. Rivers E. The outcome of patients presenting to the emergency department with severe sepsis or septic shock. Crit Care 2006;10:154.

31. Jones AE, Stiell IG, Nesbitt LP, et al. Nontraumatic out-of-hospital hypotension predicts in hospital mortality. Ann Emerg Med 2004;43:106.
32. Jones AE, Yiannibas V, Johnson C, et al. Emergency department hypotension predicts sudden unexpected in-hospital mortality: a prospective cohort study. Chest 2006;130:941.
33. Nguyen HB, Rivers EP, Knoblich BP, et al. Early lactate clearance is associated with improved outcome in severe sepsis and septic shock. Crit Care Med 2004;32:1637.
34. Rady MY, Smithline HA, Blake H, et al. A comparison of the shock index and conventional vital signs to identify acute, critical illness in the emergency department. Ann Emerg Med 1994;24:685.
35. Wo CC, Shoemaker WC, Appel PL, et al. Unreliability of blood pressure and heart rate to evaluate cardiac output in emergency resuscitation and critical illness. Crit Care Med 1993;21:218.
36. Brasel KJ, Guse C, Gentilello LM, et al. Heart rate: is it truly a vital sign? J Trauma 2007;62:812.
37. Toosi MS, Merlino JD, Leeper KV. Prognostic value of the shock index along with transthoracic echocardiography in risk stratification of patients with acute pulmonary embolism. Am J Cardiol 2008;101:700.
38. Hasdai D, Holmes DR Jr, Califf RM, et al. Cardiogenic shock complicating acute myocardial infarction: predictors of death. GUSTO Investigators. Global Utilization of Streptokinase and Tissue-Plasminogen Activator for Occluded Coronary Arteries. Am Heart J 1999;138:21.
39. Lima A, Jansen TC, van Bommel J, et al. The prognostic value of the subjective assessment of peripheral perfusion in critically ill patients. Crit Care Med 2009;37:934.
40. Bailey JM, Levy JH, Kopel MA, et al. Relationship between clinical evaluation of peripheral perfusion and global hemodynamics in adults after cardiac surgery. Crit Care Med 1990;18:1353.
41. Kaplan LJ, McPartland K, Santora TA, et al. Start with a subjective assessment of skin temperature to identify hypoperfusion in intensive care unit patients. J Trauma 2001;50:620.
42. Thompson MJ, Ninis N, Perera R, et al. Clinical recognition of meningococcal disease in children and adolescents. Lancet 2006;367:397.
43. Baron BJ, Dutton RP, Zehtabchi S, et al. Sublingual capnometry for rapid determination of the severity of hemorrhagic shock. J Trauma 2007;62:120.
44. Schmiechen NJ, Han C, Milzman DP. ED use of rapid lactate to evaluate patients with acute chest pain. Ann Emerg Med 1997;30:571.
45. Shapiro NI, Howell MD, Talmor D, et al. Serum lactate as a predictor of mortality in emergency department patients with infection. Ann Emerg Med 2005;45:524.
46. Abramson D, Scalea TM, Hitchcock R, et al. Lactate clearance and survival following injury. J Trauma 1993;35:584.
47. Lavery RF, Livingston DH, Tortella BJ, et al. The utility of venous lactate to triage injured patients in the trauma center. J Am Coll Surg 2000;190:656.
48. Weil MH, Michaels S, Rackow EC. Comparison of blood lactate concentrations in central venous, pulmonary artery, and arterial blood. Crit Care Med 1987;15:489.
49. Baron BJ, Sinert R, Zehtabchi S, et al. Diagnostic utility of sublingual PCO2 for detecting hemorrhage in penetrating trauma patients. J Trauma 2004;57:69.
50. Cohn SM, Nathens AB, Moore FA, et al. Tissue oxygen saturation predicts the development of organ dysfunction during traumatic shock resuscitation. J Trauma 2007;62:44.

51. Husain FA, Martin MJ, Mullenix PS, et al. Serum lactate and base deficit as predictors of mortality and morbidity. Am J Surg 2003;185:485.
52. Martin MJ, FitzSullivan E, Salim A, et al. Discordance between lactate and base deficit in the surgical intensive care unit: which one do you trust? Am J Surg 2006; 191:625.
53. Smith I, Kumar P, Molloy S, et al. Base excess and lactate as prognostic indicators for patients admitted to intensive care. Intensive Care Med 2001;27:74.
54. Shapiro NI, Trzeciak S, Hollander JE, et al. A prospective, multicenter derivation of a biomarker panel to assess risk of organ dysfunction, shock, and death in emergency department patients with suspected sepsis. Crit Care Med 2009; 37:96.
55. Pernat A, Weil MH, Tang W, et al. Effects of hyper- and hypoventilation on gastric and sublingual PCO(2). J Appl Phys 1999;87:933.
56. Povoas HP, Weil MH, Tang W, et al. Comparisons between sublingual and gastric tonometry during hemorrhagic shock. Chest 2000;118:1127.
57. Weil MH, Nakagawa Y, Tang W, et al. Sublingual capnometry: a new noninvasive measurement for diagnosis and quantitation of severity of circulatory shock. Crit Care Med 1999;27:1225.
58. Marik PE. Sublingual capnography: a clinical validation study. Chest 2001;120: 923.
59. Marik PE, Bankov A. Sublingual capnometry versus traditional markers of tissue oxygenation in critically ill patients. Crit Care Med 2003;31:818.
60. Creteur J. Muscle StO2 in critically ill patients. Curr Opin Crit Care 2008;14:361.
61. Ikossi DG, Knudson MM, Morabito DJ, et al. Continuous muscle tissue oxygenation in critically injured patients: a prospective observational study. J Trauma 2006;61:780.
62. Wan JJ, Cohen MJ, Rosenthal G, et al. Refining resuscitation strategies using tissue oxygen and perfusion monitoring in critical organ beds. J Trauma 2009; 66:353.
63. Shoemaker WC, Belzberg H, Wo CC, et al. Multicenter study of noninvasive monitoring systems as alternatives to invasive monitoring of acutely ill emergency patients. Chest 1998;114:1643.
64. Shoemaker WC, Wo CC, Chan L, et al. Outcome prediction of emergency patients by noninvasive hemodynamic monitoring. Chest 2001;120:528.
65. Tatevossian RG, Wo CC, Velmahos GC, et al. Transcutaneous oxygen and CO2 as early warning of tissue hypoxia and hemodynamic shock in critically ill emergency patients. Crit Care Med 2000;28:2248.
66. Yanagawa Y, Sakamoto T, Okada Y. Hypovolemic shock evaluated by sonographic measurement of the inferior vena cava during resuscitation in trauma patients. J Trauma 2007;63:1245.
67. Jones AE, Tayal VS, Sullivan DM, et al. Randomized, controlled trial of immediate versus delayed goal-directed ultrasound to identify the cause of nontraumatic hypotension in emergency department patients. Crit Care Med 2004;32:1703.
68. Moore CL, Rose GA, Tayal VS, et al. Determination of left ventricular function by emergency physician echocardiography of hypotensive patients. Acad Emerg Med 2002;9:186.

Pediatric Emergencies Associated with Fever

Ilene Claudius, MD[a], Larry J. Baraff, MD[b],*

KEYWORDS

- Serious bacterial infection • Fever • Emergency department

Fever, defined as a temperature greater than 38.0°C, is a ubiquitous complaint among pediatric patients in emergency departments (EDs) and pediatric practice. It rarely represents life-threatening pathology; however, a handful of less common serious causes of pediatric fever exist with the potential for morbidity and mortality, and also legal action. For example, when medicolegal claims against pediatricians from 1985 to 2005 were reviewed, meningitis ranked second among pediatric diagnoses resulting in litigation.[1] The authors discuss the approach to the febrile child and significant etiologies that present potential pitfalls for the emergency physician.

Important components of the physical examination of febrile children are vital signs, behavioral state, and state of hydration (**Box 1**).[2] Much of the literature regarding pediatric fever has focused on the well-appearing child, but the distinction between a well- and ill-appearing child is not always obvious. Fear of medical personnel and fatigue can make infants and children difficult to assess. Social response and response to parents, hydration status, color, arousability, and strength of cry can be used to stratify a child as either ill or well. These factors compose the Yale Observation Score, which is designed to quantify "toxicity" in pediatric patients.[3] When tested in febrile infants aged 3 to 36 months, a high Yale Observation Score has reasonable specificity but low sensitivity for detecting bacteremia.[4] Although a normal behavioral state does not exclude bacteremia, ill appearance is certainly concerning for it. Other important components of the physical examination include assessment of neck mobility, fontanel, and presence of rash. Although nuchal rigidity with meningitis is not a consistent finding until the age of 18 months, it is possible to note limitation of neck flexion, irritability when being picked up, or a bulging fontanel in younger infants. Rashes play an important role in the diagnosis of meningococcemia and Kawasaki disease (KD), both of which are discussed later. Particularly in the very young or developmentally delayed child, vital signs may be the only sign of a serious bacterial infection (SBI). Lack of recognition of significant vital sign abnormalities is common in missed cases

[a] Department of Emergency Medicine, University of Southern California and Children's Hospital, 1200 State Street 1011, Los Angeles, CA 90033, USA
[b] UCLA Emergency Medicine Center, David Geffen School of Medicine at UCLA, 924 Westwood Boulevard, Suite 300, Los Angeles, CA 90024, USA
* Corresponding author.
E-mail address: lbaraff@mednet.ucla.edu (L.J. Baraff).

Emerg Med Clin N Am 28 (2010) 67–84
doi:10.1016/j.emc.2009.09.002
0733-8627/09/$ – see front matter © 2010 Elsevier Inc. All rights reserved.

emed.theclinics.com

Box 1
Symptoms and signs of dehydration

Symptoms

    Decreased urine output

    Decreased tear production

    Decreased activity level

Signs

    Dry mucous membranes

    Decreased skin elasticity

    Sunken fontanel

    Sunken eyes

    Tachycardia

    Cool skin

    Capillary refill for more than 2 seconds

    Hypotension (late finding)

---

of SBIs. The normal vital signs by age are summarized in **Table 1**.[5] When an infant's vital signs fall outside of these normal values, it may be difficult to know if this is due to anxiety or fever or is a sign of more serious pathology. Fever with a temperature greater than 38.0°C can raise a child's heart rate by 10 beats per minute for each degree Fahrenheit. Rectal temperatures are required in infants younger than 2 years. Routine antipyretics should reduce the temperature within 20 to 30 minutes, allowing a more accurate assessment of heart rate. Overcoming anxiety to obtain accurate vital signs is more difficult. Taking the heart rate using a pulse oximeter probe may minimize agitation, allowing medical personnel to follow data while providing some distance from the child's immediate environment. Children maintain a normal blood pressure until late in the course of sepsis, so a persistently elevated heart rate, even without hypotension, must be taken seriously, and a low blood pressure may be a sign of imminent need for significant resuscitation.

Febrile infants and toddlers between 3 and 36 months of age are at risk for occult bacterial infections, including urinary tract infections (UTIs) and occult bacteremia. Before the widespread introduction of the 7-valent conjugate pneumococcal vaccine (PCV7; Prevnar, Lederle Laboratories/Wyeth-Ayerst, NY, USA) in 2000, a well-appearing child in this age group with a fever without source (FWS) of a temperature greater than 39.0°C had a 2% to 3% risk of occult bacteremia. The white blood cell (WBC) count was used to stratify infants, with the risk of bacteremia found to be approximately 10% if the WBC count was greater than 15,000 and 1% if less than 15,000.[6] The risk of pneumococcal meningitis in infants with occult pneumococcal bacteria is 4% to 5%.

Table 1
Acceptable vital signs in infants and children

Age	Neonate	2 mo–1 y	1–2 y	2–10 y
Heart rate	120–160	100–150	100–150	65–120
Respiratory rate	40–60	30–40	22–30	16–24
Systolic blood pressure	60–90	70 + 2 (age in years) = 2 SD below the mean		

Therefore, it was recommended to obtain a blood culture on infants at higher risk of bacteremia and to treat with ceftriaxone. Now, routine vaccinations beginning at 2 months of age include conjugate bacterial vaccine for *Haemophilus influenzae* type B (Hib) and PCV7. The pneumococcal vaccine is 89% effective in decreasing invasive infections caused by all strains of *Pneumococcus* and 97.4% effective in the serotypes covered by the vaccine.[7] Herd immunity provides protection to unimmunized infants and older adults. In the post-PCV7 era the occult bacteremia rate is 0.25% to 0.91% with common pathogens including *Streptococcus pneumoniae, H influenzae, Escherichia coli,* group A streptococci, *Neisseria meningitidis, Staphylococcus aureus,* and *Salmonella.*[8] A recent study found no cases of pneumococcal bacteremia in immunized children and a 2.4% rate in unimmunized children. Only 2 of 833 immunized patients had bacteremia of any cause, both associated with UTIs.[9] Nonpathogenic (contaminant) blood culture rates have remained high at 1.89% to 9.1%.[9,10] Analysis done on the cost of repeat cultures/treatment associated with false positive cultures indicated that at an occult bacteremia rate less than 0.5% it is not cost-effective to pursue a workup on a well-appearing infant aged 3 to 36 months with a fever.[11]

Managing well-appearing children aged 3 to 36 months is now more challenging than ever. With an overall decrease in bacteremia and the change in causative pathogens, the predictive value of a WBC count greater than 15,000/μL has fallen to 3.2%. An absolute neutrophil count greater than 15,000/μL has a higher predictive value at 11%.[12] A study examining a population of infants with temperatures greater than 40°C found an equivalent predictive value between a C-reactive protein level of 4.4 or more (positive predictive value [PPV] = 30%) and a WBC count greater than 17.1 (PPV = 31%). This study was selected for infants at higher risk of occult bacteremia by using a high temperature cutoff and including ill-appearing children.[13] Procalcitonin values greater than or equal to 0.12 ng/mL have a sensitivity of 95% and specificity of 25%.[14] With these test characteristics, it is difficult to find a laboratory test that predicts which patients would benefit from parenteral antibiotics with sufficient accuracy to recommend their use. Therefore, the authors suggest that a complete blood count (CBC) and blood culture are no longer necessary in the well-appearing FWS infant who has received 2 doses of conjugate bacterial vaccines (recommended at 2 months and 4 months of age). This testing should be reserved for infants who have received less than 2 doses of PCV7 or are ill appearing.

Other common occult bacterial infections include pneumonia and UTI. For pneumonia, tachypnea and abnormal pulse oximetry are the most sensitive signs, with a PPV as high as 74.5 listed in one study.[15] Rales, hypoxemia, cough lasting beyond 10 days, and fever lasting beyond 5 days suggest pneumonia as well.[16] Even in the absence of respiratory symptoms, children with fever with a temperature greater than 39°C and WBC counts greater than 20,000 have a 19% incidence of occult pneumonia.[17] Occult UTIs occur in 10% of febrile girls and uncircumcised boys younger than 1 year and in 5% of girls between 1 and 2 years.[18] Risk factors for occult UTI include female sex, uncircumcised boys, FWS, and fever with a temperature greater than 39°C.[19] The American Academy of Pediatrics recommendations suggest a catheterized urine specimen in all febrile girls and uncircumcised boys younger than 2 years without an obvious alternative cause for their fever.[20]

HERPES SIMPLEX ENCEPHALITIS

Herpes simplex virus (HSV) infections of the central nervous system (CNS) can manifest in different ways. Aseptic meningitis is uncommon, occurring in adolescents and adults with primary genital herpes. Prognosis is excellent. Neonates, primarily those with intrapartum exposure, can develop encephalitis via either neuronal migration or hematogenous dissemination of HSV-2. Affected infants present with fever and/or seizures with or without cutaneous manifestations of vesicles. Prognosis is poor, with mortality of 60% in treated patients with disseminated disease. Most survivors suffer significant neurologic sequelae. Treatment is by administering acyclovir 20 mg/kg/dose every 8 hours for 14 to 21 days.[21] Neonates presenting with isolated fever and those who were found to have cerebrospinal fluid (CSF) pleocytosis on lumbar puncture have a 1% incidence of HSV.[22] Practice varies from treatment of all neonates with fever to treatment of only those with signs and symptoms suspicious for HSV or positive HSV PCR (polymerase chain reaction). The authors recommend treatment of all infants with fever and CSF pleocytosis until an alternate diagnosis is made or PCR is negative.

Herpes encephalitis caused by HSV-1 is the most common nonepidemic, sporadic encephalitis in the United States, occurring in 1 of 250,000 to 500,000 individuals annually.[21,23] Although it can occur in any age, one-third of affected individuals are between 6 months and 20 years.[24] Clinical presentation can include fever, focal seizures, altered mental status or abnormal behavior, headache, vomiting, hemipare-sis, and/or dysphasia. Neck rigidity is frequently absent. Relapses after a treated episode of HSV encephalitis can occur from days to years after treatment cessation.[25]

As with all CNS infections, diagnosis requires examination of CSF, including a sample for HSV PCR (sensitivity 94%). False negatives occur early in the disease course and require a repeat lumbar puncture in high-risk patients with an initially nega-tive result. Lumbar punctures that are done late (10–14 days) after disease onset can also yield false negative PCR results.[26] 95% of patients have CSF pleocytosis, typi-cally in the 10 to 200 cell/mm^3 range, with a lymphocytic or monocytic predomi-nance.[26] Other classic findings include an elevated protein level in 80% of the patients (average 100 mg/dL),[27] elevated CSF red blood cell count, and normal glucose. Electroencephalography can be helpful, with a sensitivity of 84% and spec-ificity of 32.5%.[24] Nearly half of patients have computed tomographic (CT) abnormal-ities, which are poor prognostic factors; however, CT is frequently normal in the first 4 to 6 days.[27] Magnetic resonance imaging (MRI) is much more sensitive with reports to 100% of children having abnormalities in the diffusion image sequence, usually in the temporal lobe.[28] HSV causes 50% of all instances of temporal lobe encephalitis; Ep-stein-Barr virus (EBV) accounts for an additional 25%. Therefore, EBV PCR should also be done if MRI suggests temporal lobe encephalitis.[29]

Treatment includes acyclovir 20 mg/kg/dose every 8 hours for 2 to 3 weeks,[27] which has decreased mortality from 70% to 19%.[21] Morbidity and mortality rates are lower in patients younger than 30 years, in patients who receive acyclovir within 2 to 4 days of disease onset, and in those with an initial Glasgow Coma Score more than 6.[30] Neurologic sequelae are common, occurring in about 63% of children[31] and include developmental delay and seizures. Adjunctive use of corticosteroids is controversial.

INVASIVE METHICILLIN-RESISTANT *S AUREUS* DISEASE

Methicillin-resistant *S aureus* (MRSA) infections increased 12-fold during the early 2000s[32] and now account for about 40% to 67% of all pediatric *S aureus* infec-tions.[33,34] Seventy-seven to ninety-five percent of MRSA infections involve the skin and soft tissue,[35,36] and these are generally obvious on clinical examination. No iden-tifiable risk factors (recent health care contact, chronic disease, age, previous MRSA infections or antibiotic use, and tympanostomy tube placement) are found in 89% of pediatric patients with MRSA.[37] Treatment of mild skin and soft tissue infections includes incision and drainage of abscesses and antibiotic therapy. Clindamycin is a reasonable option for patients in areas where resistance rates have remained low. Overall, there is a 15% risk of inducible resistance of MRSA isolates to clindamycin, which can be determined by a positive D-test. Rates of inducible resistance vary geographically between 8% and 94%.[37] Insurance coverage of clindamycin varies, and the taste is not palatable to many children. Trimethoprim-sulfamethoxazole (Bactrim) is a tolerable medication with a low resistance rate; however, in cases where the diagnosis is presumptive, a second agent (usually cephalexin) should be added because of the poor activity of trimethoprim-sulfamethoxazole (Bactrim) against Streptococcus. Doxycycline and minocycline have efficacy against most MRSA strains but are contraindicated in children younger than 9 years. Small abscesses usually resolve with incision and drainage alone.[38]

MRSA bacteremia can occur in the absence of skin findings and can progress to sepsis, bone and joint infections, pyomyositis, toxic shock syndrome, pneumonia, necrotizing fasciitis, or meningitis. Rates of occurence of MRSA bacteremia in North America are at 19.7/100,000 population. Dialysis, human immunodeficiency virus (HIV) infection, cancer, diabetes, and organ transplantation are known risk factors but these conditions can occur in otherwise healthy children.[39] The virulence of MRSA is believed primarily to be due to the Panton-Valentine leukocidin toxin. Morbidity and mortality in pediatric patients is lower than that of adults.[40] In a study limited to infants younger than 121 days, 40% of infants with S aureus bacteremia had MRSA. Of these infants, 19% died and 20% of the survivors had neurologic impairment on follow-up.[41] Castaldo and Yang[33] reported a small case series of children with MRSA sepsis, who presented with joint pains (75%), fever (63%), myalgia (50%), and diffuse rash (25%). Their patients had a bimodal age distribution (younger than 2 years and adolescence) and 25% had a history of minor, nonpenetrating trauma. In neonates, MRSA may be acquired in the neonatal intensive care unit or nursery and should be considered in a newborn presenting with pustulosis. Pyomyositis, a hematogenous acquired infection of skeletal muscle, can cause fever and pain in a specific muscle frequently with overlying induration and redness. Once radiographically confirmed, surgical drainage is recommended in conjunction with antimicrobials. Necrotizing fasciitis may begin as mild pain over an area, then progress to intense pain and systemic toxicity. Physical findings can be minimal, even in advanced stages of the disease. Mortality is high and early surgical drainage and antibiotic therapy is required. Diagnostically, WBC count is of questionable utility: in one study of patients with MRSA bacteremia, 38% of patients had leukocytosis, 30% had leukopenia, and 29% had normal WBC counts. In patients with these severe infections, intravenous vancomycin is recommended as a first-line medication, with linezolid being an option in allergic patients.

When treating pneumonia, it is important to consider MRSA infections due to their resistance to antibiotics that are traditionally used for this condition. Some centers have reported such an increase in the incidence of MRSA pneumonia that it has surpassed S pneumoniae as the prevalent pathogen in patients with complicated pneumonia. One such center in Houston studied 92 patients with invasive MRSA disease, 21 of whom had a primary diagnosis of pneumonia. Of these patients, 14 had accompanying empyema, and 4 had lung abscesses. An additional 26 of the 71 patients with other primary sites of infection (bacteremia, osteomyelitis, etc) had findings of pneumonia, septic emboli, or other pathology on chest radiography.[42] S aureus is recognized as a common pathogen causing superinfection of influenza, and MRSA superinfections have also been reported.

KAWASAKI DISEASE

KD is a vasculitis of small and medium vessels that primarily affects children younger than 5 years. If untreated, 20% of patients will develop coronary aneurysms, which can lead to myocardial ischemia. The exact causative factor remains unknown but it is believed to be, and treated as, an immune-mediated disorder.

The hallmark of KD is a fever lasting for 5 or more days. To meet the classic diagnostic criteria, the fever must be found in conjunction with at least 4 of the following symptoms: conjunctival injection, oropharyngeal mucous membrane changes, extremity changes, polymorphous rash, or cervical lymphadenopathy greater than or equal to 1.5 cm. Specifically, the conjunctivitis is nonexudative, bilateral, and tends to spare the limbus. Children may report photophobia because of a concurrent anterior uveitis. Mucous membrane changes frequently take the form of cracked lips and a "strawberry tongue." Oral vesicles or ulcerations are not typically found in KD and may indicate enteroviral disease. The rash is most frequently morbilliform but can take any form except vesicular. Occasionally, the rash fades before the ED visit, and a history for the rash should be elicited. Extremity changes appear late in the course of the disease and begin as palmar erythema and extremity swelling, eventually progressing to periungual desquamation. Although significantly less common, acute myocarditis, pulmonary, or gastrointestinal involvement (including gallbladder hydrops) can occur. It is important to recognize that children, particularly those younger than 1 year, can present with atypical features.

Although not definitive, certain laboratories are supportive of a diagnosis of KD. C-reactive protein level, sedimentation rate, and WBC counts generally increase within the first week. Platelet counts tend to increase in the second week of illness, and normocytic anemia may develop. Evidence of sterile pyuria and transaminitis are also suggestive.

Prompt recognition and treatment of KD is instrumental in reducing the risk of coronary aneurysm formation. Patients are admitted for an 8 to 12 hour infusion of intravenous immunoglobulin (IVIG) at a dose of 2 g/kg. High-dose acetylsalicylic acid (Aspirin) is started at 80 mg/kg/d, which is decreased after defervescence. Most children respond well to these measures, but there is a risk of recurrence. Any patient returning to the ED with a fever shortly after stopping IVIG for KD should be presumed to have a recurrence until proven otherwise.[43]

SICKLE CELL ANEMIA

Infection is the leading cause of death in patients with sickle cell anemia (SCA),[44] with children aged 6 months to 3 years at greatest risk. The new PCV7 has decreased invasive pneumococcal disease by as much as 93.4% from previous levels of 7.98 per 100 patient years.[45] National Institutes of Health recommendations include a CBC, blood culture, chest radiograph and/or oxygen saturation, urinalysis and urine culture, and throat culture in the SCA patient with FWS. Temperatures greater than 40.0°C, ill appearance, poor perfusion, hypotension, WBC count greater than 30,000 or less than 5000, platelet count less than 100,000, hemoglobin level less than 5 g/dL, infiltrate of chest radiograph, or history of pneumococcal sepsis increase the risk of bacteremia. Children with 1 or more of these conditions should promptly receive parenteral antibiotics and be admitted for continued therapy and close observation.[46] Typically, febrile infants younger than 6 to 12 months are also admitted. Splenic dysfunction reduces IgG antibody formation to polysaccharides; therefore, serious infections are usually associated with encapsulated organisms, including *H influenzae*,

S pneumoniae, E coli, and Salmonella. Patients not at high risk can be discharged from the ED after treatment with a long-acting parenteral antibiotic such as ceftriaxone.

In the child with SCA, reasons for fever other than bacteremia also merit consideration. Fever coupled with cough, chest pain, and dyspnea is suggestive of either acute chest crisis (ACC) or pneumonia that may precipitate an ACC. A normal chest radiograph does not exclude ACC in a patient with concerning symptoms and clinical findings. Treatment includes supportive care, hydration, and antibiotic coverage for the leading causes of infection, including *S pneumoniae, S aureus, H influenzae, Chlamydia, or Mycoplasma*. Respiratory symptoms can also be caused by influenza, which is associated with significant morbidity in patients with SCA. Meningitis, arthritis, and osteomyelitis are also more common in patients with SCA, and they should be considered in the appropriate clinical context.

Parvovirus deserves consideration in children with SCA. It can present asymptomatically, with upper respiratory tract infection symptoms, arthralgias, or with certain febrile syndromes. Erythema infectiosum is characterized by fever, headache, nausea, coryza, and slapped cheek appearance with circumoral pallor followed by diffuse maculopapular rash. Gloves and socks syndrome describes well-demarcated painful erythema and edema of the hands and feet eventually evolving into petechiae, purpura, vesicles, and skin sloughing. In children with SCA, parvovirus can cause a transient aplastic crisis. Typically, the reticulocyte count drops 5 days after infection, followed by the hemoglobin level. These children require close monitoring of hemoglobin level and often need packed red blood cell transfusions pending spontaneous recovery of red blood cell precursors. Once infected, children should have lifelong immunity for parvovirus B19.

MENINGOCOCCEMIA

N meningitidis is a gram-negative diplococcus that can colonize the upper respiratory tract. Upper respiratory infections or tobacco smoke exposure provides the opportunity for invasion of respiratory mucosa and development of disease. The incidence of invasive disease in the United States is 1.1/100,000 population with peak incidence in the late winter and early spring.[47] Most cases occur in children, with young infants and teens being most often infected. Nearly half of infections occur in children younger than 2 years. There are 2 vaccines against *N meningitidis* that are available in the United States: meningococcal polysaccharide vaccine (MPSV4; Menomune, Sanofi Pasteur Inc, Swiftwater, PA), and meningococcal conjugate vaccine (MCV4; Menactra, Sanofi Pasteur Inc, Swiftwater, PA). These vaccines include the serogroups A, C, Y, and W-135, but do not completely eliminate the possibility of contacting meningococcemia because the uncovered serogroup B is responsible for 30% of infections.[48]

N meningitidis causes 2 life-threatening clinical syndromes: meningococcemia and meningococcal meningitis; both may occur in the same patient. Presenting symptoms often include fever, headache, myalgia, abdominal pain, and vomiting.[49] The hallmark of meningococcemia is the rash: nonblanching hemorrhagic skin lesions that are more prominent on the extremities. The purpuric rash may be preceded by a maculopapular rash and arthralgia.[50,51] A febrile patient with a nonblanching petechial rash has an 11% to 15% chance of suffering from meningococcemia.[52] In meningococcemia the individual lesions generally progress and become larger than classic petechiae, and 15% to 25% of the lesions will progress to purpura fulminans if not promptly treated. Purpura fulminans is characterized by widespread ecchymosis and disseminated intravascular coagulopathy, and frequently leads to the need for multiple skin grafts and deforming amputations.[53] Cool extremities, extremity pain, and abnormality of skin color can be early signs of meningococcal sepsis.[54,55] Extremity symptoms can range from pain to frank arthritis. Therefore, a blood culture and empiric antibiotics should be considered in any patient with fever and petechiae that extend below the level of the nipples. Approximately 50% of patients with invasive meningococcal infections present with meningitis, generally with classic signs.[48,52] These infections, if not accompanied by systemic signs of meningococcemia, are clinically indistinguishable from other bacterial meningitides.

Additional complications of meningococcal infections include pneumonia, conjunctivitis, otitis media, epiglottitis, arthritis, urethritis, and pericarditis. Seizures occur in up to 20% of cases. Adrenal hemorrhage, myocardial dysfunction, stroke, and acute respiratory distress syndrome may all complicate meningococcemia. Rarely children develop chronic meningococcemia with prolonged intermittent fevers, rash, arthralgia, and headache.[48]

Gram stain of spinal fluid is often diagnostic, as is PCR when available. Because meningococcus is very sensitive to antibiotic therapy, cultures may be negative in the setting of antibiotic pretreatment.[56] Rapid bacterial antigen detection is not reliable and generally not clinically useful.[57] In this situation, diagnosis relies on clinical suspicion in the setting of CSF pleocytosis.

Aggressive antibiotic therapy and fluid resuscitation has reduced the fatality rate from 90% to 10%.[58] A recent pediatric study reported mortality of 9% and nonfatal adverse outcomes in 3.6% of patients.[55] Penicillin (500,000 U/kg/d q4h), ceftriaxone (100 mg/kg/d), or cefotaxime (200 mg/kg/d intravenously in 3 divided doses) are preferred. Chloramphenicol is an option for penicillin-allergic patients. Shock should be managed aggressively with fluids and pressers. Recent advances in the understanding of inflammatory mechanisms that lead to disseminated intravascular coagulation has resulted in strategies aimed at the inhibition of coagulation activation, which were found beneficial in initial experimental and clinical studies. These strategies included administration of recombinant human activated protein C or antithrombin III.[59–61] Additional antiendotoxin and anticytokine therapies are in the experimental phase.[47]

Adrenal hemorrhage can result from meningococcemia, and septic shock may be associated with relative adrenal insufficiency. There is conflicting evidence of the benefit of adrenal cortical hormone replacement in patients with septic shock,[62,63] but steroids are indicated in the setting of possible adrenal hemorrhage. Recent evidence suggests that the combination of low-dose vasopressin and corticosteroids is associated with decreased mortality and organ dysfunction in septic shock.[64] Electrolyte abnormalities associated with meningococcemia, including hypoglycemia, hypocalcemia, hypokalemia, hypomagnesemia, and metabolic acidosis, should be recognized and appropriately addressed.

Patients with meningococcal infection require isolation with droplet precautions. Household and close clinical contacts should receive chemoprophylaxis with ciprofloxacin (500 mg once for adults), rifampin (10 mg/kg q12h for 2d), or ceftriaxone (125 mg intramuscularly for children <12 years and 250 mg intramuscularly for children >12 years).[49] This includes those exposed to oral secretions, household contacts, and day care contacts.[47] Ciprofloxacin-resistant N meningitidis have been recently reported in North America.[65]

NEONATAL FEVER

Unlike older children and adults, infants younger than 3 months lack diurnal temperature variation and have less normal temperature variability. The general appearance and physical examination of the febrile neonate and young infant cannot be relied on to exclude an SBI. The most common current ED practice management of even a well-appearing febrile infant aged 28 days or younger is a "full sepsis evaluation," including a CBC; blood culture; urinalysis and urine culture; and evaluation of CSF, ED administration of antibiotics (ampicillin and cefotaxime or gentamicin), and hospitalization pending culture results. HSV PCR of CSF should be obtained if CSF pleocytosis is present with a negative Gram stain. Acyclovir should be considered based on CSF results. ED practice may differ from that of some general practitioners who have the advantage of a long-standing family relationship and the ability to provide ongoing care.[66] Identification of 1 SBI does not obviate the need to look for others in this age group. In a study of 45 febrile neonates with SBI, 10 had 2 SBIs concurrently.[67]

ED practice patterns vary in well-appearing infants aged 1 to 3 months. Children who meet clinical and laboratory low-risk criteria are candidates for outpatient therapy. In 1992, the "Boston criteria" were published, defining children aged 28 to 90 days with temperatures greater than or equal to 38.0°C and no otitis media or skin/soft tissue infection, with normal CSF, with negative urinalysis, and with a peripheral WBC count less than 20,000 as low-risk. All patients were given a dose of ceftriaxone in the ED and at 24 hours. Although the low-risk group had a 5.4% incidence of SBI, all infants were well on day 7.[68] The following year, the "Philadelphia criteria" were published, defining infants aged 29 to 56 days with temperatures greater than or equal to 38.2°C as low-risk if they had a peripheral WBC count less than 15,000, a band to neutrophil ratio of less than 0.2, an infant observation score of less than or equal to 10, no focal infection on examination, and a normal urinalysis and lumbar puncture. These criteria missed 1 SBI (bacteremia) in 747 infants.[69] The "Rochester criteria" included all children younger than 60 days with temperatures greater than or equal to 38.0°C. The criteria considered patients with no history of prematurity or significant past medical problems, no evidence of otitis media or skin/soft tissue infection, a peripheral WBC count from 5000 to 15,000, a band count less than 1500, and a urinalysis with less than 10 WBCs. A lumbar puncture and examination of CSF is not included in these criteria, which identified all but 5 of 1057 infants with SBI.[70] The latter results in a missed case of bacterial meningitis in 1 in 1000 infants.[71] All infants aged 1 to 3 months with FWS should have a catheterized urine specimen obtained for urinalysis and culture and for a CBC and blood culture. There are 3 options for the lumbar puncture. From most to least conservative the options are (1) lumbar puncture in all infants aged 1 to 3 months, (2) lumbar puncture in infants aged 1 to 2 months, and (3) no lumbar puncture in well-appearing infants aged 1 to 3 months if all other low-risk criteria are met or if a probable UTI is identified. Generally, patients in whom an infection is identified or suspected are admitted and managed on intravenous antibiotics, with the exception of the well-appearing infant with a UTI. These infants can be treated as outpatients with ceftriaxone in the ED and cefixime at home if close follow-up is assured.[72] Several studies have attempted to apply low-risk criteria to febrile neonates younger than 1 month of age and have found overall SBI rates of 4.6%–6.3%.[73,74] Addition of the C-reactive protein resulted in only slightly improved sensitivity for SBI, with rates of 2.7% in one study and 0.8% in another.[75,76] Therefore, the authors do not advocate the use of low-risk criteria to determine disposition for febrile infants aged 28 days or younger.

Infants afebrile in the ED with a documented fever at home should be treated as febrile infants. In one retrospective study of 27 infants aged 28 days or younger with a documented temperature greater than or equal to 38°C at home but no fever in the ED, 10 infants had identifiable infections including 3 who received antipyretics at home and 7 who defervesced without intervention.[77] Another retrospective review of 292 infants who were younger than 2 months with a history of fever included 244 with documented fever and 48 with tactile fever. Ninety-two percent of those with documented fever and 46% of those with tactile fever were febrile in the ED. The 26 infants with tactile fever at home and no fever in the ED were observed for the ensuing 48 hours. None developed a fever and 1 had a positive urinary culture.[78] Tactile fever is an unreliable indicator of fever and one for which there is little literature to guide interpretation.

Children with proven viral respiratory infections are at lower risk of SBI. Among 1,248 infants younger than 60 days, the 22% which tested positive for respiratory syncytial virus (RSV) had overall lower rates of SBIs (7% vs 12.5%), UTI (5.4% vs 10.1%), bacteremia (1.1% vs 2.3%), and meningitis (0% vs 0.9%).[79] A subsequent study found an even lower rate of SBI among RSV positive infants (2.2% vs 9.6%).[80] Similarly, febrile patients aged 0 to 36 months with influenza A have been assessed for SBI rates and were found to be significantly less likely to have SBI. In 163 influenza positive patients, 0.6% were bacteremic, 1.8% had UTIs, and 25.4% had radiographic evidence of pneumonia.[81] It is important to note that in the early neonatal period, enteroviral infections can cause a sepsis-like syndrome, requiring supportive care. In 68 infants aged younger than 12 weeks with acute otitis media, 45 of whom were febrile, no cases of meningitis or bacteremia were found, but 8.8% were found to have a UTI.[82]

FEVER OF UNKNOWN ORIGIN

Fever of unknown origin (FUO) is defined as a fever without an obvious cause lasting beyond 3 weeks, although some investigators use 10 or 14 days of unexplained fever as criteria. Often the history of a prolonged fever represents nothing more serious than a series of viral illnesses, and careful questioning often uncovers a period of wellness between 2 or more discreet febrile episodes.

The leading causes of FUO fall into 3 categories: infections, immune-mediated inflammatory diseases, and malignancy. Infection is the most common, accounting for 40% to 60% of FUO, particularly in children younger than 6 years. EBV is the most common infection followed by osteomyelitis and bartonella ("cat scratch disease").[83] Other infections include chronic UTI, pneumonia, HIV, and bacteremia, which was found in one study to compose 1.4% of FUO cases.[84] Second most common are the immune-mediated diseases, particularly in children 6 years and older. Of these, juvenile inflammatory arthritis (also called juvenile rheumatoid arthritis) is the most common. Malignancies compose 1.5% to 6% of FUO diagnoses, led in frequency by leukemia. Disorders such as KD should also be considered. There are also several periodic fever syndromes, such as PFAPA (periodic fever, aphthous stomatitis, pharyngitis and adenitis), in which children get fevers with aphthous ulcers and lymphadenopathy recurring every 3 to 6 weeks.[83] These syndromes usually cause fevers of shorter duration but can lead to more prolonged fever.

Recent travel should prompt consideration of malaria, dengue, or typhoid fever. Fever with 2 spikes per day is associated with gonococcal endocarditis, leishmaniasis, malaria, juvenile rheumatoid arthritis, and miliary tuberculosis. Bradycardia relative to the height of fever is seen in drug fever, leishmaniasis, typhoid fever, Legionnaire disease, psittacosis, and brucellosis. Elevations in alkaline phosphatase may indicate tuberculosis. Free blood anywhere, including intracranial hemorrhage, is another cause for FUO and can occur without contributory history in the setting of nonaccidental trauma. Recurrent fever with erythema multiforme often indicates HSV, while recurrent fever with joint pain and petechiae may indicate chronic meningococcemia.

Low-grade fever with anemia and abnormal liver function tests may have been associated with Wilson disease.[85]

Unless a child with FUO seems to be either unstable or likely to have an etiology associated with rapid decompensation, they should be referred to their primary care provider or an infectious disease consultant, rather than undergo an extensive workup in the ED. Their evaluation usually begins with careful history including ill contacts, travel, animal exposures, and medication exposure. Physical examination findings related to final diagnosis are present in 59% of patients.[86] Useful laboratory tests include CBC, sedimentation rate, C-reactive protein test, urinalysis, and cultures of the blood, urine, and throat. Other diagnostic tests include bartonella titers in patients with a history of a cat scratch, EBV serology, and HIV serology. In an ill-appearing child or in one with localizing signs, lumbar puncture for chronic meningitis may be warranted.[87] Additional recommended tests include chest radiograph and a purified protein derivative placed with a tetanus or candida control. In up to 30% of cases no diagnosis is ever established.[88,89] Two long-term studies were conducted on children in whom an extensive workup yielded no diagnosis. One study showed resolution without contributory diagnosis in 17 of the 19 patients, with 2 eventually diagnosed with juvenile rheumatoid arthritis.[90] Another found that of the 40 patients studied, 4 eventually received contributory diagnoses: 2 with inflammatory bowel disease, 1 uveitis, and 1 mitochondrial encephalopathy. Six of the 40 patients also received a diagnosis of developmental delay or attention-deficit/hyperactivity disorder.[91]

EXTREME HYPERPYREXIA

A temperature greater than 40°C is often concerning to parents and health care providers alike. Literature on the hyperpyrexic children and their risk of SBI is inconsistent. In 2006, a prospective study of children with rectal temperatures greater than or equal to 41.1°C (106°F) identified 20 of 103 children (19.4%) with SBI. Diagnoses included bacteremia (11/20), UTI (8/20), and 1 of 20 each of tracheitis, enteritis, and epidural abscess. Pneumonia was not considered an SBI in this particular study, but 17% of hyperpyrexic children had an abnormal chest radiograph, including 5 with other SBI. Of the remaining hyperpyrexic children, 11 had otitis media, 1 had neuroleptic malignant syndrome, and 1 was diagnosed with lupus. In total, 45% of the children were diagnosed with a condition that required antibiotic therapy or other significant intervention. Neither age nor WBC count was helpful in determining which patients had SBI. Their conclusions included the recommendation of empiric antibiotic therapy for all patients with extreme hyperpyrexia.[92] These results are comparable to the largest retrospective set on this topic by McCarthy and Dolan in 1974.[93] In children with lower temperatures, fever with temperatures greater than or equal to 102°F was a risk factor for bacteremia in the 3 to 36 months age group.[94] Temperatures greater than 40°C (104°F) were associated with a bacteremia rate of 7% to 10% in children younger than 24 months.[95]

FEVER IN THE MEDICALLY FRAGILE PATIENT

Fever in children who are neurologically impaired or dependent on technology, such as ventilator assistance, is perhaps the greatest challenge. In children with developmental delay it is important to establish with the family how the child has deviated from their baseline when assessing for conditions such as meningitis and encephalitis. Parents are helpful allies in assessing these patients. However, an ill-appearing child must be treated as just that, even if parents believe that the deviation from baseline is minimal. Vital signs can also be difficult to interpret. Few neurologic syndromes cause alteration in the vital signs as part of the syndrome itself, but these children may be easily agitated by medical providers. Therefore, every effort should be made to establish normal vital signs for the patient. If this is not possible, tachycardia or hypotension must be considered a sign of significant illness. There is little literature advising on the care of these patients; therefore, an approach of potential overtesting and observation is the safest option. Neurologically impaired children, particularly those with a tracheostomy, are at increased risk of pneumonia, and a low threshold should be used for obtaining a chest radiograph. Also, they are at increased risk of morbidity and mortality from influenza. In a study of 745 patients with influenza, 12% of patients requiring admission had an underlying neurologic disorder. These patients were at higher risk for influenza-related morbidity (including intubation) and prolonged hospital stay.[96]

In patients with underlying malignancy and central venous catheters, bacterial infections are often accompanied by few signs and symptoms other than fever. A history of fever or chills immediately after flushing of the catheter or the presence of erythema at the catheter exit site increases the risk of bacteremia. The overall catheter-associated infection rate for oncology patients is 0.87 to 1.3 events per 1000 use days.[97,98] In one study, line-associated bacteremia was present in 24% of nonneutropenic children with cancer and fever.[99] This risk increases 25-fold during hospitalization. Common pathogens include gram-positive bacteria, including coagulase-negative staphylococci, enterococci, α-hemolytic streptococci, viridans streptococci, *Stomatococcus*, and gram-negative organisms including *Pseudomonas aeruginosa*, *Burkholderia cepacia*, *Klebsiella*, *Stenotrophomonas maltophilia*, *Acinetobacter baumannii*, and fungi including *Candida* and *Aspergillus*.[100]

Although paired blood culture from the line and periphery are ideal, the sensitivity of a single blood culture from the line is 84%.[101] Cultures are positive quickly in true infections, with a mean of 14 hours.[102] Broad-spectrum antibiotics with antistaphylococcal and antipseudomonal coverage such as vancomycin plus cefepime or piperacillin/tazobactam should be used when suspicion is high for a line-related infection. Patients with significant intestinal pathology on home parental nutrition are at increased risk of translocation of intestinal flora to their central line and are therefore at high risk of line sepsis.

Spina bifida represents the most common major birth defect, and recent advances have provided these patients with significant improvements in long-term survival. In addition to a meningomyelocele, many have hydrocephalus requiring a ventriculoperitoneal shunt (VPS). These children usually have normal intellectual development. Their spinal cord dysfunction may render them incontinent and dependent on assist devices for ambulation. Patients with spina bifida presenting febrile to an ED have a 55% risk of UTI. Other infections include cellulitis (generally related to a decubitus ulcer) at 24% and pneumonia at 15%.[103] VPS infections usually occur within 4 months of shunt placement or revision. When shunt infection occurs after 4 months then it is generally due to either an obstruction or an ascending infection from the abdominal cavity. All patients with VPS and fever should be fully undressed and examined for skin infection and should have urinalysis and culture and also undergo any additional tests that are directed by the history and physical examination.

SUMMARY

The authors would like to reemphasize some of the important points regarding the management of febrile infants and children. Fever is defined as a rectal temperature greater than 38.0°C (>100.4°F). A recently documented fever at home should be considered the same as a fever in the ED and should be managed similarly. All febrile infants younger than 28 days should receive a "full sepsis workup" and be admitted for parenteral antibiotic therapy. Clinical and laboratory criteria can be used to identify a low-risk population of febrile infants aged 1 to 4 months who have not received 2 doses of conjugate vaccines for bacterial meningitis. Occult UTIs occur often in children with FWS; therefore, a catheterized urine specimen should be obtained for urine testing in girls and uncircumcised boys younger than 2 years and in circumcised boys younger than 1 year with FWS. Fever with petechiae below the nipples should lead to consideration of meningococcemia. Children with sickle cell disease are at high risk and require special evaluation. MRSA infections are now common and should be considered in all patients with pyoderma, severe pneumonia, and catheter-related sepsis. HSV infection of the CNS should be considered whenever a patient has altered mental status and CSF findings are not diagnostic of bacterial meningitis.

REFERENCES

1. Carroll AE, Buddenbaum JL. Malpractice claims involving pediatricians: epidemiology and etiology. Pediatrics 2007;120(1):10–7.
2. Nager A. Pediatric emergency medicine. In: Baren, Brennan, Brown, et al, editors. Dehydration and Disorders of Sodium Balance. Chapter 110. 2007. p. 782–5.
3. McCarthy PL, Lembo RM, Baron MA, et al. Predictive value of abnormal physical examination findings in ill-appearing and well-appearing febrile children. Pediatrics 1985;76(2):167–71.
4. Teach SJ, Fleisher GR. Efficacy of an observation scale in detecting bacteremia in febrile children three to thirty-six months of age, treated as outpatients. J Pediatr 1995;126(6):877–81.
5. Silverman B. Practical information. In: Fleisher GR, Ludwig S, Henretig F, editors. Textbook of pediatric emergency medicine. 5th edition. Philadelphia: Lippincott Williams & Williams; 2006. p. 2013.
6. Baraff LJ. Management of infants and children 3 to 36 months of age with fever without source. Pediatr Ann 1993;22(8):501–4.
7. Black S, Shinefield H, Fireman B, et al. Efficacy, safety, and immunogenicity of heptavalent conjugate pneumococcal vaccine in children. Northern California Kaiser Permanente Vaccine Study Center Group. Pediatr Infect Dis J 2000;19:187–95.
8. Wilkinson M, Bulloch B, Smith M. Prevalence of occult bacteremia in children aged 3 to 36 months presenting to the emergency department with fever in the post-pneumococcal conjugate vaccine era. Acad Emerg Med 2008;16:1–6.
9. Carstairs KL, Tanen DA, Johnson AS, et al. Pneumococcal bacteremia in febrile infants presenting to the emergency department before and after the introduction of the heptavalent pneumococcal vaccine. Ann Emerg Med 2007;49(6):772–7.
10. Norberg A, Christopher NC, Ramundo ML, et al. Contamination rates of blood cultures obtained by dedicated phlebotomy vs intravenous catheter. JAMA 2003;289(6):726–9.
11. Lee GM, Fleisher GR, Harper MB. Management of febrile children in the age of the conjugate pneumococcal vaccine: a cost-effectiveness analysis. Pediatrics 2001;108(4):835–44.
12. Stoll ML, Rubin LG. Incidence of occult bacteremia among highly febrile young children in the era of the pneumococcal conjugate vaccine; a study from

a children's hospital emergency department and urgent care center. Arch Pediatr Adolesc Med 2004;158(7):671–5.

13. Issacman DJ, Burke B. Utility of the serum C-reactive protein for detection of occult bacterial infection in children. Arch Pediatr Adolesc Med 2002;156:905–9.

14. Maniaci V, Duaber A, Weiss S, et al. Procalcitonin in young febrile infants for the detection of serious bacterial infections. Pediatrics 2008;122(4):701–10.

15. Dai Y, Foy HM, Zhu Z, et al. Respiratory rate and signs in roentgenographically confirmed pneumonia among children in China. Pediatr Infect Dis 1995;14(1):48–50.

16. Murphey CG, van de Pol AC, Harper MB, et al. Clinical predictors of occult pneumonia in the febrile child. Acad Emerg Med 2007;14(3):243–9.

17. Bachur R, Perry H, Harper MB. Occult pneumonias: empiric chest radiographs in febrile children with leukocytosis. Ann Emerg Med 1999;33(2):166–73.

18. Hoberman A, Chao HP, Keller DM, et al. Prevalence of urinary tract infection in febrile infants. J Pediatr 1993;123(1):17–23.

19. Hoberman A, Wald ER. Urinary tract infections in young febrile children. Pediatr Infect Dis J 1997;16(1):11–7.

20. Committee on quality improvement, subcommittee on urinary tract infection. Practice parameter: the diagnosis, treatment, and evaluation of the initial urinary tract infection in febrile infants and young children. Pediatrics 1999;103(4 Pt 1): 843–52.

21. Whitley RJ, Kimberlin DW. Viral encephalitis. Pediatr Rev 1999;20:192.

22. Caviness AC, Demmler GJ, Almendarez Y, et al. The prevalence of neonatal herpes simplex virus compared to serious bacterial illness among hospitalized febrile neonates. J Pediatr 2008;153(2):164–9.

23. Meyer MH, Johnson RT, Crawford IP, et al. Central nervous system syndromes of viral etiology. Am J Med 1960;29:334–47.

24. Whitley RJ. Herpes simplex encephalitis: adolescents and adults. Antiviral Res 2006;71:141–8.

25. De Tiege X, Rozenberg F, Des Portes V, et al. Herpes simplex encephalitis relapses in children: differentiation of two neurologic entities. Neurology 2003;61:241–3.

26. Kennedy PGE, Chaudhuri A. Herpes simplex encephalitis. J Neurol Neurosurg Psychiatr 2002;73:237–8.

27. Steiner I, Kennedy PG, Pachner AR. The neurotropic herpes viruses: herpes simplex and varicella-zoster. Lancet Neurol 2007;6(11):1015–28.

28. Teixeira J, Zimmerman RA, Haselgrove JC, et al. Diffusion imaging in pediatric central nervous system infections. Neuroradiology 2001;43:1031–9.

29. Eeg-Olofsson O, Bergstrom T, Andermann E, et al. Herpesviral DNA in brain tissue from patients with temporal lobe epilepsy. Acta Neurol Scand 2004; 109(3):169–74.

30. Whitley RJ. Therapeutic advances for severe and life-threatening herpes simplex virus infections. In: Lopez C, Roizman B, editors. Human herpes virus infections. New York: Raven Press; 1986. p.153–64.

31. Elbers JM, Bitnun A, Richardson SE, et al. A 12-year prospective study of childhood herpes simplex encephalitis: is there a broader spectrum of disease? Pediatrics 2007;119:e399–407.

32. Purcell K, Fergie JE. Exponential increase in community-acquired methicillin-resistant *Staphylococcus aureus* infections in South Texas children. Pediatr Infect Dis J 2002;21(10):988–9.

33. Castaldo ET, Yang EY. Severe sepsis attributable to community-associated methicillin-resistant *Staphylococcus aureus*: an emerging fatal problem. Am Surg 2007;73:684–7.

34. Zaoutis TE, Toltzis P, Chu J, et al. Clinical and molecular epidemiology of community-acquired methicillin-resistant *Staphylococcus aureus* infections among children with risk factors for health care-associated infections: 2001–2003. Pediatr Infect Dis J 2006;25(4):343–8.

35. Gonzalez BE, Kaplan SL. Severe staphylococcal infections in children. Pediatr Ann 2008;37(10):686–93.

36. Fridkin SK, Hageman JC, Morrison M, et al. Methicillin-resistant *Staphylococcus aureus* disease in three communities. N Engl J Med 2005;352:1436–44.

37. Paintsil E. Pediatric community-acquired methicillin-resistant *Staphylococcus aureus* infection and colonization: trends and management. Curr Opin Pediatr 2007;19:75–82.

38. Lee MC, Rios AM, Aten MF, et al. Management and outcome of children with skin and soft tissue abscesses caused by community-acquired methicillin-resistant *Staphylococcus aureus*. Pediatr Infect Dis J 2004;23(2):123–7.

39. Laupland KB, Ross T, Gregson DB. *Staphylococcus aureus* bloodstream infections: risk factors, outcomes, and the influence of methicillin resistance in Calgary, Canada, 2000–2005. J Infect Dis 2008;198(3):336–43.

40. Denniston S, Riordan FA. *Staphylococcus aureus* bacteraemia in children and neonates: a 10 year retrospective review. J Infect 2006;53:387–93.

41. Cohen-Wolkowiez M, Benjamin DK, Fowler VG, et al. Mortality and neurodevelopment after *Staphylococcus aureus* bacteremia in infants. Pediatr Infect Dis J 2007;26(12):1159–61.

42. Gonzalez BE, Hulten KG, Dishop MK, et al. Pulmonary manifestations in children with invasive community-acquired *Staphylococcus aureus* infection. Clin Infect Dis 2005;41:583–90.

43. Woodward AL, Sundel RP. Rheumatologic emergencies. In: Fleisher GR, Ludwig S, Henretig F, editors. Textbook of pediatric emergency medicine. 5th edition. Philadelphia: Lippincott Williams & Williams; 2006. p. 1305–10.

44. Manci EA, Culberson DE, Yang YM, et al. Causes of death in sickle cell disease: an autopsy study. Br J Haematol 2003;123(2):359–65.

45. Halasa NB, Shankar SM, Talbot TR, et al. Incidence of invasive pneumococcal disease among individuals with sickle cell disease before and after the introduction of the pneumococcal conjugate vaccine. Clin Infect Dis 2007;44(11):1428–33.

46. Wilimas JA, Flynn PM, Harris S, et al. A randomized study of outpatient treatment with ceftriaxone for selected febrile children with sickle cell disease. N Engl J Med 1993;329(7):472–6.

47. Kirsch EA, Barton RP, Kitchen L, et al. Pathophysiology, treatment and outcome of meningococcemia: a review and recent experience. Pediatr Infect Dis J 1996; 15(11):967–79.

48. Rosenstein NE, Perkins BA, Stephens DS, et al. The changing epidemiology of meningococcal disease in the United States, 1992–1996. J Infect Dis 1999;180: 1894–901.

49. Singh J, Arrieta A. Management of meningococcemia. Indian J Pediatr 2007;71: 909–13.

50. Brandtzaed P, Dahle JS, Hoiby EA. The occurrence and features of hemorrhagic skin lesions in 115 cases of systemic meningococcal disease. NIPH Ann 1983;6: 183–90.

51. Lodder MC, Schildkamp RL, Biljmer HA, et al. Prognostic indicators of the outcome of meningococcal disease: a study of 562 patients. J Med Microbiol 1996;45:16–20.

52. Stephans DS, Greenwood B, Brantzaeg P. Epidemic meningitis, meningococ-ceamia, and *Neisseria meningitidis*. Lancet 2007;369:2196–210.

53. Herrera R, Hobar PC, Ginsburg CM. Surgical intervention for the complications of meningococcal-induced purpura fulminans. Pediatr Infect Dis J 1994;13: 734–7.

54. Thompson MJ, Ninis N, Perera R, et al. Clinical recognition of meningococcal disease in children and adolescents. Lancet 2006;367:397–403.

55. Inkelis SH, O'Leary D, Wang V, et al. Extremity pain and refusal to walk in chil-dren with invasive meningococcal disease. Pediatrics 2002;110:e3.

56. Wylie PA, Stevens D, Drake W, et al. Epidemiology and clinical management of meningococcal disease in west Gloucestershire: retrospective, population based study. BMJ 1997;315:774–9.

57. Perkins MD, Mirrett S, Reller LB. Rapid bacterial antigen detection is not clini-cally useful. J Clin Microbiol 1995;33(6):1486–91.

58. Flexner S. The results of the serum treatment in thirteen hundred cases of epidemic meningitis. J Exp Med 1913;17:553–76.

59. White B, Livingstone W, Murphy C, et al. Recombinant human protein C world-wide evaluation in severe sepsis (PROWESS) study group. Efficacy and safety of recombinant human activated protein C for severe sepsis. N Engl J Med 2001;344:699–709.

60. Levi M, de Jonge E, van der Poll T. New treatment strategies for disseminated intravascular coagulation based on current understanding of the pathophysi-ology. Ann Med 2004;36:41–9.

61. Afshari A, Wetterslev J, Brok J, et al. Antithrombin III in critically ill patients: systematic review with meta-analysis and trial sequential analysis. BMJ 2007; 335:1248–51.

62. Annane D, Sébille V, Charpentier C, et al. Effect of treatment with low doses of hydrocortisone and fludrocortisone on mortality in patients with septic shock. JAMA 2002;288(7):862–71.

63. Sprung CL, Annane D, Keh D, et al. Hydrocortisone therapy for patients with septic shock. N Engl J Med 2008;358(2):111–24.

64. Russell JA, Walley KR, Gordon AC, et al. Interaction of vasopressin infusion, corticosteroid treatment, and mortality of septic shock. Crit Care Med 2009; 37(3):811–8.

65. Wu HM, Harcourt BH, Hatcher CP, et al. Emergence of ciprofloxacin-resistant *Neisseria meningitidis* in North America. N Engl J Med 2009;360(9):886–92.

66. Pantell RH, Newman TB, Bernzweig J, et al. Management and outcomes of care of fever in early infancy. JAMA 2004;291(10):1203–12.

67. Kadish HA, Loveridge B, Tobey J, et al. Applying outpatient protocols in febrile infants 1–28 days of age: can the threshold be lowered? Clin Pediatr 2000;39: 81–8.

68. Baskin MN, O'Fourke EJ, Fleisher GR. Outpatient treatment of febrile infants 28 to 89 days with intramuscular administration of ceftriaxone. J Pediatr 1992;120: 22–7.

69. Baker MD, Bell LM, Avner JR. Outpatient management without antibiotics of fever in selected infants. N Engl J Med 1993;329:1437–41.

70. Jaskiewicz JA, McCarthy CA, Richardson AC, et al. Febrile infants at low risk for serious bacterial infections- an appraisal of the Rochester criteria and implica-tions for management. Pediatrics 1994;94:390–6.

71. Baraff LJ. Management of infants and young children with fever without source. Pediatr Ann 2008;37(10):673–9.

72. Hoberman A, Wald ER, Hickey RW, et al. Oral versus intravenous therapy for urinary tract infections in young febrile children. Pediatrics 1999;104(1 Pt 1): 79–86.
73. Baker MD, Bell LM. Unpredictability of serious bacterial illness in febrile infants from birth to 1 month of age. Arch Pediatr Adolesc Med 1999;153:508–11.
74. Ferrera PC, Bartfield JM, Snyder HS. Neonatal fever: utility of Rochester criteria in determining low risk for serious bacterial infections. Am J Emerg Med 1997; 15:299–302.
75. Wu W, Chen H, Chung P, et al. Ambulatory care of selected febrile outpatient neonates unlikely to have bacterial infections. Int Pediatr 2004;19(1):52–6.
76. Chiu C, Lin T, Bullard M. Identification of febrile neonates unlikely to have bacterial infections. Pediatr Infect Dis J 1997;16(1):59–63.
77. Brown L, Shaw T, Moynihan JA, et al. Investigation of afebrile neonates with a history of fever. CJEM 2004;6(5):343–8.
78. Bonadio WA, Hegenbarth M, Zachariason M. Correlating reported fever in young infants with subsequent temperature patterns and rate of serious bacterial infections. Pediatr Infect Dis J 1990;9(3):158–60.
79. Levine DA, Platt SL, Dayan PS, et al. Risk of serious bacterial infection in young febrile infants with respiratory syncytial virus infections. Pediatrics 2004;113: 1728–34.
80. Bilavsky E, Shouval DS, Yarden-Bilavsky H, et al. A prospective study of the risk for serious bacterial infections in hospitalized febrile infants with or without bronchiolitis. Pediatr Infect Dis J 2008;27(3):269–70.
81. Smitherman HF, Caviness AC, Macias CG. Retrospective review of serious bacterial infections in infants who are 0 to 36 months and have influenza A infection. Pediatrics 2005;115(3):710–8.
82. Sakran W, Makary H, Colodner R, et al. Acute otitis media in infants less than three moths of age: clinical presentation, etiology and concomitant diseases. Int J Pediatr Otorhinolaryngol 2006;70(4):613–7.
83. Van der Jagt EW. Fever of unknown origin. In: AAP textbook of pediatric care, 2008: Available at: http://www.pediatriccareonline.org/pco/ub/pview/AAP-Textbook-of-Pediatric-Care/394181/all/Chapter_181:_Fever?q=occult%20bacteremia. Accessed October 16, 2009.
84. Berezin EN, Iazzetti MA. Evaluation of the incidence of occult bacteremia among children with fever of unknown origin. Braz J Infect Dis 2006;10(6): 396–9.
85. Tolia J, Smith LG. Fever of unknown origin: historical and physical clues to making the diagnosis. Infect Dis Clin North Am 2007;21:917–36.
86. Lohr JA, Hendley JO. Prolonged fever of unknown origin: a record of experiences with 54 childhood patients. Clin Pediatr 1977;16:768–73.
87. Akpede GO, Akenzua GI. Management of children with prolonged fever of unknown origin and difficulties in the management of fever of unknown origin in children in developing countries. Paediatr Drugs 2001;3(4):247–62.
88. Gaeta G, Fusco F, Nardiello S. Fever of unknown origin: a systemic review of the literature for 1995–2004. Nucl Med Commun 2006;27:205–11.
89. Mackowiak P, Durack D. Fever of unknown origin. In: Mandell GL, Bennett JE, Dolin R, editors. Mandell, Douglas and Bennett's Principles and Practice of Infectious Disease. 6th edition. Philadelphia (PA): Elsevier; 2005. p. 718–29.
90. Talano JM, Kazt BZ. Long-term follow-up of children with fever of unknown origin. Clin Pediatr 2000;39:715.

91. Miller LC, Sisson BA, Tucker LB, et al. Prolonged fevers of unknown origin in children: patterns of presentation and outcome. J Pediatr 1996;12:419–23.

92. Trautner BW, Caviness C, Gerlacher GR, et al. Prospective evaluation of the risk of serious bacterial infection in children who present to the emergency department with hyperpyrexia. Pediatrics 2006;118:34–40.

93. McCarthy PL, Dolan TF Jr. Hyperpyrexia in children. Eight-year emergency room experience. Am J Dis Child 1976;130(8):849–51.

94. Jamuma R, Srinivasan S, Hariah BN. Factors predicting occult bacteremia in young children. Indian J Pediatr 2000;67(10):709.

95. McCarthy PL, Bass JW, Steele RW, et al. Antimicrobial treatment of occult bacteremia: a multicenter cooperative study. Pediatr Infect Dis J 1993;12: 466–73.

96. Coffin SE, Zaoutis TE, Rosenquist AB, et al. Incidence, complications, and risk factors for prolonged stay in children hospitalized with community-acquired influenza. Pediatrics 2007;119:740–8.

97. Fratino G, Molinari AC, Parodi S, et al. Central venous catheter-related complications in children with oncological/hematological diseases: an observational study of 418 devices. Ann Oncol 2005;16:1510–3.

98. Cesaro S, Corro R, Pelosin A, et al. A prospective survey on incidence and outcome of Broviac/Hickman catheter-related complications in pediatric patients affected by hematologic and oncologic diseases. Ann Hematol 2004;83:183–8.

99. Gorelick MH, Owen WC, Seibel NL, et al. Lack of association between neutropenia and the incidence of bacteremia associated with indwelling central venous catheters in febrile pediatric cancer patients. Pediatr Infect Dis J 1991;10: 506–10.

100. Sinom A, Bode U, Beutel K. Diagnosis and treatment of catheter-related infections in paediatric oncology: an update. Clin Microbiol Infect 2006;12:606–20.

101. Robinson JL. Sensitivity of a blood culture drawn through a single lumen of a multilumen, long-term, indwelling, central venous catheter in pediatric oncology patients. J Pediatr Hematol Oncol 2002;24(1):72–4.

102. Shah SS, Downes KJ, Elliot MR, et al. How long does it take to "rule out" bacteremia in children with central venous catheters. Pediatrics 2008;121:135–41.

103. Caterino JM, Scheatzle MD, D'Antonio JA. Descriptive analysis of 258 emergency department visits by spina bifida patients. Ann Emerg Med 2001;38(4): S74–5.

High-Risk Pediatric Orthopedic Pitfalls

Jennifer C. Laine, MD, Scott P. Kaiser, MD, Mohammad Diab, MD*

KEYWORDS

- Pediatric fracture • Limp • Septic arthritis • Abuse
- Compartment syndrome • Slipped capital femoral epiphysis

Key points

- For pediatric fractures, intra-articular injury, which can lead to osteoarthritis, is of even greater concern than physeal involvement, which can lead to growth disturbance but is correctable.
- For type I open fractures, in which the bone pokes through the skin creating a puncture from inside outward, treatment includes cleaning the wound, oral antibiotics, splinting and referral to an orthopedic surgeon within 24 hours.
- With supracondylar fractures, loss of pulse is not always an emergency as long as the hand is acceptably perfused, which is defined as warm and pink with less than 2 second capillary refill. In consultation with an orthopedist, such a fracture may be splinted in place and referred the next office day for evaluation and management.
- With supracondylar fractures, neural injury occurs in approximately 10% to 15% of cases. The outcome of such neurapraxia is recovery, which may take up to 6 months and therefore does not require immediate surgery.
- Compartmental syndrome in children differs from that in adults. Physical examination findings can be milder, children can be more difficult to examine, and they may not be able to describe their pain as clearly as adults. This difficulty can result in delayed diagnosis, so the level of suspicion should remain high.
- Axial joint septic arthritis (shoulder and hip) is treated with incision, drainage, irrigation, and debridement.
- Appendicular joint septic arthritis can often be diagnosed and treated by serial aspiration and antibiotics.
- Osteomyelitis with radiographic change will need operation and may wait until evaluation by an orthopedic surgeon within a week.

The authors have no disclosures to declare.

University of California San Francisco, Department of Orthopaedic Surgery, 500 Parnassus Avenue, MU-320W, San Francisco, CA 94143, USA

* Corresponding author.

E-mail address: Diab@orthosurg.ucsf.edu (M. Diab).

Emerg Med Clin N Am 28 (2010) 85–102

doi:10.1016/j.emc.2009.09.008

0733-8627/09/$ – see front matter © 2010 Published by Elsevier Inc.

emed.theclinics.com

- Osteomyelitis without radiographic change should not be treated with antibiotics (unless patients are in distress) until an osseous specimen is obtained.
- Articular hip disorders typically manifest as groin pain but may present as knee or thigh pain.
- In pediatric patients who have a limp, the prone position is optimal for examination, which allows uncoupling of the knee from the hip, in which the pathology of one may masquerade as the other.
- If the diagnosis of slipped capital femoral epiphysis (SCFE) is suspected, both hips should be imaged.
- Fifteen percent of children who have SCFE have mostly knee or distal thigh pain. Children who have SCFE who present with primarily knee pain are more likely to receive a misdiagnosis and have slips of greater severity.

Children are not small adults: they are peculiar and may confound even the experienced emergency provider who is more familiar with adults. The authors have selected some pediatric orthopedic pitfalls based upon frequency of occurrence, difficulty of diagnosis, or gravity of sequelae. The authors have sacrificed quantity at the alter of quality, to teach principles rather than to catalog. The authors' goals are brevity and clarity, and they hope that the included tables may serve for quick references in busy clinical settings.

FRACTURES
General

An understanding of pediatric bone anatomy is essential to the accurate description of a fracture (**Box 1** and **Table 1**). The location of a fracture relative to the growth plate has implications for growth and the eventual risk of osteoarthritis. The fracture pattern may influence the stability of a fracture and determine the type of immobilization required, the degree of weight bearing allowed, or the technique of operative treatment. Soft-tissue injury may impact risk of infection, healing, and functional outcome.

Displacement at a fracture has two components. Translation is measured in percentage of bone diameter; however, it is measured in millimeters when articular. Angulation is defined by the direction of the distal fragment (eg, dorsal in the sagittal plane, varus in the coronal plane) or by the direction of the apex of the fracture (eg, apex volar in the sagittal plane, apex lateral in the coronal plane). Rotational angulation (in the transverse plane) may be difficult to determine in standard anterior-posterior and lateral radiographs. Angulation is measured in degrees.

Fractures in children may be divided into non-physeal versus physeal. Physeal fractures have been classified by Salter and Harris (**Fig. 1**).[1] Although the Salter-Harris classification is venerable and widely established, physeal fractures may be divided according to treatment and prognosis into nonarticular versus articular (**Fig. 2**). Fractures are treated based upon acceptable criteria, as illustrated in **Table 2**. The most important factors that determine acceptable displacement are percent contribution of adjacent physis to growth and planes of motion of the adjacent joint. As a result, the fracture where the greatest amount of displacement is acceptable is the proximal humerus; the proximal physis accounts for 80% of total growth of the humerus (the highest contribution in the skeleton), and the shoulder joint allows motion in all planes.

Physeal/articular fractures require anatomic reduction, defined as within 2 mm of normal alignment, based upon the increased incidence of posttraumatic osteoarthritis seen in patients who have articular displacement greater than 2 mm.[2] Because the physis distinguishes bones in children from those in adults, it is often the focus of

---

Box 1
How to describe a fracture patient

1. Age

2. Mechanism

3. Date/time of injury

4. Bone involved

5. Location within bone

   - diaphyseal

   - metaphyseal

   - epiphyseal

6. Pattern of fracture

   - transverse

   - oblique

   - spiral

   - comminuted

7. Physeal involvement (±)

8. Articular involvement (±)

9. Soft tissue/skin:

   - open versus closed

   - swelling

   - neurovascular examination

---

discussions between parents and providers. However, in the balance of growth disturbance (with physeal injury) versus osteoarthritis (with articular displacement >2 mm), the latter is of greater concern to the surgeon. Growth disturbance is treatable (physeal bridge excision, corrective osteotomy, bone lengthening), whereas there is no effective reconstruction for osteoarthritis. An illustration of this principle is that, during open reduction and internal fixation of physeal/articular fractures, articular stability is never sacrificed for physeal preservation; trans-physeal (eg, with a plate or threaded implant), stable articular fixation is preferable to extra-physeal, less stable articular fixation.

Open fractures traditionally have been considered an emergency requiring operative treatment within 6 hours of injury. However, open fractures associated with a small skin laceration less than 1 cm, minimal surrounding soft-tissue injury, and minimal contamination are no longer considered to require emergent treatment.[3] Such fractures are classified as type I.[4] Types II and III describe increasing wound size and soft-tissue injury, including vascular and neural injury and need for reconstruction in addition to osseous fixation.[5] In type I open fractures, deformation of the limb allows the bone to poke through the skin creating a cutaneous puncture from inside outward. This type of puncture contrasts with an external object creating a large devitalized wound that brings contaminants from the outside inward, as in types II and III, necessitating irrigation, debridement, and fracture stabilization with internal fixation to optimize the environment for soft-tissue healing. Treatment for type I open fractures

Table 1 Osseous definitions	
Open fracture	Skin and soft-tissue wound that allows communication between the outside environment and the bone; also known as compound fracture
Comminuted fracture	Broken into multiple pieces
Greenstick fracture	A break in the convex cortex under tension caused by the bending of malleable bone
Torus fracture	A buckle in the concave cortex of malleable bone under compression; *Latin torus = buckle*
Epiphysis	End of long bone; secondary center of ossification; articular; separated from the rest of the bone by the physis
Metaphysis	Segment of bone between diaphysis and physis; most common site of infection
Diaphysis	Shaft of long bone; primary ossification center
Apophysis	Secondary center of ossification; site of insertion of muscle (eg, greater trochanter)
Condyle of bone	Paired articular swelling at the end of a long bone
Head of bone	Singular articular swelling at the end of a long bone

includes cleaning the wound, oral antibiotics, splinting, and referral to an orthopedic surgeon within 24 hours (**Table 3**).

Table 4 lists screening radiographic views for imaging of the skeleton. These radiographic views may be augmented by oblique views when a fracture is suspected (eg, based upon history, mechanism, severity of physical examination findings) or when there is a low tolerance for displacement (eg, in articular fractures [≤ 2 mm]).

The most frequent long bone fracture in a child involves the distal metaphysis of the radius; most of these are treated with a cast. The fracture in a child that is most frequently fixed operatively involves the supracondylar region of the humerus. Supracondylar humerus fracture may be associated with vascular injury and neural injury.

Neurovascular Injury

Vascular injury in the setting of a supracondylar humerus fracture may occur when there is sufficient displacement to require operative fixation. Physical examination findings include loss of palpable pulse at the wrist, loss of pulse on ultrasound testing at the wrist, and loss of perfusion of the hand. The majority of vascular injuries in supracondylar humerus fractures result from stretch of the brachial artery by the proximal fragment. Although this may lead to loss of pulse, measured either by palpation or ultrasound, the vascular net around the elbow allows for collateral flow distal to the fracture. As a result, loss of pulse is not an emergency as long as the hand is acceptably perfused, which is defined as warm and pink with less than 2 second capillary refill. A fracture with an acceptably perfused hand may be splinted in place and referred the next office day for evaluation and management by an orthopedic surgeon. A fracture associated with a dysvascular hand, defined as cool, blue, greater than 2 mm capillary refill, is an emergency that must be addressed within 6 hours of injury. The treatment of all such fractures is reduction and internal fixation by the orthopedic surgeon. There is no role for preoperative diagnostic arteriography.[6]

Neural injury occurs in approximately 10% to 15% of supracondylar humerus fractures. Most frequently involved are median and radial nerves. The child is tested by

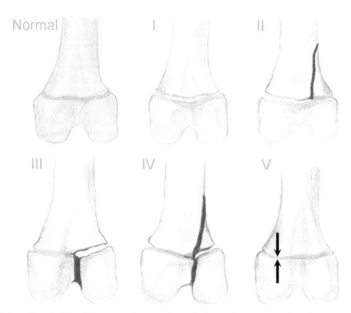

Fig. 1. Salter-Harris Classification. Illustration of the Salter-Harris classification of physeal fractures.* Normal: illustration of a normal pediatric distal femur. I: fracture through the physis. II: fracture through the physis that exits through the metaphysis. III: intra-articular fracture through the physis that exits through the epiphysis. IV: intra-articular fracture that involves the metaphysis and epiphysis, crossing the physis. V: crush injury to the physis. *Illustration by artist Joan R. Kaiser.

asking them to form the "OK sign" with the index and thumb (anterior interosseous branch of the median nerve) and the "thumbs up" sign (posterior interosseous branch of the radial nerve). The mechanism of this injury is stretched across the proximal fragment, and it represents neurapraxia and not nerve palsy. The usual outcome of such neurapraxias is full recovery that may take up to 6 months.[7–10] As a result,

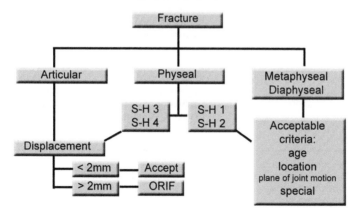

*S-H: Salter Harris classification
**ORIF: Open reduction internal fixation

Fig. 2. Fracture Algorithm. ORIF; open reduction internal fixation; S-H, Salter Harris classification.

Table 2
Pediatric fracture limits

Pediatric Fracture Limits[a]			
Bone	**Age**	**Angulation (°)**	**Translation**
Hand			
Phalanx	<10	25 apex dorsal/volar	Articular displacement <2 mm
Phalanx	>10	15 apex dorsal/volar	Articular displacement <2 mm
5th Metacarpal neck fracture (Boxer's or Brawler's)	All	30–40	
1st Metacarpal base (thumb)	All	30–40	
Wrist			
Distal radius physeal (Salter-Harris)	<10	30	2 mm articular; 50% displacment at physis in sagittal plane
Distal radius physeal (Salter-Harris)	>10	20	2 mm articular
Distal radius metaphyseal	<10	30 sagittal/20 coronal	Bayonette acceptable up to age 10 years
Distal radius metaphyseal	>10	20 sagittal	50% in coronal plane
Forearm			
Shaft	<10	30	Bayonette accepted
Shaft	>10	20	Bayonette accepted
Radial neck	All	30	30%
Humerus diaphysis	All	15–30 varus/valgus, 15–20 anterior/posterior	Bayonette accepted
Proximal humerus	<10	90	100%
Proximal humerus	>10	45	
Femur			
Femoral shaft	0–1[b]	30 varus/valgus, 30 anterior/posterior	2.5 cm shortening
Femoral shaft	1–5	15 varus/valgus, 20 anterior/posterior	2.5 cm shortening
Femoral shaft	>5[c]	minimal	minimal
Tibia			
Tibia diaphysis	<10	10 valgus, 10 varus, 10 anterior, 10 posterior.	10 mm shortening, evaluate subcutaneous border
Tibia diaphysis	>10	10 valgus, 10 varus, 10 anterior, 10 posterior.	5 mm shortening, evaluate subcutaneous border

[a] Authors' recommendations.
[b] Most deformity is accepted; these fractures are treated in a Pavlik harness with only the soft-tissue forces being corrective.
[c] All are treated surgically.

Table 3
Open fractures

Treatment of Open Fractures		
G/A Type	I	II, III
Wound Size	Small	Large
Mechanism	Inside out	Outside in
Agent	Bone	Foreign
Contamination	Clean	Dirty
Tetanus toxoid	YES	YES
Antibiotics	Oral	IV: cephalosporin, aminoglycoside
Irrigation	Local treatment	Operative I & D
Fixation	Immobilize	ORIF

Abbreviations: G/A, Gustillo Anderson classification; I & D, irrigation and debridement; ORIF, open reduction and internal fixation.

supracondylar humerus fracture with nerve out is not an emergency. The fracture may be referred the next office day and is treated by the orthopedic surgeon according to fracture principles uninfluenced by the neural status. Ulnar nerve injury is most often iatrogenic, from insertion of a medial distal humerus fixation wire at operation. Even in such cases, recovery is universal after removal of the wire.

FRACTURE: COMPARTMENTAL SYNDROME

In the steady state of limb perfusion, arterial inflow equals venous outflow (**Fig. 3**). In compartmental syndrome, this equilibrium is lost. Muscles, nerves, and vessels that

Table 4
Appropriate initial radiologic studies[a]

Proximal humerus	AP glenohumeral joint (Grashey) Axillary lateral
Humeral shaft fracture	AP/lateral humerus
Supracondylar humerus	AP/lateral distal humerus
Lateral condyle fracture	AP/lateral/two 45 degree obliques distal humerus
Proximal radius fracture	AP/lateral elbow Radiocapitellar view
Forearm fracture	AP/lateral forearm
Wrist fracture	AP/lateral wrist (clenched and unclenched fist)
Scaphoid fracture	AP/lateral/oblique hand or wrist Scaphoid view
Proximal femur fracture/SCFE	AP pelvis Frog leg or cross-table lateral hip
Femoral shaft	AP/lateral femur
Acute knee injury	AP/lateral/notch/Merchant knee
Tibial shaft	AP/lateral tibia
Ankle fracture	AP/lateral/mortise ankle
Foot fracture	Weight bearing AP/lateral/oblique foot

[a] Fracture-specific radiographs are listed only. In general, the joint immediately above and below the fracture should also be imaged (eg, the elbow and wrist should also be imaged in a forearm fracture). If injury or displacement is unclear, imaging the contralateral side may be of use.
Abbreviation: AP, anteroposterior.

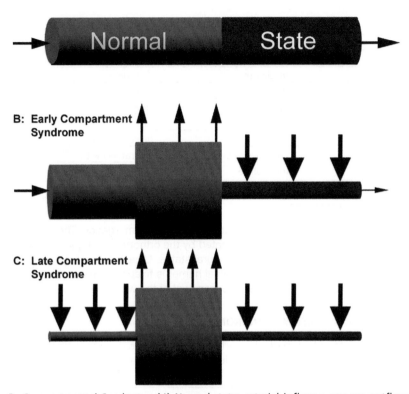

Fig. 3. Compartmental Syndrome. (*A*) Normal state: arterial inflow = venous outflow. (*B*) Early compartment syndrome: increase in compartment pressure decreases venous outflow. Arterial inflow preserved/augmented by inflammatory cascade and increased vascular permeability. Symptoms/signs: pressure (tense limb), pain (out of proportion). (*C*) Late compartment syndrome: decreased venous outflow leads to rapid increase in pressure, arterial flow compromised = ISCHEMIA. Symptoms/signs: paresthesias, lack of pulse, pallor.

course through the extremity do so within inelastic fascial membranes. Ischemia results when pressure in these compartments increases to become greater than the perfusion pressure. The forearm (especially after supracondylar humerus fracture) and leg (after tibia fracture) are most commonly affected.

Compartmental syndrome is characterized by the following sequence.[11] In the setting of the fracture, increased arterial inflow and hemorrhage from the ends of the fracture fragments cause increased pressure within the compartment. Increased pressure leads to compression followed by occlusion of venous outflow, which further increases compartmental and intra-arterial pressure. Increased intra-arterial pressure increases hemorrhage. When the intra-compartmental pressure approaches the arterial pressure, arterial inflow decreases and ischemia results. Transition to anaerobic metabolism in the setting of ischemia leads to the buildup of lactic acid, loss of the osmolar gradient, and leaky capillary membranes, which leads to a cascade of neutrophil activation, free-radical generation, and intravascular coagulation.[12] The result is a feedback loop that progresses to muscle necrosis.

The physical examination findings in compartmental syndrome are a tense limb and pain, and when advanced, paresthesias, lack of pulse, polar (coolness), and pallor. Pain is the most sensitive sign and is characteristically severe, out of proportion to the injury, and refractory to routine analgesia. Pain with passive stretch of a tendon that runs through the compartment is most suggestive of compartment syndrome.

A tense limb with firm compartments on palpation is worrisome for compartmental syndrome. Invasive pressure measurement can be a useful adjunct to clinical examination, with an intra-compartmental pressure greater than 30 mmHg and a calculated difference between the diastolic blood pressure and intra-compartmental pressure less than 30 mmHg both suggestive of compartment syndrome with sensitivity of greater than 80%.[13–15]

Pressure and pain are associated with venous obstruction, although the latter three (paresthesias, lack of pulse, and pallor) are characteristic of arterial insufficiency. Intervention initiated after onset of paresthesias, lack of pulse, or pallor may be too late to avoid permanent muscular necrosis, with its attendant loss of function and risk of infection. Plaster cast univalving can reduce compartment pressure by 40% to 60% and release of the underlying padding may reduce pressure by an additional 10%.[16] When external restrictive pressure generators are removed and compartment pressures remain unacceptable, surgical fasciotomy to allow dissipation of pressure becomes necessary. For full recovery from muscular injury, fasciotomy must be instituted within 6 hours of onset. In adults, intervention after 36 hours is not recommended; muscle recovery is sufficiently unlikely to be outweighed by a high risk for infection caused by exposure of dead tissue.

Compartmental syndrome in children differs from that in adults. Physical examination findings can be milder and children can be more difficult to examine and may not be able to describe their pain as clearly as adults. This difficulty can result in delayed diagnosis, so the level of suspicion should remain high.

BONE AND JOINT INFECTION

Joints may be divided into axial, including hip and shoulder, or appendicular, including elbow, wrist, knee, and ankle. Appendicular joints are distinguished by being visible and palpable, making them easier to access for aspiration and easier to follow for response to treatment. The knee is the most frequently infected pediatric joint. Pyarthritis of the hip is known to have the most severe consequences.

Appendicular infections often present with swelling, erythema, tenderness, and decreased joint range of motion. This decreased range of motion is often caused by swelling and splinting by patients. Axial infections are more difficult to diagnose clinically, and therefore supplemental tests are often necessary. One study that reviewed children diagnosed with either transient synovitis or septic arthritis of the hip found four predictive criteria for septic arthritis. These criteria were fever greater than 38.5°C, inability to bear weight on the affected limb, leukocyte count greater than 12,000/mm³, and erythrocyte sedimentation rate greater than 40 mm/h. The predicted probability of septic hip arthritis in these subjects was approximately 10% for one predictor, approximately 35% for two, approximately 73% for three, and approximately 93% for four.[17] In addition, C-reactive protein less than 1 mg/dL has an 87% negative predictive value,[18] and a repeat visit to the doctor may have positive predictive value.[19] The neonate may not demonstrate the same immune response to infection, so these criteria should be applied cautiously to this population.

Axial joint infection is treated with incision, drainage, irrigation and débridement. This treatment may be performed emergently if the child is systemically in distress or to avoid destruction of articular cartilage. Multiple studies have shown the destructive action of bacterial infection on articular cartilage. Poor prognosis has been associated with a delay in diagnosis/treatment greater than 4 days.[20] Children who have an unclear diagnosis of joint infection may be brought back within 4 days for a repeat assessment and surgical treatment, if necessary, without significant long-term consequence.

For appendicular joints, aspiration is central to diagnosis and treatment. Aspiration provides fluid for analysis, including cell count, Gram stain, culture and sensitivity, and crystals, and may be sufficient treatment when supplemented with antibiotics.[21] The following is an ideal sequence:

1. Joint aspiration in the emergency department, which is often the best setting for such a procedure in children
2. Admission to hospital for intravenous antibiotics
3. Immobilization of the joint
4. Modification of antibiotics according to culture and sensitivity analysis
5. Ensuring clinical response, including defervescence greater than 24 hours and reduced pain with improved range of motion
6. Ensuring laboratory response, including C-reactive protein less than 2 mg/dL
7. Discharge to home on oral antibiotics
8. Cessation of antibiotics when erythrocyte sedimentation rate is less than 20 mm/hr

In this sequence, the typical duration of intravenous antibiotics is less than 1 week, and the overall antibiotic course is less than the traditional 6 weeks.

Bone infections may be divided into those that are with and without change seen on radiograph. In the absence of radiographic change, the bone infection may be treated in the same manner as an appendicular joint infection, beginning with aspiration when the infected bone is accessible. Accessibility is associated with the following: metaphyseal location (the most common site) where the cortex is thin; hyperemia that softens bone; or the presence of periosteal abscess that obviates the need to penetrate the bone. Correct location for needle insertion may be determined by point of maximal tenderness, overlying erythema, and a mini fluoroscope to locate the nearest metaphysis.

Radiographic change requires greater than or equal to 50% bone loss. In addition, a "hole in bone" appearance represents an intraosseous abscess that is walled off by a sclerotic margin (known by the Latin involucrum, "wrapper"), and that may contain a central fragment of necrotic bone (known by the Latin sequestrum, "isolated thing"). The involucrum and sequestrum are impenetrable by antibiotics. This fact, together with extent of bone loss, make surgical intervention for débridement essential when there is radiographic change. After adequate surgical treatment, which may require multiple débridements, treatment resembles that for bone infection without radiographic change.

A bone or joint infection is only an emergency if children manifest signs of systemic infection (eg, cutaneous flushing, hypotension). Pyarthritis is regarded as urgent and is treated ideally within 6 hours with evacuation, either by way of a needle or incision. However, gray-zone presentations may be observed and reassessed within 4 days of onset without significant clinical sequela. Osteomyelitis with radiographic change will need operation and may wait until evaluation by an orthopedic surgeon within a week. Osteomyelitis without radiographic change should not be treated with antibiotics (unless patients are in distress) until an osseous specimen is obtained.

LIMPING CHILD

Disturbance of gait producing a limp may result from pain, weakness, neuromuscular imbalance, or deformity. An understanding of the gait cycle, a careful history, thorough physical examination, appropriate radiographic imaging, and laboratory studies can help the emergency physician greatly narrow the possible diagnoses causing the limp.

Gait may be divided into a swing phase, during which the referenced limb is off the ground, and a stance phase, which may be further divided into heel strike, flat foot, and push off. An antalgic gait is defined by a shortened stance phase, which in the extreme is manifested by a refusal to walk. A common theme in hip deformities that produce a limp is a Trendelenburg gait. This gait results from a shift of the body over the affected hip to reduce the momentum exerted on weak abductor muscles, which aids them in maintaining a horizontal pelvis during stance phase. In milder deformities, the gait may be apparent only after several cycles and may give way to pain as the hip abductors increasingly fatigue. This type of pain may be distinguished by its more lateral location, where the hip abductors are attached to the ilium and greater trochanter. By contrast, pain in articular hip disorders is typically referred anteriorly in the region of the groin and less frequently in the anteromedial thigh and knee. This obeys the law of Hilton, which states that a nerve supplying a muscle that acts upon a joint will supply the given joint and the skin over the distal attachment of the given muscle.[22] In the hip, the obturator and femoral nerves supply motor innervation to the adductors and rectus femoris respectively, and sensory innervation of the hip joint and the anteromedial thigh.

During physical examination the child should be undressed fully and the resting position of the limbs should be noted. The examination should be performed in supine and prone positions. The supine position may show hip obligate lateral rotation with flexion as seen in hip pyarthritis or SCFE. The prone position has the distinct advantage of allowing uncoupling of the knee from the hip, in which the pathology of one may masquerade as the other. In the prone position, the knee may be ranged from extension to flexion without moving the hip. In the supine position, moving the knee requires flexion of the hip, making it difficult at times to tell which joint is the offender. In addition, as in examination for torsion, the prone position allows simultaneous comparison of hip rotation (especially medial), which is the most sensitive to disease. Finally, the prone position can reveal a hip flexion contracture that may be concealed by lumbar hyperlordosis.

Studies of the limping child show that the cause is not always identified; no definitive diagnosis is made in up to 30% of cases.[23]

Most Common Cause: Transient Synovitis

Although the cause remains uncertain, transient synovitis may be thought of as a reactive arthritis that affects the hip. Often there is a history of antecedent infection and the condition occurs most frequently in the infant or young child. Transient synovitis is characterized by an antalgic gait, normal temperature to low fever, reduced range of motion of the hip, and normal to mildly elevated serologic markers of inflammation. Ultrasound shows a non-echogenic effusion. Treatment consists of symptomatic care, including activity modification and nonsteroidal antiinflammatory agents. In the majority of patients, symptoms and signs resolve over 1 week without sequelae.

Transient synovitis is a diagnosis of exclusion and must be distinguished from hip pyarthritis (*vide supra*). Typically in transient synovitis, patients do not appear to be systemically ill, are able to walk, motion of the hip is supple in the mid range while restricted at the extremes, and improvement begins within 72 hour. Temperature less than 37.5°C and a erythrocyte sedimentation rate less than 40 mm/hr may be used to help exclude pyarthritis.[24] It is essential to recognize that these distinctions are guidelines; the two disorders present on a continuum and may overlap. Where doubt exists, ultrasound-guided or fluoroscopically-guided diagnostic aspiration of the hip with fluid analysis for white blood cell count and bacterial staining and culture should be performed.

Discitis

Discitis represents infection of the metaphysis of the body of a vertebra that manifests in the intervertebral disk. It presents as a triad of pain, fever, and reduced intervertebral disk height on spinal radiograph. Pain in the infant typically manifests as refusal to walk; the child may complain of vague abdominal pain and often it is not until adolescence that the process can be localized to the back. Access to the intervertebral disk occurs through vascular channels that traverse the ring epiphyses in the immature skeleton.

The radiographic signs of discitis, intervertebral disk space narrowing and osseous erosion of the endplates, may be absent up to 2 to 6 weeks after the onset of symptoms.[25] In cases of clinical suspicion with negative radiographs, technetium bone scan can confirm the diagnosis and increased uptake can be seen as early as 7 days after symptom onset.[25] MRI can also assist in the diagnosis, but should usually be reserved for patients who have negative radiographs and bone scans, and for patients whose clinical course has not responded to antibiotics. Discitis may be diagnosed and treated before and without radiographic change.

The most common offending organism is *Staphylococcus aureus*. Biopsy is usually not performed because the cultures are often negative. Patients should be started on antistaphylococcal intravenous antibiotic therapy empirically and are typically transitioned to oral therapy with clinical resolution. Bracing is controversial.

Slipped Capital Femoral Epiphysis (SCFE)

SCFE is the second most commonly missed time-sensitive pediatric orthopedic problem, secondary to fracture, with frequent delays in diagnosis and treatment.[26] The disorder is characterized by disruption of the proximal femoral physis. The metaphysis displaces anteriorly and superiorly relative to the epiphysis, which remains tethered in the acetabulum by the ligamentum teres. SCFE is often likened to an ice cream scoop (epiphysis) falling off its cone.

Boys are affected more often than girls, and black and Hispanic children are affected more frequently than white children.[27] The diagnosis usually correlates with the rapid growth spurt of puberty. The average age of diagnosis is 11.2 years in girls and 12.7 years in boys, and the age at onset is declining.[27] SCFE is often associated with obesity; over half of these patients are above the 95th percentile for weight.[28]

Bilateral SCFE is common, and approximately 50% of the cases of bilateral SCFE present with simultaneous bilateral involvement.[29] If the diagnosis is suspected, both hips should be imaged. The risk of contralateral involvement is 2335 times higher in patients with the diagnosis of a unilateral slip than those who have not had a slip.[30]

There is an increased incidence of SCFE in patients who have endocrinopathies, such as hypothyroidism, hypogonadism, and growth hormone therapy.[28] Most children who have SCFE do not have a diagnosed endocrinopathy, but because of the high prevalence of a common somatotype (eg, obese, male, hypogonadal, pubescent), many think that these children have a subtle underlying endocrine disorder.[28]

Adolescents typically present with pain and a limp. Approximately 85% complain primarily of hip, groin, or proximal thigh pain, but 15% have mostly knee or distal thigh pain.[31] Patients who present with primarily knee pain are more likely to receive a misdi-agnosis and to have slips of greater severity.[31] The vast majority of patients will report symptoms lasting weeks to months, or even years.

On examination, patients who are ambulatory will have an antalgic or Trendelenburg gait, and the affected extremity may appear externally rotated and short. There is a loss of hip range of motion, especially internal rotation, but also flexion and abduc-tion. On hip flexion, there is an obligate external rotation of the hip because the proximal metaphysis abuts and slides along the anterior acetabular rim.

The diagnosis can usually be made with anteroposterior (AP) and frog-leg lateral pelvis radiographs. The frog-leg lateral film demonstrates subtle displacement more clearly than the standard AP pelvis. The physis will appear widened and blunted, and in cases of chronic SCFE, may show signs of remodeling. Klein's line, drawn along the anterosuperior aspect of the femoral neck on the AP radiograph, should intersect the epiphysis in the normal hip.[32] This line is tangential to or distant from the slipped epiphysis (**Fig. 4**). In cases of high clinical suspicion and negative radiographs, the diagnosis of a pre-slip can be made with bone scintigraphy.

There are three characteristics of SCFE that are especially useful to the orthopedic consultant:

Chronicity: symptoms for less than 3 weeks are described as acute and greater than 3 weeks as chronic.

Stability: a patient who is able to walk on a SCFE has a stable condition, whereas if they are unable, it is described as an unstable condition.

Severity: this refers to the angle subtended by the capital epiphysis and shaft of the femur, and is described as mild when this is less than 30°, moderate between 30° to 60°, and severe when greater than 60°.

Complications of SCFE, notably osteonecrosis of the head of the femur and chon-drolysis (loss of articular cartilage) of the hip-joint (defined as joint width ≤2 mm), are associated with acute, unstable, and severe presentations.[33]

Treatment in the emergency setting is removal of weight bearing from the affected limb. Although crutches may achieve this goal, a wheel chair in an over-weight and noncompliant teenager may be safer, with consultation with an orthopedic surgeon in less than 8 hours.

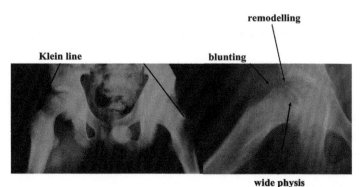

Fig. 4. Radiographic signs of SCFE.

NON-ACCIDENTAL TRAUMA

Child abuse has an unacceptably high rate of morbidity and mortality; 35% of children who are returned to their environment without intervention will be reinjured and 5% will die of abuse.[34] Thirty percent of physically abused children will require orthopedic treatment.[35]

The US Department of Health and Human Services reported that approximately 794,000 children were victims of abuse in 2007.[36] The following are risk factors for non-accidental trauma: **Box 2**

- Young age: children younger than 4 years make up 30% of total child abuse victims and 75% of the fatalities.[36]
- Single parent: this increases risk of child abuse by 77% compared with two-parent homes.[37]
- Low economic status: annual family income less than $15,000 increases risk for abuse by 22 times compared with income greater than $30,000.[37]
- Comorbidity: nearly 50% of non-accidental trauma victims older than 3 years have psychiatric or neurologic conditions.[38]

Whether race correlates with a difference in maltreatment is debatable.[36,37] There is no significant gender difference.[36]

The most frequent physical manifestation of child abuse is soft-tissue injury (>90%).[39] It is therefore imperative that the child be undressed fully for an inspection of the skin in its entirety. Although a characteristic lesion may indicate the method or instrument used (eg, iron mark, cigarette burn, scalded/dipped baby), most soft-tissue injuries are in an unremarkable pattern. The incidence of musculoskeletal injury in non-accidental trauma correlates with age. Eighty percent of fractures in abused children occur before 18 months of age; by contrast, 85% of accidental fractures occur after 5 years of age.[40]

High-risk fracture patterns are listed in **Table 5**. The diaphysis of a long bone is the most common site of fracture in physical abuse.[41] Approximately 80% of femur fractures in children younger than 2 years are associated with abuse.[42] A humeral diaphysis fracture before 3 years of age represents non-accidental trauma until proven otherwise.[40,43] In contrast to diaphyseal humerus fracture, supracondylar humerus fracture is the most frequent indication for operative fixation of a fracture in a child. Associated features that increase the significance of diaphyseal fractures are exuberant callus caused by inadequate immobilization, multiple fractures and fractures in various stages of healing, inappropriate clinical history, and delay in seeking medical attention.[35,43]

Metaphyseal-epiphyseal fractures of the distal femur, tibia, and proximal humerus usually heal with no consequence but are highly clinically relevant for their association

---

Box 2 **Risk factors for abuse**
Risk Factors:
Young age
Single-parent home
Income <$15,000
Neurologic/Psychiatric condition

Table 5
Characteristic injuries of non-accidental trauma

Most Common	Suspicious
Soft-tissue injury	Metaphyseal-epiphyseal fractures: corner fracture bucket handle fracture
—	Distal humerus transphyseal fracture
—	Femur fracture in child before walking
—	Humerus diaphyseal fracture in child <3y
—	Rib fractures, especially posterior
—	Fractures in various states of healing

with abuse. Children evaluated with these fractures should be evaluated for shaking injuries, such as head trauma. Because of indirect force (eg, shaking), the periosteum avulses the immature bone near the physis in a planar fashion, resulting in the radiologic finding of a corner fracture or bucket handle fracture (**Fig. 5**).[44] In contrast, accidental trauma usually produces metaphyseal fractures that are closer to the diaphysis, such as in a Salter-Harris type II fracture or torus fracture.

Other fractures that should cause a high level of suspicion are posterior rib fractures and scapula fractures. The mobility of the ribs makes them difficult to break accidentally. Their posterior aspect is struck directly as the child flees. The scapula is a dense, flat bone embedded in muscle on all sides, and the energy required to fracture it is high and rarely occurs with everyday childhood trauma.

The principal morbid entity in the differential diagnosis of non-accidental fracture is osteogenesis imperfecta. This may be distinguished by

- Osseous quality (eg, gracility, osteopenia, global deformation)
- Presence of wormian bones, which represent multiple non-coalesced centers of ossification in the skull
- Family history
- Blue sclera, caused by thinning and translucency exposing the subjacent choroid
- Short stature
- Possible associated broken and yellow-brown teeth, caused by fragility of the dentin
- Possible associated hearing loss

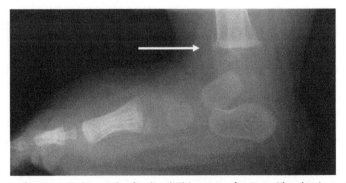

Fig. 5. Corner fracture. Radiograph of a distal tibia corner fracture. The classic metaphyseal-epiphyseal injury can be seen clearly in this radiograph.

Abused children continue to be inadequately treated. Physeal-metaphyseal fractures can have a mild clinical presentation, characterized by less pain and less displacement than other fracture patterns.[43] Up to 90% of children who have clinical evidence of abuse do not receive radiographs.[39] A radiographic skeletal survey should be performed in all children younger than 3 years in whom abuse is suspected:

- AP imaging of the appendicular skeleton: femur, tibia-fibula, foot, humerus, radius-ulna, and hand
- AP and lateral imaging of the axial skeleton: spine, chest, and skull
- A survey 10 to14 days after the initial evaluation may reveal occult fracture based upon periosteal new bone formation.[45]

Every family must be evaluated equally, regardless of socioeconomic status, appearance, or other biasing trait. Evaluation is multidisciplinary, including physician, social worker, nurse, mental health professional, and a representative from Child Protective Services.[46] Document every aspect of the presentation fully; approximately 40% of charts do not contain adequate information to determine the cause of fracture in children.[47] If there is uncertainty, admit patients.

SUMMARY

Pediatric fractures, compartment syndrome, limp, infection, SCFE, and non-accidental trauma can all be a challenge to diagnose and treat for the emergency room physician and orthopedic surgeon. Missed diagnoses and mismanagement of these conditions can have disastrous consequences for patients and family members. A high level of awareness and the proper diagnosis are the first steps in management. With the described treatment algorithms in this review article, physicians can better avoid the associated pitfalls of these urgent orthopedic conditions.

ACKNOWLEDGMENTS

Illustrations by Joan R. Kaiser.

REFERENCES

1. Salter RB, Harris WR. Injuries involving the epiphyseal plate. J Bone Joint Surg Am 1963;45:587–622.
2. Knirk JL, Jupiter JB. Intra-articular fractures of the distal end of the radius in young adults. J Bone Joint Surg Am 1986;68(5):647–59.
3. Skaggs DL, Friend L, Alman B, et al. The effect of surgical delay on acute infection following 554 open fractures in children. J Bone Joint Surg Am 2005;87(1): 8–12.
4. Gustilo RB, Anderson JT. Prevention of infection in the treatment of one thousand and twenty-five open fractures of long bones: retrospective and prospective analyses. J Bone Joint Surg Am 1976;58:453–8.
5. Gustilo RB, Mendoza RM, Williams DN. Problems in the management of type III (severe) open fractures: a new classification of type III open fractures. J Trauma 1984;24:742–6.
6. Shaw BA, Kasser JR, Emans JB, et al. Management of vascular injuries in displaced supracondylar humerus fractures without arteriography. J Orthop Trauma 1990;4(1):25–9.
7. Cramer KE, Green NE, Devito DP. Incidence of anterior interosseous nerve palsy in supracondylar humerus fractures in children. J Pediatr Orthop 1993;13(4):502–5.

8. Campbell CC, Walters PM, Millis MB. Neurovascular injury and displacement in type III supracondylar humerus fractures. J Pediatr Orthop 1995;15:47–52.

9. Culp RW, Osterman AL, Davidson RS, et al. Neural injuries associated with supracondylar fractures of the humerus in children. J Bone Joint Surg Am 1990;72(8): 1211–5.

10. Dormans JP, Squillante R, Sharf H. Acute neurovascular complications with supracondylar humerus fractures in children. J Hand Surg Am 1995;20(1):1–4.

11. Matsen FA III, Hargens AR. Compartment syndromes and Volkmann's contracture. Philadelphia: WB Saunders; 1981.

12. Matsson-Hultén L, Holmström M, Soussi B. Harmful singlet oxygen can be helpful. Free Radic Biol Med 1999;27:1203–7.

13. Janzing HM, Broos PL. Routine monitoring of compartment pressure in patients with tibial fractures: beware of overtreatment!. Injury 2001;32(5):415–21.

14. Heppenstall RB, Sapega AA, Scott R, et al. The compartment syndrome. An experimental and clinical study of muscular energy metabolism using phosphorus nuclear magnetic resonance spectroscopy. Clin Orthop Relat Res 1998; 226:138–55.

15. Matsen FA 3rd, Winquist RA, Krugmire RB Jr. Diagnosis and management of compartmental syndromes. J Bone Joint Surg Am 1980;62(2):286–91.

16. Halanski M, Noonan KJ. Cast and splint immobilization: complications. J Am Acad Orthop Surg 2008;16(1):30–40.

17. Kocher MS, Mandiga R, Zurakowski D, et al. Validation of a clinical prediction rule for the differentiation between septic arthritis and transient synovitis of the hip in children. J Bone Joint Surg Am 2004;86(8):1629–35.

18. Levine MJ, McGuire KJ, McGowan KL, et al. Assessment of the test characteristics of C-reactive protein for septic arthritis in children. J Pediatr Orthop 2003;23: 373–7.

19. Luhmann SJ, Jones A, Schootman M, et al. Differentiation between septic arthritis and transient synovitis of the hip in children with clinical prediction algorithms. J Bone Joint Surg Am 2004;86:956–62.

20. Choi IH, Pizzutillo PD, Bowen JR, et al. Sequelae and reconstruction after septic arthritis of the hip in infants. J Bone Joint Surg Am 1990;72:1150–65.

21. Herndon WA, Knauer S, Sullivan JA, et al. Management of septic arthritis in children. J Pediatr Orthop 1986;6:576–8.

22. Hilton J. On rest and pain: a course of lectures on the influence of mechanical and physiological rest in the treatment of accidents and surgical diseases, and the diagnostic value of pain. In: Jacobson WHA, editor. Lectures delivered at the Royal College of Surgeons of England 1860–1862. New York: William Wood and Company; 1879. p. 191–210.

23. Fischer SU, Beattie TF. The limping child: epidemiology, assessment and outcome. J Bone Joint Surg Br 1999;81:1029–34.

24. Del Beccaro MA, Champoux AN, Bockers T, et al. Septic arthritis versus transient synovitis of the hip: the value of screening laboratory tests. Ann Emerg Med 1992; 21:1418–22.

25. Szalay EA, Green NE, Heller RM, et al. Magnetic resonance imaging in the diagnosis of childhood discitis. J Pediatr Orthop 1987;7(2):164–7.

26. Skaggs DL, Roy AK, Vitale MG, et al. Quality of evaluation and management of children requiring timely orthopaedic surgery before admission to a tertiary pediatric facility. J Pediatr Orthop 2002;22:265–7.

27. Lehmann CL, Arons RR, Loder RT, et al. The epidemiology of slipped capital femoral epiphysis: an update. J Pediatr Orthop 2006;26(3):286–90.

28. Aronsson DD, Loder RT, Breur GJ, et al. Slipped capital femoral epiphysis: current concepts. J Am Acad Orthop Surg 2006;14:666–79.
29. Loder RT, Aronson DD, Greenfield ML. The epidemiology of bilateral slipped capital femoral epiphysis. A study of children in Michigan. J Bone Joint Surg Am 1993;75:1141–7.
30. Schultz WR, Weinstein JN, Weinstein SL, et al. Prophylactic pinning of the contralateral hip in slipped capital femoral epiphysis: evaluation of long-term outcome for the contralateral hip with use of decision analysis. J Bone Joint Surg Am 2002; 84:1305–14.
31. Matava MJ, Patton CM, Luhmann S, et al. Knee pain as the initial symptom of slipped capital femoral epiphysis: an analysis of initial presentation and treatment. J Pediatr Orthop 1999;19(4):455–60.
32. Klein A, Joplin RJ, Reidy JA, et al. Slipped capital femoral epiphysis: early diagnosis and treatment facilitated by "normal" roentgenograms. J Bone Joint Surg Am 1952;34:233–9.
33. Loder RT, Richards BS, Shapiro PS, et al. Acute slipped capital femoral epiphysis: the importance of physeal stability. J Bone Joint Surg Am 1993;75:1134–40.
34. Schmitt B, Clemmens M. Battered child syndrome. In: Touloukin R, editor. Pediatric trauma. St Louis (MO): Mosby-Year Book; 1990. p. 161–87.
35. Akbarnia B, Torg JS, Kirkpatrick J, et al. Manifestations of the battered-child syndrome. J Bone Joint Surg Am 1974;56:1159–66.
36. US Department of Health and Human Services. Child maltreatment 2007. Available at: http://www.acf.hhs.gov/programs/cb/pubs/cm07/cm07.pdf. Accessed May 10, 2009
37. Sedlak AJ, Broadhurst DD. Executive summary of the third national incidence study of child abuse and neglect. US Department of Health and Human Services. Available at: http://www.childwelfare.gov/pubs/statsinfo/nis3.cfm. Accessed May 10, 2009.
38. Loder RT, Feinberg JR. Orthopaedic injuries in children with nonaccidental trauma. J Pediatr Orthop 2007;27(4):421–6.
39. McMahon P, Grossman W, Gaffney M, et al. Soft-tissue injury as an indication of child abuse. J Bone Joint Surg Am 1995;77:1179–83.
40. Worlock P, Stower M, Barbor P. Patterns of fractures in accidental and non-accidental injury in children: a comparative study. Br Med J (Clin Res Ed) 1986;293: 100–2.
41. Merten DF, Radowski MA, Leonidas JC. The abused child: a radiological reappraisal. Radiology 1983;146:377–81.
42. Anderson WA. The significance of femoral fractures in children. Ann Emerg Med 1982;11(4):174–7.
43. Carty HM. Fractures caused by child abuse. J Bone Joint Surg Br 1993;75: 849–57.
44. Kleinman PK. Diagnostic imaging in infant abuse. AJR Am J Roentgenol 1990; 155(4):703–12.
45. Kleinman PK, Nimkin K, Spevak MR, et al. Follow-up skeletal surveys in suspected child abuse. AJR Am J Roentgenol 1996;167(4):893–6.
46. McDonald KC. Child abuse: approach and management. Am Fam Physician 2007;75(2):221–8.
47. Oral R, Blum KL, Johnson C. Fractures in young children: are physicians in the emergency department and orthopedic clinics adequately screening for possible abuse? Pediatr Emerg Care 2003;19(3):148–53.

Pitfalls in Appendicitis

Robert J. Vissers, MD[a,b,*], William B. Lennarz, MD[c,d]

KEYWORDS

- Appendicitis • CT • Abdominal pain • Ultrasound
- Appendectomy • Pediatrics

Appendicitis, first characterized in 1886 by the pathologist Reginald Fitz, remains one of the most common causes of abdominal pain presenting to the emergency department. More than 250,000 cases of appendicitis are diagnosed in the United States each year, and appendectomy is the most frequent emergent surgery performed worldwide. The lifetime risk for appendicitis is slightly higher for men than for women (8.6% and 6.7%, respectively). In emergency patients with acute abdominal pain less than a week in duration, the incidence of appendicitis varies from 12% to 28%, and although the incidence peaks in the second and third decades of life, it can occur at any age. Despite its prevalence, the diagnosis of appendicitis can be elusive and fraught with pitfalls because of the absence of a pathognomonic sign or symptom, the poor predictive value of associated laboratory testing, and its varied presentation.[1,2] Although there have been significant advances in imaging accuracy, appendicitis remains a high-risk disease for delayed or missed diagnosis in the emergency department.

The overall mortality rate for appendicitis is less than 1%, but it increases to 3% if the appendix is ruptured and approaches 15% in the elderly.[3] The diagnosis of appendicitis is more difficult in the extremely young and the elderly, resulting in a higher incidence of delayed diagnosis and rupture in these populations. Most children aged less than 4 years have an already ruptured appendix at the time of diagnosis. Because a ruptured appendix can be associated with increased morbidity and mortality, it is felt that a certain number of negative laparotomies is acceptable (approximately 15% in the United States). However, negative laparotomies are twice as common in young women as in men (20% vs 9%, respectively).[4,5]

---

[a] Department of Emergency Medicine, Legacy Emanuel Hospital, 2801 North Gantenbein Avenue, Portland, OR 97227, USA
[b] Department of Emergency Medicine, Oregon Health Sciences University, USA
[c] Pediatric Emergency Medicine, Legacy Health System, Legacy Emanuel Hospital, 2801 North Gantenbein Avenue, Portland, OR 97227, USA
[d] Legacy Health Pediatric Emergency Medicine Fellowship, Oregon Health and Science University, USA
* Corresponding author.
E-mail address: rvissers@comcast.net (R.J. Vissers).

Emerg Med Clin N Am 28 (2010) 103–118
doi:10.1016/j.emc.2009.09.003
0733-8627/09/$ – see front matter

PATHOPHYSIOLOGY

The common process in the development of acute appendicitis is the luminal obstruction of the appendix. The cause of obstruction varies with age. In children, lymphoid hyperplasia, possibly exacerbated by infection and dehydration, is thought to be the primary cause. In adults, fecaliths are a more frequent cause, and neoplasm can cause obstruction in the elderly. Once obstructed, the appendix becomes inflamed, ischemic, and necrotic. Bacterial overgrowth occurs and eventually leads to gangrenous and perforated appendicitis. Most patients experience inflammation only in the first 24 hours, whereas patients with perforation typically have symptoms for more than 48 hours.[6]

MEDICAL LEGAL RISK

Because of its atypical presentation, appendicitis has been described as being a particular risk for misdiagnosis and subsequent litigation.[7] Appendicitis is the leading cause of litigation against emergency physicians in the case of patients with abdominal pain and one of the leading causes overall. In a review of closed malpractice claims involving mistaken or delayed diagnoses, appendicitis was the sixth most common missed diagnosis.[8] In children aged between 6 and 17 years, appendicitis is the second most common cause of malpractice lawsuits against emergency physicians.[9] Common features in cases of missed diagnosis of appendicitis leading to litigation include lack of distress, no rebound or guarding on examination, a discharge diagnosis of gastroenteritis, and lack of timely follow-up.

DIAGNOSIS

The gold standard for the diagnosis of appendicitis is pathologic confirmation after appendectomy. However, to balance an acceptable positive laparotomy rate with minimal delayed or missed diagnoses, the clinician must take into account all the available historical and physical findings, laboratory data, and appropriate imaging. There is no single sign, symptom, or laboratory test to reliably identify or exclude appendicitis. A positive radiographic result can be helpful, but may also be costly, time intensive, and potentially associated with unwanted radiation or contrast exposure. Even the best studies are imperfect. To optimize the diagnostic accuracy in acute appendicitis, the clinician must be familiar with the limitations and pitfalls associated with each sign, symptom, and laboratory or imaging study.

History and Physical Exam

No individual sign or symptom can be relied on to diagnose or exclude appendicitis. Rather, the clinician must rely on cumulative features of the history and physical examination to try to increase or decrease the posttest probability of possible appendicitis. It is important to understand the relative importance of specific signs and symptoms, best expressed as the associated likelihood ratio (LR), that represent the increased likelihood of the disease being present if the result is positive, or conversely, absent if the result is negative. A common pitfall is to include or exclude the diagnosis because of 1 sign or symptom.

The finding of right lower quadrant pain seems to be the most useful clinical sign in possible appendicitis (LR, 7.31–8.46).[3,10] The absence of right lower quadrant pain makes the diagnosis less likely. Pain migration to the right lower quadrant and pain preceding vomiting may increase the possibility of appendicitis (**Table 1**). In other meta-analyses, pain migration was found to be less clinically significant.[11] The

Table 1
LRs for specific symptoms in appendicitis

Historical Symptom	Positive LR	Increase in Posttest Probability	Negative LR
RLQ pain	7.31–8.46	Moderate probability	0–0.28
Migration	3.18	Small increase	0.50
Pain before vomiting	2.76	Small increase	—
No past similar pain	1.50	Not helpful	0.323
Anorexia	1.27	Not helpful	0.64
Nausea	0.69–1.20	Not helpful	0.70–0.84
Vomiting	0.92	Not helpful	1.12

LR of 5–10, presence moderately increases probability of disease.
LR of 2–5, may increase probability of the disease.
LR of <2, not likely to change the probability of the disease.
Abbreviation: RLQ, right lower quadrant.
Data from Wagner JM, McKinney WP, Carpenter JL. Does this patient have appendicitis? JAMA 1996;276(19):1589–94; and Yeh B. Does this adult patient have appendicitis? Ann Emerg Med 2008;52:301–3.

presence or absence of anorexia is not likely to be clinically significant and should not influence the clinicians' diagnosis of appendicitis. The historical features of nausea, vomiting, or the absence of prior pain are also not useful in making the diagnosis of appendicitis. However, the presence of a similar prior pain may reduce the probability of appendicitis.

Similar to the symptoms, no single physical finding is clinically significant enough to definitively make or exclude the diagnosis of appendicitis.[10] When present, the physical signs of rigidity, right lower quadrant tenderness, the psoas sign, and rebound tenderness may slightly increase the probability of appendicitis (**Table 2**). The presence or absence of fever does not significantly change the probability of appendicitis. It is not unusual for patients with appendicitis to be afebrile; however, this also reflects the poor specificity associated with the finding of fever. Guarding and rectal

Table 2
LRs for specific signs in appendicitis

Physical Sign	Positive LR	Increase in Posttest Probability	Negative LR
Rigidity	3.76	Small increase	0.82
Tender RLQ	2.30	Small increase	0.0–0.1
Psoas sign	2.38	Small increase	0.90
Rebound tenderness	3.70	Small increase	0.43
Fever	1.94	Not helpful	0.58
Guarding	1.65–1.78	Not helpful	0.27
Rectal tenderness	0.83–5.34	Not helpful	0.76

LR of 5–10, presence moderately increases probability of disease.
LR of 2–5, may increase probability of the disease.
LR of less than 2, not likely to change the probability of the disease.
Abbreviation: RLQ, right lower quadrant.
Data from Refs.[3,11,19]

tenderness are not clinically significant. The absence of right lower quadrant tenderness reduces the likelihood of appendicitis.

Localization of pain to the right lower quadrant, or McBurney point, is secondary to the inflammation progressing to the overlying parietal peritoneum. However, an abnormal location of the appendix may alter the localization of the pain. A retrocecal appendix may not cause peritoneal inflammation and can present with milder, less-localized pain. A pelvic appendix may cause tenderness below the McBurney point and can be associated with urinary symptoms or tenesmus and diarrhea. The obturator sign, pain with internal rotation of the hip, may suggest a pelvic appendix. Pain with extension of the hip, the iliopsoas sign, suggests a retrocecal appendicitis.

Laboratory Tests

There is no laboratory test specific for appendicitis. Although the white blood cell (WBC) count is usually obtained, it is not a reliable independent predictor of appendicitis. This is consistent with several studies, which have found a relatively unimpressive positive LR between 1.59 and 2.7 and a negative ratio between 0.25 and 0.50 for the WBC count in appendicitis.[11–14] Repeating WBC counts is not beneficial. A significantly elevated WBC count does not preclude the diagnosis of appendicitis but does suggest that rupture may be present.

A urinalysis is usually obtained to rule out possible urinary tract infection. However, the urinalysis can also represent a potential pitfall, because the proximate location of the appendix to the ureter and bladder can cause microscopic pyuria or hematuria in up to a third of patients with appendicitis. A beta-human chorionic gonadotropin is helpful in excluding pregnancy-related conditions, such as ectopic pregnancy, but pregnancy does not exclude the possibility of appendicitis (see discussion later in the article).

C-reactive protein alone also demonstrates poor specificity; however, when combined with a WBC count, it may be more useful. In one study, C-reactive protein alone had a LR of 4.24 but when combined with an elevated WBC count, the positive LR of the combination was a significant 23.32.[11] Other studies have found a high negative predictive value when the combination of the WBC count, C-reactive protein, and the neutrophil count were normal.[15] Similar results were obtained when phospholipase A2 was combined with the white cell count and C-reactive protein; however, large prospective studies are lacking.[16]

Scoring Systems

There are several scoring systems that have been created in an attempt to improve the clinical accuracy of the diagnosis of appendicitis by attaching an aggregate value to specific signs, symptoms, and laboratory results. The most common is the Alvarado score, also known as the MANTRELS (Migration of pain, Anorexia, Nausea/vomiting, Tenderness in the right lower quadrant, Rebound tenderness, Elevated temperature, Leukocytosis, Shift to the left).[17] There are several variants, some specifically designed for pediatrics, which exclude the WBC count or replace rebound tenderness with pain on coughing or hopping. None have shown increased accuracy. The Ohmann score uses a combination of clinical variables and the WBC count to predict appendicitis in adults and in children older than 6 years.[18] In a prospective validation study, the Ohmann score was able to identify patients at low, moderate, and high risk for appendicitis. None of the scoring systems are accurate enough to reliably predict appendicitis, but they have been described as a useful tool to decide on further management, such as observation, imaging, or direct surgical intervention.[19–22]

Imaging

In the past decade, imaging has been increasingly used for suspected appendicitis and has a significant added benefit to clinical assessment alone.[23–25] Although indirect signs of appendicitis may be found on plain abdominal radiographs, they no longer have a role in the diagnosis of appendicitis because of their poor sensitivity and specificity. Ultrasound can be helpful in possible appendicitis, particularly in children, pregnant women, and women of childbearing age. However, computed tomography (CT) has a greater accuracy than ultrasound and has seen a dramatic increase in use. Despite its widespread use, associated cost, time delay, and exposure to contrast and radiation need to be considered. The optimal role for CT in suspected appendicitis is currently in debate.

CT

Many studies, including a meta-analysis, have demonstrated the superiority of CT over ultrasound in appendicitis.[26] Although the specificity was similar between CT and ultrasound (94% and 93%, respectively), the sensitivity was better for CT (94% vs 83%) and therefore, the overall accuracy. CT has a demonstrated accuracy of 92% to 97% and positive LRs ranging from 11 to 96 for the diagnosis of appendicitis.[27–29]

The CT findings suggestive of appendicitis include an appendix greater than 6 mm; wall thickening; right lower quadrant inflammatory changes, such as fat stranding; and the presence of appendicoliths.[25]

It remains unclear which type of CT study (with or without contrast) is best in suspected appendicitis. The type of contrast to be used (intravenous [IV], oral, rectal, or some combination thereof) further complicates the question. A systematic review of 23 studies of CT in suspected appendicitis found a weighted sensitivity and specificity of 93% and 98%, respectively, for noncontrast CT compared with CT with IV and oral contrast (93% and 93%) and CT with rectal contrast (97% and 97%).[29] The addition of oral contrast did not improve the diagnostic accuracy of CT in appendicitis. The described advantage of oral contrast is the ability to better differentiate the appendix from surrounding structures. IV contrast highlights inflammation of the appendix and surrounding tissues.[30] The addition of oral and IV contrast likely increases the ability to identify other conditions that may be causing abdominal pain. But there are disadvantages with oral contrast, including the significant time delay associated with administration and bowel transit, the challenge of oral contrast in someone with nausea and vomiting, and the possible increased risk of aspiration in surgery. IV contrast can cause serious allergic reactions and renal toxicity. In the only prospective randomized study that compared 3 different techniques, CT with oral and IV contrast, CT with rectal contrast, and CT without contrast, CT with oral and IV contrast was more sensitive than CT with rectal contrast and not significantly different from noncontrast CT.[31]

It is uncertain if there is any advantage to the addition of IV or enteric contrast in CT for suspected appendicitis. If there is an advantage, it is likely small and unlikely to outweigh the real disadvantages. Therefore, noncontrast CT may be the best strategy if appendicitis is the diagnosis in question. If the differential is broad and other pathology suspected, the addition of oral contrast should be considered. In thin patients who lack the periappendiceal fat and the associated fat stranding useful in identifying appendicitis, IV contrast may be helpful in highlighting the inflammation.

There also exists some debate over who benefits the most from CT in suspected appendicitis. In some centers, the use of CT in the diagnosis of appendicitis has resulted in a reduction in the negative appendectomy rate to 3%, with no increase in the rate of perforation.[23] However, several studies have challenged the benefit of routine use of CT in suspected appendicitis.[32,33] In the landmark article by Rao and colleagues,[25] which first demonstrated the diagnostic and financial benefit of CT in appendicitis, CT was used selectively. Newer articles have argued that routine CT offers no advantage in patients with a high probability of appendicitis based on clinical assessment and, in some cases, may lead to unnecessary delay and costs.[34]

As with most diagnostic studies, CT is most beneficial in patients in whom the clinical diagnosis of appendicitis remains equivocal. There are also populations, such as the very young and the elderly, that are associated with a reduced clinical accuracy and are therefore more likely to benefit from the addition of CT. The extremes of age are also associated with a much higher rate of ruptured appendix on presentation.[35] One study reported a decrease in the rate of ruptured appendicitis from 72% to 51% with the earlier use of CT in an elderly population.[36] Children also seem to benefit from a reduced negative appendectomy and perforation rate with the use of CT. However, the risks of radiation exposure are also higher in this population. Appendicitis in pediatrics and the elderly is discussed in detail later in the article. Women of childbearing age is another group that seems to benefit from preoperative imaging, both CT and ultrasound.[37] This may be secondary to the additional gynecologic conditions that can mimic appendicitis and reduce the clinical accuracy in this population. When perforation is suspected, CT can be helpful because the optimal management of these patients may initially be nonoperative.[38]

There is increasing concern over the potential link between the ionizing radiation of diagnostic radiographic procedures, such as CT, and an associated increased lifetime risk of cancer. There are no prospective studies proving a causal link, but results have been extrapolated from the increased risk of atomic bomb survivors. A lifetime risk of cancer attributable to an abdominal and pelvic CT has been estimated to be 0.14% in infants and 0.06% in adults.[39] Although the degree of risk is in debate, it is clear that children are at higher risk because of their higher sensitivity to radiation and more subsequent years to develop cancer.[40] In most cases, the known improvement in diagnostic accuracy and subsequent reduction in negative appendectomies and perforations outweigh the possible risks of radiation. However, in situations in which the risk is higher (children, pregnant women, women of childbearing age), alternative diagnostic strategies should be considered. Unfortunately, these groups of patients are those in whom clinical accuracy is reduced. This concern has led to the common strategy, in these patients, of first using ultrasound and then considering CT or observation if the ultrasound is nondiagnostic.

There are also several strategies that can be used to reduce the radiation dose in CT. Although the benefit of a medically indicated CT far outweighs the potential risks, the use of CT must be justified for the specific task and the examination should be performed using doses that are as low as reasonably achievable.[41] The guiding principle of radiation reduction in CT is making the dose specific to the size of the patient and the diagnostic task. The particular techniques are beyond the scope of discussion here; however, it is important to be aware that these strategies exist and are not always optimized. Future advances, such as better size-based adjustments and iterative reconstruction, promise similar-quality images at lower radiation exposure.

Ultrasound

Ultrasound represents a noninvasive, noncontrast imaging option that avoids the exposure to nonionizing radiation and can be less expensive than CT. Findings suggestive of appendicitis include a thickened wall, a noncompressible lumen, diameter greater than 6 mm, absence of gas in the lumen, and appendicoliths. The most sensitive sign seems to be a compressed appendix that exceeds 6 mm in diameter (up to 98% sensitive), although some centers use 7 mm to improve their specificity.[13,42] As described earlier, ultrasound is inferior to CT in sensitivity and its negative predictive value for appendicitis and may not be as useful for excluding appendicitis.[43,44] This is particularly true if the appendix was never visualized. False negatives are also more likely in patients with a ruptured appendix, and inconclusive studies are more common in obese patients and in those with significant bowel gas.[13,45] The specificity of a positive ultrasound approaches that of CT and its associated positive LRs, which usually exceed 10, particularly in pediatric studies. This threshold suggests that a positive result should be enough to support the diagnosis and the decision to operate based on the ultrasound findings.

The quality of the ultrasound examination improves with operator experience and skill, and accuracy also improves when the patient can self-localize the area of maximal tenderness.[42,46,47] Doppler examination of the appendix has been a useful adjunct to improve the sensitivity by demonstrating increased flow in an inflamed appendix.[48] But the flow diminishes in advanced necrosis and rupture. It is clear that an inflamed appendix is usually easier to identify.

If available, ultrasound may be best used as an initial study in pediatric patients, women of childbearing age, and pregnant patients when appendicitis is suspected. In women, ultrasound may be useful in identifying gynecologic causes of the pain. Depending on the preexisting clinical suspicion, a negative study should be followed by CT or close observation.

Magnetic resonance

Magnetic resonance (MR) imaging has a limited role in the diagnosis of appendicitis. Although MR avoids any ionizing radiation and is deemed to be safe in pregnancy, it is more costly, time consuming, and of limited availability in most emergent settings. Also, gadolinium contrast may be used, which should be avoided in the first trimester of pregnancy. Although studies with MR are limited, they suggest that MR may be superior to ultrasound in its sensitivity for appendicitis.[49] One study showed that MR is superior to ultrasound in pregnant patients, and some centers have advocated using MR when the ultrasound in a pregnant patient is equivocal.[50]

MANAGEMENT AND DISPOSITION

Since its first description, the treatment of choice for appendicitis has been emergent appendectomy. In a unique study published in 1995, patients were randomized to antibiotics for 10 days or to appendectomy.[51] Although initially 95% of the antibiotic-only group were successfully treated without surgery, 35% later returned with rupture or phlegmon.

Patients with suspected appendicitis should be kept without oral food and fluids and be adequately hydrated. Antibiotics appropriate for surgical wound prophylaxis should be initiated preoperatively once the diagnosis has been made and are usually not continued postoperatively in uncomplicated appendicitis. There is some debate in the surgical literature whether appendectomy is best done by laparoscopy or traditional open technique.[52–54] Although some studies have shown no difference, it appears that laparoscopy may be associated with less postoperative pain and shorter hospital stays.[53–57] The laparoscopic approach may be advantageous in patients in whom the diagnosis is uncertain. If a ruptured appendix is identified preoperatively, broader spectrum antibiotics are started. Antibiotics should cover enteric gram-negative bacteria and anaerobes, such as a second or third generation cephalosporin or a fluoroquinolone and metronidazole for 7 to 10 days. The preferred management seems to be image-guided percutaneous drainage, continued antibiotics, and then an interval appendectomy performed at a later date. Immediate appendectomy may result in higher complication rates and a longer duration of stay.[38,58]

Ultimately, it is the decision of the surgeon regarding the timing and technique of appendectomy. It is the emergency physicians' judgment when to involve the surgeon. If appendicitis or rupture is diagnosed by imaging, surgical consultation is suggested, based on the high likelihood of disease. Not all patients require imaging to diagnose appendicitis. For patients in whom the clinical and laboratory findings suggest a high likelihood of appendicitis and alternative diagnoses are less likely, surgical consultation and operative appendectomy without imaging remains a reasonable option that can avoid unwanted delays and unnecessary testing. If patients have moderate to high likelihood of appendicitis and if there is debate over the benefit of imaging versus direct operative intervention, an early surgical opinion is also prudent.

In patients with suspected appendicitis but a broad differential, and in whom the relative risk of CT is low, CT imaging is suggested. This is particularly true in elderly patients or in cases in which a ruptured appendix is suspected. However, in some patients with suspected appendicitis, the diagnosis remains equivocal and the radiation from CT scan is less desirable (children, pregnant women, women of childbearing age). Ultrasound should be considered as the first imaging choice. If positive, surgical consultation is indicated. If the ultrasound is negative or nondiagnostic, further management may depend on the pretest likelihood of appendicitis and the quality of the ultrasound study. In low-risk patients in whom a normal appendix is visualized by an experienced operator, observation or recheck in 12 to 24 hours may be reasonable. If appendicitis is still suspected but a normal appendix is not seen, surgical consultation and possible CT imaging are suggested.

Despite the improved accuracy of imaging, false negatives occur and missed appendicitis continues to be a part of emergency practice. Therefore, even in patients with an alternative diagnosis, such as gastroenteritis or urinary tract infection, it should be emphasized that appendicitis could still be present. Any patient discharged should be cautioned about this, and a recheck in 12 to 24 hours in any patient for whom a diagnosis of appendicitis was entertained is suggested.

APPENDICITIS IN THE VERY YOUNG PATIENT

Although appendicitis is most common in the second decade of life, it occurs in all pediatric age groups. Five percent of all appendicitis occurs in children younger than 5 years. It even occurs in neonates. In children younger than 2 years, the appendix has more of a funnel or tapered morphology that, theoretically, may make it less prone to obstruction by reactive lymphoid tissue and ensuing focal infection. Childhood rates of appendicitis (and diagnostic accuracy) increase with age, whereas rates of rupture decrease at higher ages. Neonatal appendicitis has a high mortality rate. Nearly 100% of children younger than 3 years who have appendicitis are diagnosed after perforation.[59] Appendicitis is the most common surgical emergency in children, yet missed appendicitis is the second most frequent reason for medical malpractice suits in pediatric emergency medicine, only behind missed meningitis.

The diagnosis of appendicitis in young children may be considerably more challenging than in teenagers and young adults for several reasons. First, children in this age group may be preverbal and developmentally unable to accurately communicate typical historical features. Even verbal children may lack the abstract thinking needed to answer questions needed to shape the diagnostic impression, such as duration and migration over time of the pain. In addition, children may feel intimidated by the emergency department environment and therefore be less communicative and cooperative with the examination, a feature especially common in toddlers with stranger anxiety. Preschool-aged children often answer "yes" to all questions in an effort to please the adult questioner. Thus, parents have to be relied on to provide the history, and they may not be able to describe the nuances of the pain and of its development (that is needed for diagnosis) as clearly as when the patient can describe the pain himself or herself. Developmentally disabled children, who are often cared for in large numbers at pediatric referral centers, may be unable to provide verbal history at any age.

Children may also be more stoic and less verbal and/or demonstrative about their pain. Because pain is the most consistent symptom of appendicitis, this behavior complicates diagnosis. "Quiet, still, withdrawn" is often the manifestation of severe pain in a toddler or infant. Emergency department staff inexperienced in pediatrics may misinterpret this silent withdrawal as evidence of the lack of pain. Because of this, physicians often underestimate and undertreat pain in children.

The presentation of appendicitis in very young children and infants differs from that in older children and young adults. Appendicitis has earned the description of "the great masquerader," and this is especially true in young children. The signs and symptoms of appendicitis in infants, toddlers, and early school-aged children typically differ from the presentation in older children and often evolve as the disease progresses. The signs and symptoms of appendicitis also overlap with other common pediatric presentations such as gastroenteritis and constipation. One study quantified the most common initial misdiagnoses of children who ended up having acute appendicitis.[60] These diagnoses are gastroenteritis, abdominal pain, pharyngitis, otitis, sepsis, urinary tract infection, and febrile seizure.

Diagnosis in Children

Mark Twain once said that a "classic is something everyone talks about and no one reads." The same can be said for classic appendicitis, which seldom, if ever, occurs in very young children. Unlike the classic signs and symptoms of appendicitis in adults, various studies have shown the following in children[61–63]:

- No migration of pain in greater than 50% of children
- No anorexia in greater than 50% of children
- No focal tenderness elicitable in greater than 50% of children
- No demonstrable rebound tenderness in greater than 50% of children
- Reported time course of pain less than 24 hours is common

Thus, it is helpful to consider pediatric appendicitis presentation by age group.

In infancy, fever, vomiting, and abdominal distention are prominent and should be carefully evaluated. Irritability, lethargy, and grunting respirations may also indicate appendicitis. Abdominal tenderness is commonly diffuse rather than focal.

In toddlers, fever and vomiting are again most common and may precede pain. Pain may seem intermittent, which may also suggest intussusception. Right hip pain and/or limp have been reported in many cases of appendicitis in this age group. Abdominal tenderness may be either focal or generalized.

In school-aged children, abdominal pain and vomiting are common. Pain with walking or movement is highly specific. Fever is common, and abdominal wall tenderness tends to occur focally in the right lower quadrant. Involuntary guarding is often present and is quite sensitive for appendicitis.

In general, across the entire age spectrum of young children, fever, right lower quadrant pain, and pain with walking (or limp) are highly sensitive indicators for appendicitis. Right lower quadrant tenderness and guarding or rebound tenderness are the most highly sensitive physical findings. Abdominal distention is also a physical finding that is highly specific for appendicitis.[61]

Laboratory studies in children

Laboratory studies may be less useful in young children than in adults. A WBC count of less than 10,000/μL moderately decreases the likelihood of appendicitis (negative LR, 0.22), but elevation of WBC count to more than 10,000/μL only minimally increases the likelihood (positive LR, 2.0). Raising the WBC count cutoff to more than 15,000/μL is not helpful.[62–64] Similarly, C-reactive protein testing does not provide consistently useful negative or positive LRs. Urinalysis should be performed for all children with suspected appendicitis. Pyuria is reported in a significant number of adults with appendicitis but may be even more prevalent in children with appendicitis (approximately 30%). Several scoring systems have attempted to combine signs, symptoms, and laboratory findings to improve diagnostic accuracy in appendicitis. One study evaluated the Alvarado and Samuel appendicitis scoring systems in a prospective cohort.[65] Neither system demonstrated useful positive or negative LRs to significantly affect management.

The 3 most common imaging modalities have significant limitations and risks in directing the important decision on whether to perform an appendectomy on a child.

Plain radiographs are insensitive and nonspecific for appendicitis. In few patients with appendicitis, plain films will reveal an appendicolith and/or right lower quadrant focal ileus, which are suggestive but not diagnostic findings. If diffuse peritonitis is present and there is concern for bowel perforation, then plain radiographs may provide more rapid information than waiting for a CT scan. However, generally, plain radiographs are not recommended for the diagnosis of appendicitis.

Ultrasonography has great potential in its application for diagnosis of appendicitis in children. Most children are thin (relative to adults), and therefore, superior imaging may be obtained. A specific technique of graded compressions is used, and positive findings are the same as described for adults. Although specificity of ultrasonography is high, sensitivity is highly operator dependent and even in the hands of attending-level radiologists, is reported to range from 73% to 98%.[66,67] Diagnostic accuracy may be improved when the radiologist performs the graded compression directly instead of reading static images taken during a study performed by a technician. Ultrasound cannot visualize the appendix in 30% to 50% of children with a normal appendix and in more than 10% of children with appendicitis. Sensitivity is lower in cases of perforation. The most significant advantage of ultrasound as a diagnostic modality for appendicitis is its safety; ultrasound requires neither contrast nor ionizing radiation.

CT is highly specific and sensitive, with reports of 90% to 100% for both parameters.[68,69] CT can also identify alternative diagnoses in more than 80% of children with normal appendices. There are no studies that directly address the value of oral or IV contrast in pediatric abdominal CT, and the data have been extrapolated from the adult literature.

Unfortunately, abdominal CT scanning delivers ionizing radiation. Children are at higher risk for malignancy because of their more rapidly dividing cells, their proportionately greater solid organ exposure, and their proportionately greater radiation exposure for the same study. Based on the radiation dose, the science of ionizing radiation risk extrapolated from Hiroshima and Nagasaki, and current mortalities for various cancers, Brenner and Hall[39] have predicted more than a 1 in 1000 risk of fatal malignancy resulting from the typical radiation of an abdominal CT in early childhood. This should give any clinician a reason to pause before ordering abdominal CT for any reason.

As a result of this information about the implications of CT imaging, the authors recommend the following approach:

1. In patients who have a strong clinical indication of appendicitis based on history and examination, consider laparoscopy and appendectomy based on history and examination (after laboratory evaluation that includes urinalysis) alone.
2. In cases where an imaging modality is necessary, use ultrasound first.
3. Reserve CT for specialized scenarios, including:
   a. suspected perforation or
   b. intra-abdominal abscess or
   c. indeterminate ultrasonographic assessment (in the patient without high clinical suspicion)

In addition, emergency medicine leadership should advocate increased institutional ultrasound competency and availability at all hours. It is essential to confirm that the radiology department has implemented CT scanner protocols using reduced ionizing radiation for infants and children.

Another group of pediatric patients that warrant special consideration in the evaluation of appendicitis is adolescent girls. The differential of right lower quadrant pain and tenderness in pubertal and postpubertal girls includes ovarian cyst, ovarian torsion, pregnancy, and ectopic pregnancy. A urine pregnancy test should be performed on all female patients with abdominal pain who have entered puberty. Because ultrasound is particularly helpful in the diagnosis of ovarian pathology, pelvic ultrasound is usually the first choice of imaging modalities in adolescent girls, pregnant or not. In cases of right lower quadrant pain and tenderness in postpubertal girls, difficulties in distinguishing ovarian pathology from appendicitis may lead to a higher rate of laparotomy.

APPENDICITIS IN PREGNANT PATIENT

The incidence, pathophysiology, and management of appendicitis is similar to the nonpregnant patient and is the most common reason for nonobstetric surgery in pregnancy.[70] The location of the appendix during pregnancy has been described as rising in the abdominal cavity as pregnancy progresses, changing the location of symptoms. However, some studies suggest that this traditional belief may be overstated and that the location is similar to nonpregnant patients.[71,72] Regardless, the most common presenting symptom of appendicitis in pregnancy is still pain in the right lower quadrant.[70] Leukocytosis may be secondary to pregnancy. However, an increase in band cells suggests that an infection is present. Physical signs or peritonitis may be delayed because of the enlarged uterus. Delay in diagnosis is a common cause of morbidity in this population. Unruptured appendectomy is associated with a fetal loss rate of 3% to 5%. Ruptured appendicitis is associated with a fetal loss rate of 20% to 25% and maternal mortality rate of 4%.[73]

If appendicitis is suspected but clinical findings are not definitive, imaging should not be delayed in the pregnant patient. Ultrasound is often obtained first because there is no associated ionizing radiation. In some studies, ultrasound had an accuracy approaching CT; however, the study is technically more difficult and dependent upon the habitus of the patient and the experience of the radiologist.[74] A positive test is considered diagnostic, but a negative test is less reliable at excluding appendicitis and should be followed by observation or imaging with CT. A ruptured appendix is not well visualized by ultrasound, and beyond 35 weeks gestation, ultrasound is less useful because graded compression technique is not easily performed.[75] When ultrasound is not available or is nondiagnostic, CT is the study of choice for the diagnosis of appendicitis. MRI has been used in pregnant patients with suspected appendicitis, but the studies are too small to draw conclusions about its relative accuracy.[76,77] Laparoscopy is as safe as laparotomy for appendectomy in pregnancy.

APPENDICITIS IN THE GERIATRIC PATIENT

The diagnosis of appendicitis in the elderly is particularly challenging. Although appendicitis is often considered rare in the elderly, it still accounts for 7% of abdominal pain in the elderly seeking emergency evaluation. The elderly are more likely to present atypically and delay seeking medical evaluation.[36] Diagnosis is further obscured by a much broader differential and the increased likelihood of comorbidities or immunosuppression. These factors may explain the significantly higher perforation rate of up to 72%.[36,78] This population may benefit in particular from the use of CT imaging because the differential is broad, the incidence of rupture is much higher, and the risk of ionizing radiation is much lower. In one study, the ruptured appendicitis rate dropped from 72% to 51% with the use of CT imaging. Because the differential is broad, this population may benefit more from the addition of oral and, possibly, IV contrast. Appendectomy remains the treatment of choice in elderly patients with unruptured appendicitis, either by laparoscopy or traditional open technique.[79]

SUMMARY

The diagnosis of appendicitis is fraught with potential pitfalls, and despite its prevalence, appendicitis continues to be a high risk for missed and delayed diagnosis. There is no one historical or physical finding or laboratory test that can make the definitive identification of appendicitis. However, with a clear understanding of their relative strengths, a combination of findings can increase the likelihood of disease diagnosis and help guide further management, and the clinician can avoid the pitfall of ascribing too much significance to the presence or absence of 1 finding. Imaging has played an important role in increasing the diagnostic accuracy in appendicitis. Ultrasound is an excellent first study in some populations, such as children and pregnant patients. Although ultrasound is helpful when positive, it is not as reliable at excluding appendicitis or identifying rupture. CT is very accurate and can often identify alternative causes for abdominal pain. It appears that for most cases a noncontrast CT is sufficient. Because of its expense, potential delay, and ionizing radiation, CT is not always indicated in suspected appendicitis, and if appendicitis is very likely based on clinical impression, appendectomy without imaging remains an appropriate strategy. There are some populations, such as the elderly who may benefit more from routine imaging. Appendicitis continues to be a source of medical legal risk and misdiagnosis; however, a clear understanding of the strengths and limitations of all tests in suspected appendicitis can improve the diagnostic accuracy in this high-risk disease.

REFERENCES

1. Pittman-Waller VA, Myers JG, Stewart RM, et al. Appendicitis: why so complicated? Analysis of 5755 consecutive appendectomies. Am Surg 2006;66:548.
2. Addis DG, Shaffer N, Fowler BS, et al. The epidemiology of appendicitis and appendectomy in the United States. Am J Epidemiol 1990;132:910.
3. Yeh B. Does this adult patient have appendicitis? Ann Emerg Med 2008;52: 301–3.

 4. Velanovich V, Satava R. Balancing the normal appendectomy rate with the perfo-
    rated appendicitis rate. Am Surg 1992;52:264–9.
 5. Colson M, Skinner KA, Dunnington G. High negative appendectomy rates are no
    longer acceptable. Am J Surg 1997;174:723–7.
 6. Hale DA, Jaques DP, Molloy M, et al. Appendectomy: improving care through
    quality improvement. Arch Surg 1997;132:153–7.
 7. Rusnak RA, Borer J, Faston JS. Misdiagnosis of acute appendicitis in emergency
    department patients: an analysis of common error discovered after litigation. Am
    J Emerg Med 1991;20:503–7.
 8. Kachalia A, Gandhi TK, Puopolo AL, et al. Missed and delayed diagnoses in the
    emergency department: a study of closed malpractice claims from 4 liability
    insurers. Ann Emerg Med 2007;49:196–205.
 9. Selbst SM, Friedman MJ, Singh SB. Epidemiology and etiology of malpractice
    lawsuits involving children in US emergency departments and urgent care
    centers. Pediatr Emerg Care 2005;21:165–9.
10. Wagner JM, McKinney WP, Carpenter JL. Does this patient have appendicitis?
    JAMA 1996;276(19):1589–94.
11. Andersson RE. Meta-analysis of the clinical and laboratory diagnosis of appendi-
    citis. Br J Surg 2004;91:28–37.
12. Cardall T, Glasser J, Guss DA. Clinical value of the total white blood cell count
    and temperature in the evaluation of patients with suspected appendicitis.
    Acad Emerg Med 2004;11:1021–7.
13. Kessler N, Cyteval C, Gallix B, et al. Appendicitis: evaluation of sensitivity,
    specificity, and predictive values of US, Doppler US, and laboratory findings.
    Radiology 2004;230:472–8.
14. Birchley D. Patients with clinical acute appendicitis should have pre-operative full
    blood count and C-reactive protein assays. Ann R Coll Surg Engl 2006;88:27–32.
15. Dueholm S, Bagi P, Bud M. Laboratory aid in the diagnosis of acute appendicitis.
    Dis Colon Rectum 1989;32:855–9.
16. Gronroos JM, Gronroos P. Leukocyte count and C-reactive protein in the diag-
    nosis of acute appendicitis. Br J Surg 1999;86:501–4.
17. Alvarado A. A practical score for the early diagnosis of acute appendicitis. Ann
    Emerg Med 1986;15:557–64.
18. Ohmann C, Franke C, Yang Q, et al. Clinical benefit of a diagnostic score for appen-
    dicitis: results of a prospective interventional study. Arch Surg 1999;134:993–6.
19. Gwynn LK. The diagnosis of acute appendicitis: clinical assessment versus
    computed tomography evaluation. J Emerg Med 2001;21:119–23.
20. McKay R, Shepherd J. The use of the clinical scoring system by Alvarado in the
    decision to perform computed tomography for acute appendicitis in the ED. Am J
    Emerg Med 2007;25:489–93.
21. Chan MYP, Tan C, Chiu MT, et al. Alvarado score: an admission criterion in
    patients with right iliac fossa pain. Surg J R Coll Surg Edinb Irel 2003;1:
    39–41.
22. Yildirim E, Karagulle E, Kirbas I, et al. Alvarado scores and pain onset in relation
    to multislice CT findings in acute appendicitis. Diagn Interv Radiol 2008;14:14–8.
23. Rhea JT, Halpern EF, Ptak T, et al. The status of appendiceal CT in an urban
    medical center 5 years after its introduction: experience with 753 patients. AJR
    Am J Roentgenol 2005;184:1802–8.
24. Garcia Pena BM, Mandl KD, Kraus SJ, et al. Ultrasonography and limited
    computed tomography in the diagnosis and management of appendicitis in
    children. JAMA 1999;282(11):1041–6.

25. Rao PM, Rhea JT, Novelline RA, et al. Effect of computed tomography of the appendix on treatment of patients and use of hospital resources. N Engl J Med 1998;338:141–6.

26. Doria AS, Moineddin R, Kellenberger CJ, et al. US or CT for diagnosis of appendicitis in children and adults? A meta-analysis. Radiology 2006;241:83–94.

27. Lane MJ, Liu DM, Huynh MD, et al. Suspected acute appendicitis: nonenhanced helical CT in 300 consecutive patients. Radiology 1999;213:341–6.

28. Hershko DD, Sroka G, Bahouth H, et al. The role of selective computed tomography in the diagnosis and management of suspected acute appendicitis. Am Surg 2002;68:1003–7.

29. Anderson BA, Salem L, Flum DR. A systematic review of whether oral contrast is necessary for the computed tomography diagnosis of appendicitis in adults. Am J Surg 2005;190:474–8.

30. Jacobs JE, Birnbaum BA, Macari M, et al. Acute appendicitis: comparisons of helical CT diagnosis—focused technique with oral contrast material versus nonfocused technique with oral and intravenous contrast material. Radiology 2001; 220:683–90.

31. Hershko DD, Awad N, Fischer D, et al. Focused helical CT using rectal contrast material only as the preferred technique for the diagnosis of suspected acute appendicitis: a prospective, randomized, controlled study comparing three different techniques. Dis Colon Rectum 2007;50:1223–9.

32. Flum DR, Morris A, Koepsel T, et al. Has misdiagnosis of appendicitis decreased over time? A population-based analysis. JAMA 2001;286:1748–53.

33. Vadeboncoeur TF, Heister RR, Behling CA. Impact of helical computed tomography on the rate of negative appendicitis. Am J Emerg Med 2006;24:43–7.

34. Lee SL, Walsh AJ, Ho HS. Computed tomography and ultrasonography do not improve and may delay the diagnosis and treatment of acute appendicitis. Arch Surg 2001;135:556–62.

35. Korner H, Sondenaa K, Soreide JA, et al. Incidence of acute nonperforated and perforated appendicitis: age-specific and sex-specific analysis. World J Surg 1997;21:313–7.

36. Storm-Dickerson TL, Horattas MC. What have we learned over the past 20 years about appendicitis in the elderly. Am J Surg 2003;185:198–201.

37. Bendeck SE, Nino-Murcia M, Berry GJ, et al. Imaging for suspected acute appendicitis: negative appendectomy and perforation rates. Radiology 2002; 225:131–6.

38. Brown C, Abrishami M, Muller M, et al. Appendiceal abscess: immediate operation or percutaneous drainage? Am Surg 2003;69:829–33.

39. Brenner DJ, Hall EJ. Computed tomography—an increasing source of radiation exposure. N Engl J Med 2007;357:2277–84.

40. Brody AS, Frush DP, Huda W, et al. Radiation risk to children from computed tomography. Pediatrics 2007;120:677–82.

41. McCollough CH, Primak AN, Braun N, et al. Strategies for reducing radiation dose in CT. Radiol Clin North Am 2009;47:27–40.

42. Rettenbacher T, Hollerweger A, Macheiner P, et al. Outer diameter of the vermiform appendix as a sign of acute appendicitis: evaluation at US. Radiology 2001;218:757–62.

43. Balthazar EJ, Birnbaum BA, Yee J, et al. Acute appendicitis: CT and US correlation in 100 patients. Radiology 1994;190(1):31–5.

44. Terasawa T, Blackmore CC, Bent S, et al. Systematic review: computed tomography and ultrasonography to detect acute appendicitis in adults and adolescents. Ann Intern Med 2004;141:537–46.

45. Rettenbacher T, Hollerweger A, Macheiner P, et al. Ovoid shape of the vermiform appendix: a criterion to exclude acute appendicitis—evaluation with US. Radiology 2003;226:95–100.

46. Chesbrough RM, Burkhard TK, Balsara ZN, et al. Self-localization in US of appendicitis: an addition to graded compression. Radiology 1993;187:349–51.

47. Lee JH, Jeong YK, Park KB, et al. Operator-dependent techniques for graded compression sonography to detect the appendix and diagnose acute appendicitis. AJR Am J Roentgenol 2005;184:91–7.

48. Lim HK, Lee WJ, Kim TH, et al. Appendicitis: usefulness of color Doppler US. Radiology 1996;201:221–5.

49. Incesu L, Coskun A, Selcuk MB, et al. Acute appendicitis: MR imaging and sonographic correlation. AJR Am J Roentgenol 1997;168:669–74.

50. Cobben LP, Groot I, Haans L, et al. MRI for clinically suspected appendicitis during pregnancy. Am J Roentgenol 2004;183:671–5.

51. Erickson S, Granstrom L. Randomized controlled trial of appendectomy versus antibiotic therapy for acute appendicitis. Br J Surg 1995;82:166–9.

52. Chung RS, Rowland DY, Li P, et al. A meta-analysis of randomized controlled trials of laparoscopic versus conventional appendectomy. Am J Surg 1999;177:250–6.

53. Guller U, Hervey S, Purves H, et al. Laparoscopic versus open appendectomy. Outcomes comparison based on a large administrative database. Ann Surg 2004;239:43–52.

54. Martin LC, Puente I, Sosa JL, et al. Open vs laparoscopic appendectomy. A prospective randomized comparison. Ann Surg 1995;222:256–62.

55. Hellberg A, Rudberg C, Kullman E, et al. Prospective randomized multicenter study of laparoscopic versus open appendectomy. Br J Surg 1999;86:48–53.

56. Pedersen AG, Petersen OB, Wara P, et al. Randomized clinical trial of laparoscopic versus open appendectomy. Br J Surg 2001;88:200–5.

57. Marzouk M, Khater M, Elsadek M, et al. Laparoscopic vs open appendectomy. A prospective comparative study of 227 patients. Surg Endosc 2003;17:721–4.

58. Oliak D, Yamini D, Udani VM, et al. Initial nonoperative management for periappendiceal abscess. Dis Colon Rectum 2001;44:936–41.

59. Nelson DS, Bateman B, Bolte RG. Appendiceal perforation in children diagnosed in a pediatric emergency department. Pediatr Emerg Care 2000;16:233–7.

60. Rothrock SG, Skeoch G, Rush JJ, et al. Clinical features of misdiagnosed appendicitis. Ann Emerg Med 1991;20:45.

61. Bundy DG, Byerley JS, Liles EA, et al. Does this child have appendicitis. JAMA 2007;298:438.

62. Kwok MY, Kim MK, Gorelick MH. Evidence based approach to the diagnosis of appendicitis in children. Pediatr Emerg Care 2004;20:690.

63. Rothrock SG, Pagane J. Acute appendicitis in children: emergency department diagnosis and management. Ann Emerg Med 2000;36:39–51.

64. Wang LT, Prentiss KA, Simon JZ, et al. The use of white blood cell count and left shift in the diagnosis of appendicitis in children. Pediatr Emerg Care 2007;23:69.

65. Schneider C. Evaluating appendicitis scoring systems using a prospective pediatric cohort. Ann Emerg Med 2007;49:778–84.

66. Baldisserotto M, Marchiori E. Accuracy of noncompressive sonography of children with appendicitis according to the potential positions of the appendix. AJR Am J Roentgenol 2000;175:1387–92.

67. Kaiser S, Frenckner B, Jorulf HK. Suspected appendicitis in children: US and CT—a prospective randomized study. Radiology 2002;223:633–8.
68. Lowe LH, Penney MW, Stein SM, et al. Unenhanced limited CT of the abdomen in the diagnosis of appendicitis in children: comparison with sonography. AJR Am J Roentgenol 2001;176:31–5.
69. Sivit CJ, Applegate KE, Stallion A, et al. Imaging evaluation of suspected appendicitis in a pediatric population: effectiveness of sonography versus CT. AJR Am J Roentgenol 2000;175:977–80.
70. Mourad J, Elliot JP, Erikson L, et al. Appendicitis in pregnancy: new information that contradicts long-held clinical beliefs. Am J Obstet Gynecol 2000;182(5): 1027–9.
71. Oto A, Srinivisan PN, Ernst RD, et al. Revisiting MRI for appendix location during pregnancy. AJR Am J Roentgenol 2006;186(3):883–7.
72. Hodjati H, Kazerooni T. Location of the appendix in the gravid patient: a re-evaluation of the established concept. Int J Gynaecol Obstet 2003;81(3):245–7.
73. Kilpatrick CC, Monga M. Approach to the acute abdomen in pregnancy. Obstet Gynecol Clin North Am 2007;34:389–402.
74. Poortman P, Lohle PN, Schoemaker CM, et al. Comparison of CT and sonography in the diagnosis of acute appendicitis: a blinded prospective study. AJR Am J Roentgenol 2003;181(5):1355–9.
75. Lim HK, Bae SH, Seo GS. Diagnosis of acute appendicitis in pregnant women: value of sonography. AJR Am J Roentgenol 1992;159(3):539–42.
76. Pedrosa I, Levine D, Eyvazzadeh AD, et al. MR imaging evaluation of acute appendicitis in pregnancy. Radiology 2006;238(3):891–9.
77. Oto A, Ernst RD, Shah R, et al. Right-lower-quadrant pain and suspected appendicitis in pregnant women: evaluation with MR imaging-initial experience. Radiology 2005;234:445–51.
78. Hiu TT, Major KM, Avital I, et al. Outcome of elderly patients with appendicitis. Arch Surg 2002;137:995–1000.
79. Guller U, Jain N, Peterson ED, et al. Laparoscopic appendectomy in the elderly. Surgery 2004;135:479–88.

Pediatric Airway Nightmares

James D'Agostino, MD

KEYWORDS

• Pediatric airway • Airway obstruction • Croup
• Bacterial tracheitis

Pediatric disorders that involve actual or potential airway compromise are among the most challenging cases that emergency department providers face. This article discusses the diagnosis and management of common and uncommon conditions in infants and children who may present with airway obstruction.

UPPER AIRWAY OBSTRUCTIONS

Croup, or laryngotracheobronchitis, is the most common infectious cause of acute upper airway obstruction in children. Emergency physicians and pediatricians manage thousands of patients with this condition every year, commonly without radiographic evaluation. The general croup population benefits greatly from one oral dose of dexamethasone,[1] which seems as efficacious as an intramuscular dose,[2,3] and occasionally children need nebulized racemic epinephrine for persistent stridor or significantly increased work of breathing. Although croup is usually a benign and rapidly reversible condition, emergency providers must be aware of young children who present with stridor, increased work of breathing, and fever and who do not respond to croup management. The differential diagnosis for these children includes bacterial tracheitis, epiglottitis, retropharyngeal abscess, and structural lesions worsened by laryngotracheobronchitis. Airway burns may also cause rapidly progressive airway obstruction.

TRACHEITIS

Cases of bacterial tracheitis are most likely a complication of a preceding viral upper airway infection involving the trachea. Children often present with croup symptoms, such as cough, stridor, prolonged inspiratory phase breathing, retractions, and fever. Several key factors, however, differentiate young children with croup from those with bacterial tracheitis. Children with croup develop a croupy or bark-like cough soon followed by respiratory distress and stridor due to subglottic edema.

Department of Emergency Medicine, Pediatric Emergency Medicine, Upstate Medical University, 750 East Adams Street, Syracuse, NY 13210, USA
E-mail address: dagostinj@upstate.edu

Emerg Med Clin N Am 28 (2010) 119–126
doi:10.1016/j.emc.2009.09.005
0733-8627/09/$ – see front matter © 2010 Elsevier Inc. All rights reserved.

It is common for young children to be distressed at home and calm and free of stridor on presentation in an emergency department, possibly due to amelioration of the subglottic edema from a combination of the upright position and breathing cool night air on the ride to the hospital. In contrast, children with bacterial tracheitis universally present to emergency departments with stridor and fever. Common features are copious purulent sputum, high fever, and toxic appearance. Toxic-appearing children with croup-like symptoms who respond poorly to croup management should be evaluated for tracheitis.

Bacterial tracheitis is a secondary infection caused by *Staphylococcus aureus* or *Haemophilus influenzae* type b (usually in unvaccinated patients) in a trachea inflamed by an antecedent viral infection.[4] Bacterial tracheitis has features of croup and epiglottitis: stridor and croup-like coughing as in the former and high fever and toxic appearance as in the latter. Doses of dexamethasone and aerosolized racemic epinephrine, which have substantial efficacy in the symptomatic relief of stridor and respiratory distress in croup, have little to no effect in patients with tracheitis.[5,6] With the widespread use of dexamethasone for croup infections and *H influenzae* immunization, bacterial tracheitis has now eclipsed croup and epiglottitis as a cause of severe upper airway obstruction and respiratory failure requiring intubation.[5]

The management of tracheitis is airway control with intubation and intravenous (IV) antibiotic administration. Ear, nose, and throat (ENT) consultation is warranted because nearly all patients with bacterial tracheitis require tracheal intubation and, as in epiglottitis, intubation should be done in an operating suite under anesthesia. If a portable lateral neck radiograph is done in a patient with tracheitis, the epiglottis appears normal in size, and laryngoscopy and intubation confirm this finding. Copious purulent debris is found in the trachea during intubation. Every attempt at clearing the endotracheal tube of purulent material should be done via suction catheter to prevent complete obstruction. After patient stabilization and cultures of tracheal aspirate and blood are done, a broad-spectrum parenteral antibiotic, such as ceftriaxone, should immediately be started.[7] Antibiotic therapy and hospitalization may be required for up to 14 days.[4]

EPIGLOTTITIS

Over the past 20 years, there has been a dramatic decline in pediatric cases of epiglottitis. The *H influenzae* vaccine has practically eliminated invasive *H influenzae* infection, well known to have caused meningitis and epiglottitis in children under 4 years of age.[8,9] In a retrospective chart review, a large children's hospital noted a 10-fold decrease in the admission rates for pediatric epiglottitis over the past 27 years.[10] In a recent retrospective study, however, 10% of children presenting with epiglottitis were found to have invasive *H influenzae* type b infection, despite having being vaccinated.[7] These findings highlight the importance of considering acute epiglottitis in the differential diagnosis of all children presenting with upper airway obstruction. This is particularly relevant because fewer doctors today are familiar with the symptoms and signs of the disease.

Epiglottitis presents abruptly with high fever, toxicity, and significant upper airway obstruction with stridor, unlike tracheitis, which usually is preceded by a viral croup infection but can manifest as a primary infection.[11] Children with epiglottitis present in distress with muffled voices and without spontaneous coughing. They may present leaning forward (ie, tripod position) with mouth breathing and tongue and mandible protrusion. When acute bacterial epiglottitis is suspected, immediate airway management, preferably under anesthesia in an operating suite, is indicated.

RETROPHARYNGEAL ABSCESS

Retropharyngeal abscess is an uncommon disease. In a pediatric study of 64 patients under 16 years of age, 75% of retropharyngeal abscesses were found in children less than 5 years of age and 16% of this condition in infants less than 1 year of age.[13] In a mixed-group study of 19 patients, 1 to 69 years of age, with retropharyngeal abscess, 37% of retropharyngeal abscesses cases were less than 5 years of age and 47% of these cases were over 17 years of age.[13] Unlike epiglottitis, with its rapid onset, retropharyngeal abscess is commonly preceded by nasopharyngitis with development of high fever, dysphagia, severe throat pain, noisy breathing, and stiff neck. Infants under 1 year of age may present with fever, drooling, and stridor or, instead, with isolated fever and lethargy. In a study of 25 infants under 9 months of age with deep neck abscesses, 92% had a neck mass, 60% had fever, and 36% had dysphagia or poor feeding. In 13 of 17 who were scanned, the computerized tomography scan of the neck revealed some degree of airway compromise.[12]

With the exception of the abrupt onset and tripod position seen in epiglottitis, epiglottitis and retropharyngeal abscess may have strikingly similar clinical presentations. Children with retropharyngeal abscess may use mouth breathing, tongue protrusion, and mandible thrust to maintain a patent airway. They often present with fever and a toxic appearance. In the same study of 64 pediatric patients under 16 years of age with retropharyngeal abscess, however, only 5% had respiratory distress or frank stridor whereas 45% had limitation to neck extension.[14] In another study of 169 patients under 19 years of age with deep neck abscesses, only 6% had stridor and 7% had respiratory distress. The most common clinical finding in this study was neck mass in 91%.[15] The low incidence of respiratory distress and stridor in children with retropharyngeal abscesses, in contrast to the high incidence of these findings in epiglottitis and tracheitis, helps differentiate these airway disorders. An adequate portable lateral neck radiograph revealing the distended retropharyngeal space can be diagnostic of retropharyngeal abscesses (**Fig. 1**). Although the management of tracheitis and epiglottitis includes early airway control via intubation in addition to IV antibiotic administration, retropharyngeal abscesses can often be managed with IV antibiotics and close observation. The need for immediate intubation is rare. ENT consultation is warranted in all cases of retropharyngeal abscess confirmed by CT.

CONGENITAL STRUCTURAL DEFECTS

Infants with stridor beginning at birth or within 2 weeks of birth may have congenital airway abnormalities, such as laryngomalacia, tracheomalacia, and subglottic hemangioma. Infants with a history of chronic stridor suggestive of one of these disorders who present with worsened upper airway obstruction after a viral prodrome may have superimposed laryngotracheobronchitis exacerbating pre-existing airway abnormalities. These infants generally have only partial response to croup management, and a high index of suspicion for underlying structural abnormality is recommended in these clinical scenarios. ENT consultation and airway endoscopy should be considered in all suspected cases.

AIRWAY FOREIGN BODIES

Children with foreign bodies in the nasal cavity may present with rhinorrhea, malodorous breath, or an explicit history of placing an object in the nose, although they generally do not present with extreme respiratory distress. Children with foreign bodies, such as plastic candy wrappers, lodged in the oropharynx generally present

Normal upper airway.

Patient with fever, stridor and stiff neck.

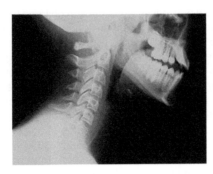
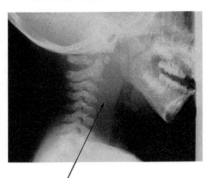

Grossly enlarged
retropharyngeal space

Fig. 1. Retropharyngeal abscess in a 3-year-old (*right*) compared with a normal upper airway (*left*).

with mouth breathing, refusal to feed, irritability, and mild drooling. These children do not usually present in respiratory distress unless the object is large and partially obstructing the glottic opening. Children who present in distress with a sudden onset of stridor, prolonged inspiratory phase, head bobbing, and excessive drooling are more likely to have foreign bodies partially obstructing the supraglottic area and proximal esophagus.

Management of nonaspirated foreign bodies in children depends on the location of the foreign bodies and the degree of resulting obstruction. Children who can cough and verbalize should be given supplemental oxygen and placed in a position of comfort. Nasal foreign bodies can generally be removed in an emergency department with a variety of instruments, such as a balloon-tipped catheter. Oropharyngeal foreign bodies in patients without extreme respiratory distress can be removed with Magill forceps. Beware of children who present with severe partial upper airway obstruction due to foreign body. If these children can cough and verbalize, give supplemental oxygen and place them in a position of comfort. Consider delaying IV line placement and other interventions that might cause agitation and worsen airway resistance. Do not try to remove foreign bodies causing severe partial upper airway obstruction because these attempts may result in complete glottic obstruction. A better course of action is immediate consultation with an otolaryngologist and operating room personnel to ensure rapid transfer to an operating suite for intubation. In children with airway obstruction that prevents cough or verbalization, basic life-support maneuvers should be initiated immediately to dislodge the foreign body.

Aspirated lower airway foreign bodies in children may be subtle, and delays of up to 4 months[16] and as long as 5 years[17] in diagnosing foreign bodies are reported. In one study, 99% of patients reporting foreign body aspiration or choking were found to have confirmed foreign body,[17] although in another study of 202 confirmed cases of airway foreign bodies, there was no history of foreign body aspiration in 15% of cases.[18] In a study of 128 patients with suspected foreign body aspirations, 28 presented later than 1 month after the event or onset of symptoms. All those who presented late had a chronic cough and 48% had a history suggestive of foreign body aspiration; 63% of the children presented with complications that included pneumonia (n = 13), bronchiectasis (n = 3), and bronchoesophageal fistula (n = 1). The diagnostic delays were variously attributed to physician misdiagnosis (n = 9), failure by parents to seek early medical advice (n = 4), patients leaving against medical advice (n = 1), and unknown cause in the remaining 14 children.[19] The most common age for foreign body aspiration is 1 to 2 years of age with up to two-thirds of cases occurring in this age group[16] and 68% of foreign body aspirations occur within the first 8 years of life.[17] Approximately 80% of aspirated foreign bodies are lodged in the lower airways,[17] leaving laryngotracheal foreign bodies less common but immediately life threatening.[16]

In 548 cases of foreign body aspiration over a 10-year period, in children 2 months to 16 years of age, the percentage of children presenting with cough was 83%, choking 4%, and wheezing 10%. Four percent of children presented asymptomatically and 16% of cases had no physical examination findings to suggest foreign body.[17] In this same study, chest radiograph was frequently abnormal with atelectasis in 35%, hyperinflation in 27%, and radiopaque foreign bodies in 13%, although chest radiograph was normal in 14% of cases. A peanut was the most common aspirated foreign body in children[16,17] whereas balloons are the most common foreign body aspirations to result in death.[16]

Management of aspirated foreign bodies in children depends on a child's age and location of the aspirated foreign body. Because the narrowest portion of the pediatric airway is at the cricoid ring, any foreign body at this level may cause severe airway resistance. Children with foreign bodies at the cricoid region generally present in extreme respiratory distress with severe retractions and stridor. Immediate intubation using rapid sequence intubation medications or immediate transfer to an operating suite is generally indicated. Children with aspirated foreign bodies in the lower airways present as diagnostic challenges. Findings suggestive of lower airway foreign bodies include air trapping leading to asymmetric hyperinflation (38%–63%), pulmonary consolidation (8%–25%), or barotrauma (7%).[16] Initial radiographic studies should include standard anteroposterior and lateral chest radiographs. Only approximately 6% to 15% of aspirated foreign bodies are radiopaque, however, and approximately 15% of radiopaque foreign bodies cases are initially seen on radiograph.[16] In suspected cases of aspirated foreign bodies, where standard radiographic studies are normal (**Fig. 2**), lateral decubitus films in young children and inspiratory and expiratory films in cooperative older children may provide more information. A lung placed on its side on a lateral decubitus film without a foreign body will compress normally due to gravity (**Fig. 3**). A lung placed on its side with a foreign body generally will not compress and will resist the forces of gravity due to the ball-valve obstruction (**Fig. 4**). Likewise, inspiratory and expiratory films may reveal hyperinflation on expiratory film if the foreign body in the lower airways causes a ball-valve obstruction and prevents full deflation of the obstructed lung on expiration. Bronchoscopy, however, remains the diagnostic tool of choice for suspected foreign body aspiration.

AIRWAY BURNS

There are many documented cases of delayed airway deterioration in young children who initially present with body scald burns.[20,21] Although compromise of the airway by direct thermal injury to the upper respiratory tract is most commonly associated with smoke or steam inhalation,[22] aspiration of microwave-heated liquids is the most common cause in infants and young children.[20,23] Heated liquid ingestions and aspiration have caused thermal epiglottitis and edematous arytenoidal tissue.[20,24]

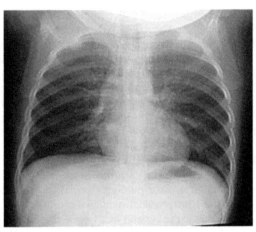

Fig. 2. Normal-appearing anteroposterior chest radiograph in a 12-month-old infant with a left mainstem foreign body.

Because thermal epiglottitis injuries in children may be clinically (and radiographically) similar to acute infectious epiglottitis,[24,25] children with these injuries are at risk for significant upper airway obstruction, which may continue to progress for several hours. Children in whom thermal epiglottitis is suspected should be approached with the same caution and preparedness for emergency airway management as those with acute infectious epiglottitis.[24] Even superheated, microwaved hot potato ingestions have caused edematous arytenoidal tissue and acute airway deterioration requiring intubation. Patients with airway burns often progress rapidly to acute upper airway occlusion.

Judicious airway management is crucial in these children. Because the initial pharyngeal examination does not always identify patients at risk, fiberoptic visualization of the larynx provides an excellent diagnostic and prognostic tool. Because edema may continue to progress over several hours, it is essential to secure the airway

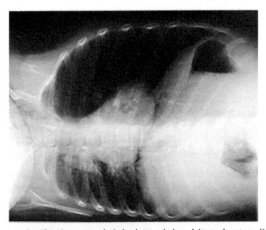

Fig. 3. Same patient as in **Fig. 2**; normal right lateral decubitus chest radiograph. Note how the right lung compresses normally due to the effects of gravity.

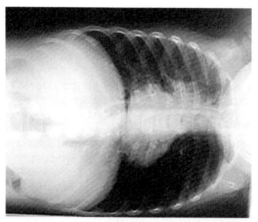

Fig. 4. Same patient as in **Fig. 2**; abnormal left lateral decubitus chest radiograph. Note how the left lung does not compress despite the effects of gravity. A large, dog-claw, foreign body was found in the left mainstem bronchus and removed by bronchoscopy.

via endotracheal intubation at the onset of any signs of laryngeal edema, including stridor, hoarseness, or change in character of a child's voice or cry.[20]

SUMMARY

Upper airway obstruction in infants and children, whether or not caused by infection, foreign body or airway burn, may present with extreme respiratory distress. Simple croup should be responsive to dexamethasone and nebulized racemic epinephrine. The incidence of epiglottitis has dramatically decreased in the pediatric population in the past decade, and bacterial tracheitis seems to have eclipsed croup and epiglottitis as the most common infectious cause of severe upper airway obstruction requiring intubation. Retropharyngeal abscess commonly presents with neck pain, stiffness, or mass and uncommonly causes respiratory distress and stridor. Airway foreign bodies in the laryngotracheal region may be immediately life threatening whereas lower airway foreign bodies may be subtle and the delay to diagnosis may be prolonged. Airway burns in infants and children may be occult on routine inspection of the oropharynx, and fiberoptic visualization of the larynx provides an excellent diagnostic and prognostic tool. Airway burns may progress rapidly to acute upper airway occlusion and intubation at the first signs of laryngeal edema is essential to prevent complete airway obstruction and respiratory failure.

REFERENCES

1. Cruz MN, Stewart G, Rosenberg N. Use of dexamethasone in the outpatient management of acute laryngotracheitis. Pediatrics 1995;96(2 Pt 1):220–3.
2. Rittichier KK, Ledwith CA. Outpatient treatment of moderate croup with dexamethasone: intramuscular versus oral dosing. Pediatrics 2000;106(6):1344–8.
3. Donaldson D, Poleski D, Knipple E, et al. Intramuscular versus oral dexamethasone for the treatment of moderate-to-severe croup: a randomized, double-blind trial. Acad Emerg Med 2003;10:16–21.
4. Al-Jundi S. Acute upper airway obstruction: croup, epiglottitis, bacterial tracheitis and retropharyngeal abscess. In: Levin DL, Morriss FC, editors. Essentials of

pediatric intensive care. 2nd edition. New York: Churchill Livingstone Inc; 1997. p. 121–9.

5. Hopkins A, Lahiri T, Salerno R, et al. Changing epidemiology of life-threatening upper airway infections: the reemergence of bacterial tracheitis. Pediatrics 2006;118(4):1418–21.

6. de Bilderling G, Bodart E, Tuerlinckx D, et al. Laryngitis revealing bacterial tracheitis in a five-year-old child. Arch Pediatr 2001;8(11):1214–7.

7. Maloney E, Meakin GH. Acute stridor in children. Cont Edu Anaesth Crit Care Pain 2007;7(6):183–6.

8. Montoya C. Pediatric immunizations. Program and abstracts of the American College of Nurse Practitioners National Clinical Symposium. Albuquerque, New Mexico. Session F21, October 9–13, 2002.

9. Leung AK, Jadavji T. Polysaccharide vaccine for prevention of *Haemophilus influenzae* type b disease. J R Soc Health 1988;108:180–1.

10. Faden H. The dramatic change in the epidemiology of pediatric epiglottitis. Pediatr Emerg Care 2006;22(6):443–4. Conclusion: the admission rate for acute epiglottitis is a large children's hospital has declined ten fold over the last 27 years.

11. Ewig JM. Croup. Pediatr Ann 2002;31:125–30.

12. Cmejrek RC. Presentation, diagnosis and management of deep neck abscesses in infants. Arch Otolaryngol Head Neck Surg 2002;128(12):1361–4.

13. Goldenberg D, Golz A, Joachims HZ. Retropharyngeal abscess: a clinical review. J Laryngol Otol 1997;111:546–50.

14. Craig FW, Schunk JE. Retropharyngeal abscess in children: clinical presentation, utility of imaging and current management. Pediatrics 2003;111:1394–8.

15. Coticchia JM, Getnick GS, Yun RD, et al. Age-, site-, and time-specific differences in pediatric deep neck abscesses. Arch Otolaryngol Head Neck Surg 2004;130(2):201–7.

16. Gausche-Hill M, Fuchs S, Yamamoto L, editors. Advanced pediatric life support. 4th edition. Academy of Pediatrics/American College of Emergency Physicians. Sudbury (MA): American Jones and Bartlett; 2004.

17. Oguzkaya F, Akcali Y, Kahraman C, et al. Tracheobronchial foreign body aspirations in childhood: a 10-year experience. Eur J Cardiothorac Surg 1998;14(4):388–92.

18. Kim GL. Foreign body in the airway: a review of 202 cases. Laryngoscope 1973;83(1):347.

19. Saquib Mallick M, Rauf Khan A, Al-Bassam A. Late presentation of tracheobronchial foreign body aspiration in children. J Trop Pediatr 2005;51(3):145–8.

20. Rosen D, Avishai-Eliner S, Borenstein A, et al. Life-threatening laryngeal burns in toddlers following hot liquid aspiration. Acta Paediatr 2000;89(8):1018–22.

21. Watts AM, McCallum MI. Acute airway obstruction following facial scalding: differential diagnosis between a thermal and infective cause. Burns 1996;22(7):570–3.

22. Jones JE, Rosenberg D. Management of laryngotracheal thermal trauma in children. Laryngoscope 1995;105(5 Pt 1):540–2.

23. Garland JS, Rice TB, Kelly KJ. Airway burns in an infant following aspiration of microwave-heated tea. Chest 1986;90(4):621–2.

24. Kulick RM, Selbst SM, Baker MD, et al. Thermal epiglottitis after swallowing hot beverages. Pediatrics 1988;81(3):441–4.

25. Harjacek M, Kornberg AE, Yates EW, et al. Thermal epiglottitis after swallowing hot tea. Pediatr Emerg Care 1992;8(6):342–4.

Pitfalls in the Management of Headache in the Emergency Department

Stuart P. Swadron, MD, FRCP(C), FAAEM, FACEP

KEYWORDS

• Headache • Cephalgia • Emergency medicine

Headache, or cephalgia, is the fifth most common primary complaint of patients presenting to an emergency department (ED) in the United States, representing more than 3 million patients each year, or 2% of all ED visits.[1] An additional number seek treatment at ambulatory care clinics, where diagnostic capabilities may be more limited. When headache coexists with certain other presenting signs and symptoms, such as alteration of mental status or hypoxia, these features may overshadow the headache and will likely direct the diagnostic and therapeutic approach. This article focuses on patients for whom headache is their most prominent presenting complaint.

The role of the emergency physician (EP) is unique in the evaluation and treatment of headache, one that differs from that of the primary care physician, the neurologist, and other specialists. The EP has 2 major responsibilities: to relieve headache pain and to ensure that life-threatening and disabling underlying causes are uncovered and treated. As with other cardinal presentations, these 2 priorities are addressed simultaneously. Because most patients with headache are subsequently discharged home, appropriate follow-up planning and patient education are also important aspects of emergency care. The pitfalls that follow are those most frequently encountered in emergency medicine practice and those with the greatest likelihood to adversely affect patient outcomes.

PITFALLS OF NOMENCLATURE
Being Too Specific

The underlying pathophysiologic mechanisms of many types of headache are still poorly defined, and diagnostic terminology is rapidly evolving. The International

Department of Emergency Medicine, Los Angeles County/USC Medical Center, Keck School of Medicine of the University of Southern California, Room G1011, 1200 North State Street, Los Angeles, CA 90033, USA
E-mail address: swadron@usc.edu

Emerg Med Clin N Am 28 (2010) 127–147
doi:10.1016/j.emc.2009.09.007
0733-8627/09/$ – see front matter © 2010 Elsevier Inc. All rights reserved.

Headache Society, a multidisciplinary group of clinicians and scholars, has attempted to provide a standard nomenclature to aid in the study and treatment of the various disorders that result in headache. The most recent edition of their classification scheme, the International Classification of Headache Disorders (ICHD-2), provides an exhaustive, categorized list of more than 200 disease entities, each with specific, detailed diagnostic criteria.[2] However, from an emergency medicine perspective, such diagnostic precision is unnecessary, and may distract the clinician from important priorities in the ED.

At the most basic level, most investigators, including those of the ICHD-2, classify headaches as primary or secondary. Primary headaches are those that cannot be attributed to another known disease or condition, and include migraine, tension, and cluster headaches. Because their underlying causes are still being elucidated, they are classified according to their symptomatology. Secondary headaches are classified according to their underlying cause. All of the specific diagnoses that require time-dependent therapies in the ED to prevent poor patient outcomes are of secondary headaches.

Several investigators have brought attention to the lack of diagnostic accuracy applied to patients with primary headache in the ED, most notably for those with migraine.[3–5] They propose that increasing accuracy would allow for therapy that is more targeted and appropriate to specific underlying diagnoses. However, there is remarkable overlap in the response of the various subclasses of primary headache to the different agents and regimens used to treat headache pain in the ED. In one recent study, a dedicated research assistant performed a detailed interview of ED patients with headache, and formally classified them into ICHD-2 categories.[6] No difference was found in their response to sumatriptan, an antimigraine therapy, regardless of whether they were classified as having migraine, probable migraine, or tension headache. Similarly, patients treated with antiemetics, opioids, and dihydroergotamine (DHE) show excellent response to therapy, regardless of their specific underlying diagnosis.[7] Moreover, it may be difficult to make a specific diagnosis in the ED; many of the diagnostic criteria involve the observation of headache patterns over time, and are best evaluated in the interval between acute episodes. In one study of ED patients, even when a structured questionnaire based on ICHD-2 was applied, no specific diagnosis could be made in more than one-third of cases.[8]

Although it may be appropriate to make specific diagnoses in individual cases, a premature diagnosis of migraine, or another subclass of primary headache, may have other adverse consequences. Such a diagnosis may inappropriately stigmatize the patient with a chronic medical condition. More importantly, such a diagnosis may result in anchoring bias, which is the tendency to ignore important data by relying too heavily on 1 trait or source of information, such as a previous diagnosis, when making decisions. Thus, it may prevent the clinician from pursuing further appropriate evaluation to reach another correct diagnosis of a secondary headache. In a recent study performed in a community ED, patients with a previous diagnosis of migraine headache did not meet widely accepted diagnostic criteria.[9] Unless all of the elements necessary for the diagnosis are present, it may be more prudent to leave definitive diagnosis to the primary care provider or specialist consultant.

Dangerous Primary Headache Diagnoses

Some of the specific primary headache diagnoses listed in the ICHD-2 are fraught with hazard for the EP and the primary care physician. Entities such as hemiplegic migraine and thunderclap headache mimic life-threatening secondary headaches such as stroke and subarachnoid hemorrhage (SAH) in their clinical presentation. For this reason, these are conditions that cannot be diagnosed without a thorough diagnostic evaluation and subsequent follow-up. It is inadvisable for the EP to make these diagnoses de novo without specialist consultation.

PITFALLS OF HISTORY AND PHYSICAL EXAMINATION
Linking Treatment Response to Diagnosis

One dangerous and common misunderstanding is that primary headaches may be differentiated from secondary headaches based on a patient's response to analgesic agents. Because headache pain seems to be mediated through a limited number of final common physiologic pathways, response to analgesia may provide few, if any, clues to the underlying cause. Life-threatening secondary headaches may resolve with antimigraine therapies, simple analgesics such as acetaminophen, or even spontaneously without treatment. A positive response to analgesics and antimigraine therapy has been reported with virtually every category of secondary headache, including carotid artery dissection, carbon monoxide (CO) exposure, brain tumor, SAH, meningitis, and venous sinus thrombosis (VST).[10-17]

Dismissing Secondary Headache Diagnoses in Patients with Known Primary Headaches

A small number of patients with headache account for a disproportionately large number of ED visits.[18,19] Many of these patients carry established specific primary headache diagnoses, most commonly migraine.[19] As every EP knows, sometimes the biggest impediment to a new, correct diagnosis is a current longstanding diagnosis. In addition, a history of migraine headache may increase the risk for some life-threatening causes of secondary headaches, such as ischemic stroke.[20] Practitioners must be careful to consider each new headache presentation for features that may distinguish it from previous headaches and warrant further investigation.

Ascribing Headaches to Increased Blood Pressure

It is common for patients to ascribe headache pain to elevated blood pressure. Although patients with hypertensive encephalopathy may suffer from headache in association with severely elevated blood pressure, this condition is rare and requires additional features for diagnosis, such as an alteration in mental status. In most cases, mild, moderate, and even severe elevations of blood pressure are likely unrelated to headaches and other acute symptomatology that is frequently ascribed to hypertension.[21] Conversely, acute pain syndromes, such as headache, may result in increases in blood pressure, and the treatment of pain should be the first approach in these patients. In the absence of acute end-organ injury, the aggressive treatment of increased blood pressure with antihypertensive agents may result in undesirable and precipitous drops in blood pressure that, in turn, may cause watershed ischemia and stroke in patients with longstanding hypertension.

Historical Features of SAH

Of all of the causes of secondary headache, SAH is of foremost concern for the EP because it commonly presents as an isolated headache in the absence of other findings, and it is highly lethal if left undiagnosed. Generations of medical students have been taught to link "the worst headache of your life" with the diagnosis of nontraumatic SAH. Although some patients who describe their headache in this way are ultimately found to have SAH or other life-threatening secondary headache, most do not.[22,23] In addition, there seems to be an inherent inconsistency in how patients answer questions related to the intensity of their headache. In one recent study, one-third of patients who stated that their headache was the worst of their life subsequently were able to identify a previous headache of equal intensity.[24] Using this single descriptor alone, without further delineation to direct a workup for secondary causes of headache, may lead to an ineffective use of resources and unnecessary complications of the various studies used.

It is more helpful to elicit descriptors that characterize the suddenness of headache onset, its intensity at onset, and how the headache compares in quality to any previous headaches. Patients who describe a headache that is sudden in onset and maximum in intensity immediately or within a few minutes of onset, the so-called thunderclap headache, are much more likely to harbor serious pathology. Two studies that prospectively examined patients with severe, sudden-onset headache found significant numbers (44% and 71%) with SAH or other serious pathologies.[25,26] This has led to the recommendation by the American College of Emergency Physicians that patients with thunderclap headache undergo emergent neuroimaging followed by cerebrospinal fluid (CSF) analysis if imaging studies do not reveal a diagnosis.[27]

The familiar descriptor of the "worst headache of your life" may also serve clinicians poorly when patients present with sudden-onset, maximal-at-onset headaches that are not necessarily perceived as severe. Studies of patients with confirmed SAH have consistently found that many had presented previously with a new symptom of headache in the days and weeks that preceded their diagnosis and admission to hospital. The initial headache is often dismissed as benign after it remits spontaneously or with analgesics.[28] In some cases, patients do not seek medical attention. This is consistent with the natural history of aneurysmal SAH, in which a small, symptomatic leak is typically followed by a more severe, disabling, and life-threatening bleed in the days and weeks that follow. Patients with aneurysmal SAH are served best if the diagnosis is made in this interval, when neurosurgical intervention can forestall disaster. Although the precise incidence of this phenomenon is difficult to ascertain, because of variable workups performed for sudden-onset headache in different clinical settings and recall bias on the part of survivors, studies have found rates of so-called sentinel leak ranging from 10% to 43%.[29] Thus, any headache that is sudden in onset, maximal at onset, and different in nature from headaches that the patient has had in the past deserves a diagnostic workup.

Other Critical History and Physical Examination Features

As with any cardinal complaint, the EP considers all causes of headache that are life threatening or disabling and for which a critical intervention may be indicated. This list of secondary headaches is summarized in **Table 1**. Each diagnosis is associated with critical features on history and physical examination, and if these features are present, a diagnostic workup is indicated. Likewise, in most patients with a primary headache diagnosis, for whom diagnostic testing is not necessary, the absence of these features should be documented.

In most patients, a simple report of the absence of trauma is sufficient to eliminate the possibility of head injury. However, in any patient dependent on others, such as children, the elderly, and those requiring assistance in their activities of daily living, the absence of suspicious clues of occult trauma, such as abnormal behavior of the caregivers, should be noted. If child abuse is suspected, computed tomography (CT) is superior to magnetic resonance (MR) imaging to detect acute injury. However, MR gives more definitive information about the nature and extent of subacute and chronic injuries, without the risks of radiation.[30]

Bacterial meningitis can present subtly, and may initially resemble a viral upper respiratory tract infection. At a minimum, patients with fever and headache should be thoroughly examined for the presence of a petechial rash and signs of meningeal irritation. Although the absence of Kernig and Brudzinski signs are often documented in patients with headache, both are rare and insensitive in meningitis.[31,32] In contrast, the jolt accentuation test, which is considered positive when headache pain is exacerbated by patients rotating their heads from side to side, has been found to be sensitive, and may be more helpful in identifying patients for further evaluation.[33] It is easy to overlook the importance of contiguous spread from surrounding head and neck structures; the absence of recent head and neck instrumentation and a full examination of the head and neck should be documented. The absence of severely ill contacts should also be noted, as should risk factors for immune compromise, both of which will lower the threshold for imaging and CSF examination.

CO poisoning is the most common poisoning in the United States and worldwide. It is life threatening and disabling, and remains commonly unrecognized and misdiagnosed. Headache that is associated with a flulike illness in the winter months when home furnaces are in use, similar symptoms in others within same residence, and a pattern of daily improvement after leaving the area of exposure are all clues that should heighten suspicion for CO poisoning.[34–37]

Temporal arteritis (TA) is a panarteritis that may be associated with polymyalgia rheumatica, a disease that results in chronic proximal muscle weakness in a predominantly older white female population. Prototypical symptoms of TA include bitemporal pain and jaw claudication, and ischemic pain with mastication that is relieved by rest. Classic physical findings include visual field deficits, temporal tenderness, and nodularity of the superficial temporal arteries on palpation. Although most patients do not present with these classic symptoms and signs, the majority do present with a new-onset headache, and almost all patients are more than 50 years of age.[38,39] Because of its natural progression to blindness that is preventable with treatment, TA should be considered in older patients with new-onset headaches.

Cervical artery dissection is a rare but potentially life-threatening cause of sudden-onset headache that may mimic SAH in its presentation. Carotid and vertebral artery dissections may occur spontaneously or may be precipitated by seemingly minor trauma, such as vigorous coughing or chiropractic manipulation. In carotid dissection, the pain may be unilateral, involving the face, and may be associated with pulsatile tinnitus or oculosympathethic palsy (miosis and ptosis).[40] In vertebral dissection, the pain is most commonly occipital or nuchal.[41] Although, in some cases, neurologic signs related to embolic events in the respective vascular territories may be present on the initial presentation, there is most commonly an interval of several days between the onset of headache and such events. Nonetheless, cervical artery dissection may be suspected clinically in a patient with new, sudden-onset headache if there is a history of a precipitating event, connective tissue disease, or a family history of unexplained ischemic stroke in younger or middle-aged relatives.[40]

Although most EPs would consider the diagnosis of preeclampsia in a pregnant woman who presents with a headache, many fail to do so in patients in the postpartum period. A large proportion of eclampsia and preeclampsia cases occur after delivery, and may result in permanent disability from cerebral infarction or death. Because headache is the most common presenting complaint in patients with postpartum preeclampsia, the onset of headache with new features at any time up to 4 weeks following delivery should prompt consideration of this diagnosis.[42]

Because it may present dramatically with severe headache, vomiting, and photophobia, acute angle-closure glaucoma is sometimes overlooked initially in the ED while time-consuming diagnostic investigations are performed to rule out SAH or meningitis. This time could be spent obtaining emergent ophthalmologic consultation

Table 1
Critical headache diagnoses for the EP

Diagnosis	Critical Clinical Features	Critical Diagnostic Tests	Critical Interventions	Comments
SAH	Sudden onset Maximal at onset Different than previous headaches	CT head LP	Neurosurgical consultation Blood pressure control Nimodipine Ventriculostomy	CT head and other neuroimaging modalities are insufficient to rule out the diagnosis
Occult trauma	Signs of abuse or neglect Anticoagulation or coagulopathy	CT head	Neurosurgical consultation Admission	Patients in at-risk populations may not volunteer a history of trauma
Bacterial meningitis	Fever Meningeal irritation Immune compromise Head and neck infection or instrumentation	CT head LP	Antibiotics Corticosteroids Isolation	Treatment should be initiated before diagnostic confirmation by CSF analysis if clinical suspicion is high. Corticosteroids should be initiated before or with the first dose of antibiotics in clinically apparent cases
TA	Jaw claudication Superficial temporal artery tenderness or nodularity Visual symptoms	Temporal artery biopsy	Systemic corticosteroids	ESR is an adequately sensitive screening test in patients without these high-risk features. Empirical corticosteroids are indicated in patients with high-risk features and findings or a markedly increased ESR
CO toxicity	Symptomatic cohabitants Flulike illness that is worse each morning Potentially toxic environment (eg, home furnace in winter)	Arterial cooximetry	HBOT	HBOT is indicated for patients with neurologic and cardiovascular signs and above certain cutoff levels
Acute glaucoma	Red eye Midrange fixed pupil Cloudy cornea	Intraocular pressure	Topical ocular therapy Systemic osmotic agents Ophthalmologic consultation	A cursory examination before neuroimaging should prevent costly delays in consultation and therapy

Condition	Clinical features	Diagnostic test	Consultation/treatment	Notes
Cervical artery dissection	SAH-like onset; Facial (carotid), neck (vertebral) pain; Cranial nerve abnormalities	Angiography	Neurologic/neurosurgical consultation; Anticoagulation	In the absence of brain hemorrhage, anticoagulation is initiated to reduce the risk of thrombus formation and embolization
Cerebral/dural VST	Hypercoagulable state (pregnancy and puerperum, oral contraceptives, malignancy); Head and neck infection; Proptosis (cavernous sinus thrombosis)	MR head Venography	Neurosurgical consultation; Systemic anticoagulation	A D-dimer may be falsely negative
Space-occupying lesion	Progressively worse over time; New onset in patient >50 years old; History of malignancy; Worse in morning; Worse in head-down position	CT head	Neurosurgical consultation; ICP-lowering therapies; Lesion-specific therapies	Emergent ICP-lowering therapies may include elevating the head of the bed, restriction of intravenous fluids, mannitol, and hyperventilation. Lesion-specific therapies may include emergent surgery/neuroradiological procedures, corticosteroids, and antimicrobial agents
Cerebellar infarction	Headache with dizziness; Cerebellar signs; Cranial nerve abnormalities	CT head	Neurologic/neurosurgical consultation	Although CT head is insensitive for infarction, it is helpful initially to rule out hemorrhage and identify life-threatening edema and mass effect
Idiopathic intracranial hypertension	Obese, young female patient; Cranial nerve 6 palsy (false localizing sign)	LP	CSF drainage; Neurologic referral	After negative neuroimaging, an LP will reveal a markedly increased opening pressure and provide temporary headache relief
Pituitary apoplexy	Thunderclap headache; Vomiting; Visual acuity, field deficits; Ocular palsies	CT head MR head	Neurosurgical consultation	Many pituitary infarctions and hemorrhages will not be easily visible on CT. MR is considered the diagnostic modality of choice
Preeclampsia	Postpartum (up to 4 weeks)	Complete blood count; Chemistry panel with Liver function tests; Coagulation studies	Intravenous magnesium; Obstetric consultation	Up to half of all patients present in the postpartum period, the majority with a chief complaint of headache

Abbreviations: CSF, cerebrospinal fluid; CT, computed tomography; ESR, erythrocyte sedimentation rate; HBOT, hyperbaric oxygen therapy; ICP, intracranial pressure; LP, lumbar puncture; MR, magnetic resonance; TA, temporal arteritis; VST, venous sinus thrombosis.

and lowering intraocular pressure with topical and systemic therapy. Patients with acute angle-closure glaucoma will have ocular findings such as a unilateral red eye with decreased visual acuity, a fixed, midrange pupil, and corneal edema. A cursory examination before diagnostic studies that take the patient out of the ED are performed will prevent delays to critical interventions.

Space-occupying lesions include primary and secondary neoplasms, infectious processes such as brain abscesses and cysts, and vascular lesions such as unruptured giant cerebral aneurysms and arteriovenous malformations. Although this is a heterogeneous group of pathologies, headaches caused by space-occupying lesions share common features in their presentation; the sine qua non being a progressive and unremitting course as the lesion expands in volume and increases intracranial pressure (ICP). Headaches also tend to be worse with the head-down position, and in the morning after waking, when ICP is higher. The specific location of the lesion and its adjacent structures within the calvarium will determine other features of the presentation. Whether or not it is critical for the EP to uncover the presence of a space-occupying lesion differs from case to case. In the absence of neurologic findings on examination, a patient with a slowly progressive headache of several weeks' or months' duration may be appropriately discharged from the ED for urgent neuroimaging and follow-up in a primary care setting. On the other hand, patients at high risk for pathology, such as those with a history of malignancy, recent head and neck infection or surgery, immune compromise, or those more than 50 years of age with a new onset of headache, often receive neuroimaging in the ED. The discovery of a large lesion, or a lesion in a critical location, will sometimes lead to the initiation of emergency therapies to prevent further expansion, brain injury, and herniation. If neuroimaging is performed in the ED, CT is usually sufficient; space-occupying lesions that are only detectable on MR are unlikely to alter ED management.

Cerebral and dural VST is another rare, but life-threatening and treatable, cause of headache. The characteristics of the headache are variable, but some patients present with a thunderclap. Patients at risk for VST include those with hypercoagulable states, including pregnancy and the postpartum period, oral contraceptive use, and the nephrotic syndrome, head and neck infections, malignancies, and vasculitidies.[43–45] Patients may present with signs of increased ICP, such as papilledema, and may continue to be symptomatic despite attempts at analgesia. If untreated, the thrombosis may progress to venous infarction and hemorrhage, which results in neurologic deficits that do not conform to an arterial territorial distribution. In some cases, VST eventually leads to brain herniation and death. Unless there are positive findings on the neurologic examination, there may be few other clues to compel the EP to pursue this diagnosis, and many cases go undiagnosed on the initial presentation.[46,47]

Idiopathic intracranial hypertension (IIH), previously known as pseudotumor cerebri, is a poorly understood disease with a predilection for obese middle-aged women. In these patients, a sustained increase in ICP seems to be related to an obstruction of CSF drainage at the level of the arachnoid granulations. However, in at least some cases coexistent VST is visible on contrast imaging studies, and, in this subgroup, more emergent therapy is necessary to prevent rapid deterioration.[48,49] In the absence of macroscopic thrombosis, deterioration is more gradual, with progressive visual-field deterioration occurring if ICP is not reduced. The physical examination most often reveals papilledema, and may reveal loss of peripheral visual fields. In some cases, a unilateral or bilateral sixth cranial nerve palsy is present. This palsy is a result of increased ICP, not a localized process, and thus is considered a false localizing sign. The diagnosis of IIH should be suspected in patients with a headache pattern consistent with a space-occupying lesion who have negative neuroimaging studies. Although the diagnosis is not as time critical as with VST, it is strongly suggested by the finding of a grossly increased opening pressure during lumbar puncture (LP) that is accompanied by an immediate improvement in the patient's symptoms.

Pituitary apoplexy is an extremely rare cause of thunderclap headache. It is defined as hemorrhage or infarction of the pituitary gland, typically into a preexisting adenoma. Although headache may be the most prominent presenting complaint, pituitary apoplexy is most often accompanied by visual symptoms and signs, such as decreased acuity, reduction in visual fields, and ocular palsies.[50]

PITFALLS OF DIAGNOSTIC TESTING
Relying on Neuroimaging to Rule out SAH

Despite advances in CT technology, noncontrast CT imaging alone remains inadequate to rule out nontraumatic SAH. In all but a single published case series,[51] an LP was required after a negative CT scan to make the diagnosis of SAH in a substantial minority of cases.[52–58] Although reported sensitivities in these case series typically exceed 90%, in practice, the sensitivity of CT for SAH is likely significantly lower, for several reasons. First and foremost is the critical issue of spectrum bias. Most studies begin their analysis with a group of patients ultimately diagnosed with SAH in hospital, potentially missing patients who are discharged from the ED and other outpatient settings with less severe presentations. These are precisely the patients in whom a timely diagnosis of SAH is so important to prevent a second, more severe bleed. In addition, most studies are conducted at referral centers, at which the equipment and the expertise of the radiologists are optimal. The ability of a general radiologist to detect small amounts of hemorrhage on CT is known to be inferior to that of a subspecialist neuroradiologist.[59] Lastly, small amounts of subarachnoid blood, after an initial leak, are rapidly absorbed; following the initial 12-hour interval after symptom onset, the sensitivity of CT decreases over time.[60]

Other imaging modalities, including MR, MR angiography, CT angiography, and conventional angiography, have not eliminated the need for LP with CSF analysis in cases of suspected SAH. MR is less sensitive than CT for the presence of blood in the first several hours after the onset of bleeding.[30] Even the addition of the fluid-attenuated inversion-recovery (FLAIR) technique, with its enhanced ability to detect blood, is insufficient. In a recent study of 12 patients with a negative CT scan who subsequently had SAH confirmed by CSF analysis, MR was only able to detect bleeding in 2.[61]

Although these technologies are continuing to evolve and improve, conventional angiography, CT angiography, and MR angiography are not 100% sensitive for the detection of cerebral aneurysms.[62–65] More importantly, angiography by any method is unable to distinguish between unruptured, asymptomatic aneurysms, which have an exceedingly low likelihood of rupture throughout a patient's lifetime, and symptomatic aneurysms that have already bled, and are likely to rebleed with serious consequences.[66,67] Thus, an LP with CSF analysis to confirm SAH can be critical to determine the need for surgical intervention when aneurysms are detected on angiography. Because the overall prevalence of cerebral aneurysms in the general population ranges from 2% to 6%,[67] the indiscriminate application of angiography to an unselected population of patients with headaches could result in unnecessary and harmful invasive procedures.

Other Limitations of CT

CT is insensitive to detect VST. Although data are lacking to precisely estimate its sensitivity, in one consecutive series of 127 patients with VST, 17 patients who presented with isolated headache had normal brain CT scan and CSF examination.[46] The addition of contrast to CT will help identify some cases, but the diagnosis can only be ruled out using MR venography.[68] However, because of the rarity of this diagnosis, it is an unreasonable expectation for MR venography to be performed emergently in patients without neurologic findings unless risk factors and a strong clinical suspicion exist for VST.

Cerebellar infarction, like cerebral infarction, may not become apparent on CT scan for several hours. However, cerebellar infarction deserves special consideration by the EP because it is more likely to present as a headache without weakness or other localizing signs on neurologic examination.[69] Moreover, because of its location in the posterior fossa, there is a greater risk for brain herniation as the lesion evolves and edema ensues. Although CT is less sensitive than MR to visualize the contents of the posterior fossa, edema from cerebellar infarction is often visible. Distortion or obliteration of the fourth ventricle from the resultant mass effect should prompt neurosurgical consultation for possible decompression. Pituitary apoplexy, by contrast, is frequently not visualized on CT, and MR is advised if clinical suspicion for this entity exists.[50]

Misinterpreting CSF Results

LP with CSF examination is critical in the evaluation of headaches suspicious for SAH or meningitis. In both instances, there are several common pitfalls that may interfere with a correct diagnosis. Within hours of the onset of subarachnoid bleeding, red blood cells (RBCs) are detectable in large numbers throughout the circulating CSF. In up to 15% of cases, LPs are traumatic, and RBCs from epidural vessels contaminate the specimen, making it difficult to identify a true SAH.[70] A common misunderstanding is that a progressive decrease in RBCs across serial collection tubes eliminates the possibility of SAH. Because SAH may coexist with RBCs that arise from a traumatic LP, the possibility of SAH can only safely be eliminated if the CSF count in one of the tubes approaches zero. If blood is encountered at the beginning of the LP, wasting the first 2 or 3 mL of fluid as the CSF clears will increase the likelihood that the RBC count will approach zero. If it does not, it may be necessary to repeat the procedure at a different interspace.

In cases in which traumatic LP makes the interpretation of RBC counts difficult, the presence of xanthochromia has been used to confirm the presence of true SAH. Xanthochromia is the yellowish discoloration of CSF that occurs in the hours following SAH as RBCs break down in vivo into bilirubin and oxyhemoglobin. However, xanthochromia has also been demonstrated to occur in vitro in collected specimens, resulting in falsely positive results.[71] Moreover, the practice of waiting until 12 hours have elapsed following the onset of headache, until the xanthochromia that develops in vivo is more reliably present, is not advised. Any advantage of this technique regarding the interpretation of CSF specimens is outweighed by the risk of a second aneurysmal bleed, which occurs more frequently in the hours immediately following the initial bleed than in any time period thereafter.[72] Almost all laboratories in the United States measure xanthochromia by visual inspection after centrifugation of the CSF specimen. Using this technique, falsely negative results are also possible.[73] Nonetheless, in patients who present several days after the onset of headache pain, xanthochromia may be the only remaining sign of SAH on CSF analysis; it typically persists for 2 weeks.[74]

Although a negative LP effectively rules out the diagnosis of SAH,[75] it does not rule out other vascular emergencies that may result in a thunderclap headache, such as cervical artery dissection, cerebral and dural VST, cerebellar infarction, and pituitary apoplexy.

There are other important pitfalls of CSF interpretation in patients with a suspected central nervous system infection. It may be difficult to distinguish between bacterial and viral meningitis using the initial results of CSF analysis available in the ED. Although bacterial meningitis is more likely to result in high cell counts with a preponderance of polymorphonuclear leukocytes, a low glucose, and a positive Gram stain, none of these features is reliably present, and there is a significant overlap in CSF findings with viral meningitis. If sufficient clinical suspicion exists for bacterial meningitis, the most prudent course is to proceed with broad-spectrum antibiotic coverage until the results of bacterial cultures are available.

Certain populations, such as infants, the elderly, and those with immune compromise, may have a limited cellular response on initial CSF analysis. Moreover, in patients with suspected immune compromise, atypical pathogens, such as *Cryptococcus neoformans* and mycobacteria should be considered. Specific tests for these pathogens are necessary, and the collection of an additional tube of CSF for later use by the inpatient physician may be helpful.

In a traumatic LP, leukocytes should be present in small numbers in a fixed ratio with RBCs, typically in the range of 1 leukocyte for every 500 RBCs. This ratio may vary depending on the relative proportions of these cells in the peripheral blood. Although there is some evidence to support using such ratios to rule out meningitis in a traumatic tap, in the presence of large numbers of leukocytes and a high clinical suspicion for meningitis, it is advisable to repeat the LP at a different interspace.[76] It should also be noted that the most important treatable cause of viral encephalitis, herpes simplex encephalitis (HSE), may present with red cells and leukocytes in the CSF.[77,78]

Complications of LP

The most common complication of LP is a postural headache that can be persistent and debilitating, often resulting in repeat visits to the ED. These headaches occur in up to one-third of patients in some series, and usually occur within 3 days of the procedure. The headache is typically described as worse in the upright position, forcing patients to lie down; this is consistent with the theory that it is due to ongoing CSF leakage at the site of puncture and the resultant intracranial hypotension. Many of the traditional instructions given to patients to prevent post-LP headaches, including postprocedural bed rest, increased fluid intake, and caffeine administration, have little or no basis in evidence.[79,80] There is, however, sufficient evidence to support the practice of using a small (22 gauge), atraumatic (noncutting tip) needle to prevent post-LP headache.[81,82] Epidural blood patch, the injection of 5 to 30 mL of the patient's own blood into the epidural space at the site of the prior procedure, has been found to be an effective treatment of post-LP headache refractory to other therapies.[83]

The most feared complication of LP is brain herniation. Although it is rare, a strong temporal correlation between the procedure and subsequent herniation lends strength to a causal relationship.[84] Most investigators recommend performing a CT scan before LP to minimize this risk. Although a normal CT scan does not completely eliminate the risk of brain herniation with LP, in patients with mass lesions or other structural changes, an LP is not advised. Although there may be a small increase in the risk of deterioration or herniation from an unsuspected lesion, it may be acceptable to omit the CT scan in selected patients with headache, such as those less than 60 years of age with no significant neurologic history and a normal neurologic examination.[85,86]

Other Laboratory Pitfalls

CO cooximetry values may be misleading. Low or undetectable levels may not rule out CO poisoning in the patient who presents many hours after exposure, as CO clears from the blood over time. Even in toxic patients with high tissue levels that have accumulated over a long period of exposure, the administration of high-flow supplemental oxygen will accelerate clearance from the blood and may lead to levels in the normal or near-normal range.[34,37] If the diagnosis is strongly suspected, removal of the patient from the suspected toxic environment, and repeat testing with any recurrent symptoms, is advised.

Although erythrocyte sedimentation rate (ESR) is an invaluable screening test for TA in older adult patients with headache, in the presence of an extremely high pretest probability it is inadequately sensitive to rule out the diagnosis. Thus, in patients with jaw claudication, nodularity or tenderness over the superficial temporal artery, or diploplia, the diagnostic evaluation should not end with a normal, or only mildly increased, ESR. In patients with such suggestive clinical features, or those with less specific features but a highly increased ESR, empirical corticosteroids should be administered in the interval before a definite diagnostic determination is made with temporal artery biopsy.[39]

The dimerized plasmin fragment D (D-dimer) test may help to identify some patients with VST. However, its lack of specificity has been well documented, most notably in patients with identified risk factors for VST, such as women in the peripartum period, and patients with malignancy, vasculitis, and other chronic inflammatory conditions.[87] D-dimer is also falsely negative in a significant number of cases of VST diagnosed definitely with contrast neuroimaging studies, especially in patients who present with isolated headache.[88–90]

PITFALLS OF TREATMENT
Poor Analgesic Agent Choices

Several investigators have been critical of the patterns of analgesic use for headache in the ED setting. One criticism is directed at the lack of specificity of the agents used with respect to the underlying diagnoses, especially for migraine. Another is in regard to the frequency of opioid use, which is said to be too high and inconsistent with published consensus guidelines.[3,91,92] Many agents have been proven to be highly effective for acute headache in the ED, including migraine, and, in any given patient, there may be several acceptable choices. One of the key factors for the EP is the patient's previous response to the various agents available.

The dopamine antagonists, including droperidol, prochlorperazine, metochlopramide, and chlorpromazine, have a less well-delineated mechanism of action than the more migraine-specific DHE and triptans, which activate serotonin 1B/1D receptors. Nonetheless, these agents, when used alone[93–99] or in combination with other drugs,[100] have been shown to be equivalent or superior to drugs from all other classes in multiple controlled trials. Droperidol seems to be more efficacious than prochlorperazine,[101,102] which in turn seems to be more efficacious as a single agent than metochlopramide.[103,104] All agents are more effective when they reach the central nervous system quickly, with intravenous administration superior to the intramuscular and oral routes.[104,105]

Although not as effective overall as the dopamine antagonists, opioids are also successful at abating headache. Although they may be used in some cases for which other options are available, the treatment guidelines set forth by nonemergency medicine societies may not be an appropriate standard against which to evaluate ED practices. The patient population in the ED is unique. The more severe spectrum of acuity in the ED, the lower likelihood of diagnostic precision, and the fact that many patients have already tried 1 or more medications before being evaluated, all suggest that different practice patterns are to be expected. Nonetheless, wide regional differences among EPs, and the discrepancy between their responses to hypothetical scenarios and actual practices observed, indicate that other factors also play a role.[106,107]

Patients who visit the ED frequently with a chief complaint of headache are often stigmatized by EPs and ED staff. These patients, who make up a larger proportion of patients in the ED than in office-based and specialty clinic settings are often labeled as drug-seekers.[18] They often request specific medications and are more frequently prescribed opioids. They also have a higher frequency of chronic headaches, and a large proportion use symptomatic headache therapies on a daily or almost daily basis, especially combination preparations containing opioids and caffeine, a syndrome known as medication overuse headache. Higher rates of opioid use in the ED may reflect, in part, the refractoriness of such patients to other therapies.[18]

With so many efficacious therapies available, pitfalls are more commonly related to medication side effects. The EP must therefore be mindful of a few key contraindications and complications of the commonly used agents. The dopamine antagonists are notable for prolonging the QT interval on the electrocardiogram (ECG). Moreover, it is not uncommon for 2 agents to be used that each cause some degree of QT prolongation, such as ondansetron for nausea, combined with a dopamine antagonist. Although this is rarely of clinical consequence, in patients with preexisting conduction or electrolyte abnormalities, or those who are already receiving therapy with other agents that prolong the QT interval, it can sometimes lead to torsades de pointes (TdP), a potentially fatal dysrhythmia. Women, who are disproportionately represented among patients with migraine headache, are at higher risk than men.[108] The relationship between QT-prolonging agents and TdP is unclear, and seems to be nonlinear. Agents that cause only minimal prolongation of the QT interval may cause TdP at higher rates than those that cause more marked prolongation.[108] Because patients with cardiac or electrolyte abnormalities are known to be at higher risk, it may be prudent to avoid dopamine antagonists in these patients, or to monitor them with telemetry or serial ECGs during therapy.

The other, more common but less life-threatening, concern with the dopamine antagonists is akathisia, an uncomfortable sensation of not being able to sit still. It occurs with varying severity in a substantial minority of patients.[109] In general, it has not limited the ability of this class of agents to be effective, and when severe, it is reliably abated by the use of anticholinergic agents such as diphenhydramine.[109] The incidence of akathisia may be decreased by the use of slower infusion rates,[110] or by using an anticholinergic premedication.[111]

The triptans offer greater selectivity for serotonin receptors, and are available for administration by oral and subcutaneous routes. They have largely replaced DHE in the primary care and neurology specialty clinic settings. However, DHE is still in use in many EDs, possibly because of its low cost and availability as an intravenous preparation. Most investigators recommend avoiding DHE in patients with cardiovascular disease, uncontrolled hypertension, and in pregnancy.[112] Although triptans have been shown to be more efficacious than DHE,[113] many EPs have lingering concerns about their cardiovascular risk, and are concerned about the frequent occurrence of chest pain and pressure that occurs after their administration. Although there is evidence that these symptoms are not cardiac related,[114] coronary vasospasm has been documented in the catheterization laboratory with the administration of triptans in patients with diseased coronary arteries.[115] Moreover, most subjects studied to establish the safety of triptans have been those without evidence of cardiac disease. It is thus recommended that these agents be avoided in patients with a history of coronary artery disease.

Withholding Empirical Antibiotics and Steroids in Suspected Meningitis

In patients clinically suspected of having bacterial meningitis, such as those who appear ill and are febrile with signs of meningeal irritation, broad-spectrum antibiotics should not be withheld pending the results of diagnostic studies. Bacterial meningitis progresses rapidly, and outcomes are most likely related to the time to antibiotic administration in patients with overt presentations.[116–118] Moreover, a short interval of antibiotics before LP is unlikely to obscure the diagnosis on CSF analysis.[119]

Corticosteroids have also been shown to reduce mortality and improve outcomes in patients with bacterial meningitis when they are administered before, or concurrently, with antibiotics. Their empirical administration should similarly be considered in patients in whom bacterial meningitis is strongly suspected.[120,121] Because many patients in the United States receive empirical antibiotics before CSF examination based on a low or moderate clinical suspicion, coadministering a large dose of corticosteroids in all of these patients may expose the majority, who do not have meningitis, to unnecessary risks. There are limited data to address this question; the best approach may be to limit empirical steroid administration to those patients in whom meningitis is most strongly suspected.

After CSF results become available, additional antimicrobial therapy may be indicated to cover specific organisms and possible drug-resistant strains, especially in special at-risk populations.[122,123] Acyclovir should be added to the empirical treatment regimen for patients with CSF pleocytosis and a negative Gram stain until the results of more definitive tests are available, such as the polymerase chain reaction test for the herpes simplex virus.[77]

PITFALLS OF DISCHARGE AND FOLLOW-UP MANAGEMENT
Poor Discharge Planning

Although many patients leave the ED pain free, recurrence of headache in the day following the ED visit is a common problem occurring in most discharged patients with a diagnosis of migraine in one study,[124] and in almost one-third of patients with primary headaches in another.[125] It is important to consider the patient's previous history of headache recurrence during discharge, as repeat ED visits can be avoided in many cases. Risk factors associated with recurrence of moderate to severe pain and functional impairment within 24 hours of discharge include incomplete resolution at discharge,[124,126] severe baseline pain, a longer duration of pain, baseline nausea, and a positive screen for depression.[125] In patients who obtain headache relief with intramuscular sumatriptan, discharge with an oral dose, to be used in the event of recurrence, is appropriate.[127] In other patients, the use of nonsteroidal antiinflammatory agents, acetaminophen, aspirin, or oral antiemetics at the first sign of recurrence may be helpful. Several randomized, controlled studies have looked at the role of oral or intravenous dexamethasone to reduce the rate of headache recurrence. Although several of these studies were negative,[126,128–130] a recent meta-analysis[131] found an overall benefit of parenteral dexamethasone at 72 hours posttreatment. Although it is difficult to recommend the routine use of corticosteroids, they seem to have a role, and may be especially useful in those patients with a headache of greater than 72 hours duration before presentation.[130]

Patients should be given follow-up care with a primary care provider. In certain cases that present a diagnostic or therapeutic challenge, neurologist or headache specialist follow-up may also be warranted. It is important for patients to be instructed to return to the ED if their symptoms worsen or if new symptoms evolve; many of the dangerous diagnoses discussed earlier may initially present as an isolated headache but go on to develop additional symptoms and signs as they progress.

Patients who visit the ED frequently with exacerbations of primary headache present a special challenge. Although there are few data to describe successful strategies for their ED management, consistency in their care among EPs and other ED staff, and regular communication among EPs, primary care providers, and specialists, may improve their outcomes.

REFERENCES

1. McCaig LF, Burt CW. National Hospital Ambulatory Medical Care Survey: 2002 emergency department summary. Adv Data 2004;340:1.
2. Headache Classification Subcommittee of the International Headache Society. The International Classification of Headache Disorders: 2nd edition. Cephalalgia 2004;24(Suppl 1):9.
3. Sahai-Srivastava S, Desai P, Zheng L. Analysis of headache management in a busy emergency room in the United States. Headache 2008;48:931.
4. Maizels M. Headache evaluation and treatment by primary care physicians in an emergency department in the era of triptans. Arch Intern Med 1969;161:2001.
5. Blumenthal HJ, Weisz MA, Kelly KM, et al. Treatment of primary headache in the emergency department. Headache 2003;43:1026.
6. Miner JR, Smith SW, Moore J, et al. Sumatriptan for the treatment of undifferentiated primary headaches in the ED. Am J Emerg Med 2007;25:60.
7. Trainor A, Miner J. Pain treatment and relief among patients with primary headache subtypes in the ED. Am J Emerg Med 2008;26:1029.
8. Friedman BW, Hochberg ML, Esses D, et al. Applying the International Classification of Headache Disorders to the emergency department: an assessment of reproducibility and the frequency with which a unique diagnosis can be assigned to every acute headache presentation. Ann Emerg Med 2007;49:409.
9. Fiesseler FW, Riggs RL, Holubek W, et al. Canadian Headache Society criteria for the diagnosis of acute migraine headache in the ED – do our patients meet these criteria? Am J Emerg Med 2005;23:149.
10. Pope JV, Edlow JA. Favorable response to analgesics does not predict a benign etiology of headache. Headache 2008;48:944.
11. Pfadenhauer K, Schonsteiner T, Keller H. The risks of sumatriptan administration in patients with unrecognized subarachnoid haemorrhage (SAH). Cephalalgia 2006;26:320.
12. Lipton RB, Mazer C, Newman LC, et al. Sumatriptan relieves migrainelike headaches associated with carbon monoxide exposure. Headache 1997;37:392.
13. Abisaab J, Nevadunsky N, Flomenbaum N. Emergency department presentation of bilateral carotid artery dissections in a postpartum patient. Ann Emerg Med 2004;44:484.
14. Leira EC, Cruz-Flores S, Leacock RO, et al. Sumatriptan can alleviate headaches due to carotid artery dissection. Headache 2001;41:590.

15. Prokhorov S, Khanna S, Alapati D, et al. Subcutaneous sumatriptan relieved migraine-like headache in two adolescents with aseptic meningitis. Headache 2008;48:1235.
16. Rosenberg JH, Silberstein SD. The headache of SAH responds to sumatriptan. Headache 2005;45:597.
17. Barclay CL, Shuaib A, Montoya D, et al. Response of non-migrainous headaches to chlorpromazine. Headache 1990;30:85.
18. Maizels M. Health resource utilization of the emergency department headache "repeater". Headache 2002;42:747.
19. Friedman BW, Serrano D, Reed M, et al. Use of the emergency department for severe headache. A population-based study. Headache 2009;49:21.
20. Katsarava Z, Rabe K, Diener HC. From migraine to stroke. Intern Emerg Med 2008;3(Suppl 1):S9.
21. Karras DJ, Ufberg JW, Harrigan RA, et al. Lack of relationship between hypertension-associated symptoms and blood pressure in hypertensive ED patients. Am J Emerg Med 2005;23:106.
22. Mitchell CS, Osborn RE, Grosskreutz SR. Computed tomography in the headache patient: is routine evaluation really necessary? Headache 1993;33:82.
23. Reinus WR, Wippold FJ 2nd, Erickson KK. Practical selection criteria for non-contrast cranial computed tomography in patients with head trauma. Ann Emerg Med 1993;22:1148.
24. Diaz M, Braude D, Skipper B. Concordance of historical questions used in risk-stratifying patients with headache. Am J Emerg Med 2007;25:907.
25. Harling DW, Peatfield RC, Van Hille PT, et al. Thunderclap headache: is it migraine? Cephalalgia 1989;9:87.
26. Lledo A, Calandre L, Martinez-Menendez B, et al. Acute headache of recent onset and subarachnoid hemorrhage: a prospective study. Headache 1994;34:172.
27. Edlow JA, Panagos PD, Godwin SA, et al. Clinical policy: critical issues in the evaluation and management of adult patients presenting to the emergency department with acute headache. Ann Emerg Med 2008;52:407.
28. Vannemreddy P, Nanda A, Kelley R, et al. Delayed diagnosis of intracranial aneurysms: confounding factors in clinical presentation and the influence of misdiagnosis on outcome. South Med J 2001;94:1108.
29. Polmear A. Sentinel headaches in aneurysmal subarachnoid haemorrhage: what is the true incidence? A systematic review. Cephalalgia 2003;23:935.
30. Hesselink JR, Dowd CF, Healy ME, et al. MR imaging of brain contusions: a comparative study with CT. AJR Am J Roentgenol 1988;150:1133.
31. Thomas KE, Hasbun R, Jekel J, et al. The diagnostic accuracy of Kernig's sign, Brudzinski's sign, and nuchal rigidity in adults with suspected meningitis. Clin Infect Dis 2002;35:46.
32. Attia J, Hatala R, Cook DJ, et al. The rational clinical examination. Does this adult patient have acute meningitis? JAMA 1999;282:175.
33. Uchihara T, Tsukagoshi H. Jolt accentuation of headache: the most sensitive sign of CSF pleocytosis. Headache 1991;31:167.
34. Kao LW, Nanagas KA. Carbon monoxide poisoning. Emerg Med Clin North Am 2004;22:985.
35. Centers for Disease Control and Prevention (CDC). Unintentional non-fire-related carbon monoxide exposures – United States, 2001–2003. MMWR Morb Mortal Wkly Rep 2005;54:36.
36. Salameh S, Amitai Y, Antopolsky M, et al. Carbon monoxide poisoning in Jerusalem: epidemiology and risk factors. Clin Toxicol (Phila) 2009;47:137.

37. Keles A, Demircan A, Kurtoglu G. Carbon monoxide poisoning: how many patients do we miss? Eur J Emerg Med 2008;15:154.
38. Hellmann DB. Temporal arteritis: a cough, toothache, and tongue infarction. JAMA 2002;287:2996.
39. Smetana GW, Shmerling RH. Does this patient have temporal arteritis? JAMA 2002;287:92.
40. Schievink WI. Spontaneous dissection of the carotid and vertebral arteries. N Engl J Med 2001;344:898.
41. Saeed AB, Shuaib A, Al-Sulaiti G, et al. Vertebral artery dissection: warning symptoms, clinical features and prognosis in 26 patients. Can J Neurol Sci 2000;27:292.
42. Matthys LA, Coppage KH, Lambers DS, et al. Delayed postpartum preeclampsia: an experience of 151 cases. Am J Obstet Gynecol 2004;190:1464.
43. Cantu C, Barinagarrementeria F. Cerebral venous thrombosis associated with pregnancy and puerperium. Review of 67 cases. Stroke 1993;24:1880.
44. Akatsu H, Vaysburd M, Fervenza F, et al. Cerebral venous thrombosis in nephrotic syndrome. Clin Nephrol 1997;48:317.
45. Ferro JM, Canhao P, Stam J, et al. Prognosis of cerebral vein and dural sinus thrombosis: results of the International Study on Cerebral Vein and Dural Sinus Thrombosis (ISCVT). Stroke 2004;35:664.
46. Cumurciuc R, Crassard I, Sarov M, et al. Headache as the only neurological sign of cerebral venous thrombosis: a series of 17 cases. J Neurol Neurosurg Psychiatr 2005;76:1084.
47. Beeson MS, Vesco JA, Reilly BA, et al. Dural sinus thrombosis. Am J Emerg Med 2002;20:568.
48. Lin A, Foroozan R, Danesh-Meyer HV, et al. Occurrence of cerebral venous sinus thrombosis in patients with presumed idiopathic intracranial hypertension. Ophthalmology 2006;113:2281.
49. Ooi LY, Walker BR, Bodkin PA, et al. Idiopathic intracranial hypertension: can studies of obesity provide the key to understanding pathogenesis? Br J Neurosurg 2008;22:187.
50. Randeva HS, Schoebel J, Byrne J, et al. Classical pituitary apoplexy: clinical features, management and outcome. Clin Endocrinol (Oxf) 1999;51:181.
51. Boesiger BM, Shiber JR. Subarachnoid hemorrhage diagnosis by computed tomography and lumbar puncture: are fifth generation CT scanners better at identifying subarachnoid hemorrhage? J Emerg Med 2005;29:23.
52. Byyny RL, Mower WR, Shum N, et al. Sensitivity of noncontrast cranial computed tomography for the emergency department diagnosis of subarachnoid hemorrhage. Ann Emerg Med 2008;51:697.
53. van der Wee N, Rinkel GJ, Hasan D, et al. Detection of subarachnoid haemorrhage on early CT: is lumbar puncture still needed after a negative scan? J Neurol Neurosurg Psychiatr 1995;58:357.
54. Sames TA, Storrow AB, Finkelstein JA, et al. Sensitivity of new-generation computed tomography in subarachnoid hemorrhage. Acad Emerg Med 1996;3:16.
55. Foot C, Staib A. How valuable is a lumbar puncture in the management of patients with suspected subarachnoid haemorrhage? Emerg Med (Fremantle) 2001;13:326.
56. Morgenstern LB, Luna-Gonzales H, Huber JC Jr, et al. Worst headache and subarachnoid hemorrhage: prospective, modern computed tomography and spinal fluid analysis. Ann Emerg Med 1998;32:297.

57. O'Neill J, McLaggan S, Gibson R. Acute headache and subarachnoid haemorrhage: a retrospective review of CT and lumbar puncture findings. Scott Med J 2005;50:151.

58. Sidman R, Connolly E, Lemke T. Subarachnoid hemorrhage diagnosis: lumbar puncture is still needed when the computed tomography scan is normal. Acad Emerg Med 1996;3:827.

59. Schriger DL, Kalafut M, Starkman S, et al. Cranial computed tomography interpretation in acute stroke: physician accuracy in determining eligibility for thrombolytic therapy. JAMA 1998;279:1293.

60. van Gijn J, van Dongen K. The time course of aneurysmal haemorrhage on computed tomograms. Neuroradiology 1982;23:153–6.

61. Mohamed M, Heasly DC, Yagmurlu B, et al. Fluid-attenuated inversion recovery MR imaging and subarachnoid hemorrhage: not a panacea. AJNR Am J Neuroradiol 2004;25:545.

62. El Khaldi M, Pernter P, Ferro F, et al. Detection of cerebral aneurysms in nontraumatic subarachnoid haemorrhage: role of multislice CT angiography in 130 consecutive patients. Radiol Med 2007;112:123.

63. White PM, Wardlaw JM, Easton V. Can noninvasive imaging accurately depict intracranial aneurysms? A systematic review. Radiology 2000;217:361.

64. Chappell ET, Moure FC, Good MC. Comparison of computed tomographic angiography with digital subtraction angiography in the diagnosis of cerebral aneurysms: a meta-analysis. Neurosurgery 2003;52:624.

65. Johnson MR, Good CD, Penny WD, et al. Lesson of the week: playing the odds in clinical decision making: lessons from berry aneurysms undetected by magnetic resonance angiography. BMJ 2001;322:1347.

66. Wiebers DO. Unruptured intracranial aneurysms: natural history and clinical management. Update on the international study of unruptured intracranial aneurysms. Neuroimaging Clin N Am 2006;16:383.

67. Rinkel GJ, Djibuti M, Algra A, et al. Prevalence and risk of rupture of intracranial aneurysms: a systematic review. Stroke 1998;29:251.

68. Cortez O, Schaeffer CJ, Hatem SF, et al. Cases from the Cleveland Clinic: cerebral venous sinus thrombosis presenting to the emergency department with worst headache of life. Emerg Radiol 2009;16:79.

69. Savitz SI, Caplan LR, Edlow JA. Pitfalls in the diagnosis of cerebellar infarction. Acad Emerg Med 2007;14:63.

70. Shah KH, Richard KM, Nicholas S, et al. Incidence of traumatic lumbar puncture. Acad Emerg Med 2003;10:151.

71. Graves P, Sidman R. Xanthochromia is not pathognomonic for subarachnoid hemorrhage. Acad Emerg Med 2004;11:131.

72. Naidech AM, Janjua N, Kreiter KT, et al. Predictors and impact of aneurysm rebleeding after subarachnoid hemorrhage. Arch Neurol 2005;62:410.

73. Sidman R, Spitalnic S, Demelis M, et al. Xanthrochromia? By what method? A comparison of visual and spectrophotometric xanthrochromia. Ann Emerg Med 2005;46:51.

74. Edlow JA, Caplan LR. Avoiding pitfalls in the diagnosis of subarachnoid hemorrhage. N Engl J Med 2000;342:29.

75. Perry JJ, Spacek A, Forbes M, et al. Is the combination of negative computed tomography result and negative lumbar puncture result sufficient to rule out subarachnoid hemorrhage? Ann Emerg Med 2008;51:707.

76. Mazor SS, McNulty JE, Roosevelt GE. Interpretation of traumatic lumbar punctures: who can go home? Pediatrics 2003;111:525.

77. Kennedy PG, Chaudhuri A. Herpes simplex encephalitis. J Neurol Neurosurg Psychiatr 2002;73:237.
78. Benson PC, Swadron SP. Empiric acyclovir is infrequently initiated in the emergency department to patients ultimately diagnosed with encephalitis. Ann Emerg Med 2006;47:100.
79. Lin W, Geiderman J. Myth: fluids, bed rest, and caffeine are effective in preventing and treating patients with post-lumbar puncture headache. West J Med 2002;176:69.
80. Ebinger F, Kosel C, Pietz J, et al. Strict bed rest following lumbar puncture in children and adolescents is of no benefit. Neurology 2004;62:1003.
81. Thomas SR, Jamieson DR, Muir KW. Randomised controlled trial of atraumatic versus standard needles for diagnostic lumbar puncture. BMJ 2000;321:986.
82. Halpern S, Preston R. Postdural puncture headache and spinal needle design. Metaanalyses. Anesthesiology 1994;81:1376.
83. Safa-Tisseront V, Thormann F, Malassine P, et al. Effectiveness of epidural blood patch in the management of post-dural puncture headache. Anesthesiology 2001;95:334.
84. Rennick G, Shann F, de Campo J. Cerebral herniation during bacterial meningitis in children. BMJ 1993;306:953.
85. Hasbun R, Abrahams J, Jekel J, et al. Computed tomography of the head before lumbar puncture in adults with suspected meningitis. N Engl J Med 2001;345:1727.
86. Schull MJ. Lumbar puncture first: an alternative model for the investigation of lone acute sudden headache. Acad Emerg Med 1999;6:131.
87. Haapaniemi E, Tatlisumak T. Is D-dimer helpful in evaluating stroke patients? A systematic review. Acta Neurol Scand 2009;119:141.
88. Squizzato A, Ageno W. D-dimer testing in ischemic stroke and cerebral sinus and venous thrombosis. Semin Vasc Med 2005;5:379.
89. Misra UK, Kalita J, Bansal V. D-dimer is useful in the diagnosis of cortical venous sinus thrombosis. Neurol India 2009;57:50.
90. Bousser MG, Ferro JM. Cerebral venous thrombosis: an update. Lancet Neurol 2007;6:162.
91. Colman I, Rothney A, Wright SC, et al. Use of narcotic analgesics in the emergency department treatment of migraine headache. Neurology 2004;62:1695.
92. Gupta MX, Silberstein SD, Young WB, et al. Less is not more: underutilization of headache medications in a university hospital emergency department. Headache 2007;47:1125.
93. Friedman BW, Corbo J, Lipton RB, et al. A trial of metoclopramide vs sumatriptan for the emergency department treatment of migraines. Neurology 2005;64:463.
94. Griffith JD, Mycyk MB, Kyriacou DN. Metoclopramide versus hydromorphone for the emergency department treatment of migraine headache. J Pain 2008;9:88.
95. Ginder S, Oatman B, Pollack M. A prospective study of i.v. magnesium and i.v. prochlorperazine in the treatment of headaches. J Emerg Med 2000;18:311.
96. Tanen DA, Miller S, French T, et al. Intravenous sodium valproate versus prochlorperazine for the emergency department treatment of acute migraine headaches: a prospective, randomized, double-blind trial. Ann Emerg Med 2003;41:847.
97. Callan JE, Kostic MA, Bachrach EA, et al. Prochlorperazine vs. promethazine for headache treatment in the emergency department: a randomized controlled trial. J Emerg Med 2008;35:247.
98. Lane PL, McLellan BA, Baggoley CJ. Comparative efficacy of chlorpromazine and meperidine with dimenhydrinate in migraine headache. Ann Emerg Med 1989;18:360.

99. Bell R, Montoya D, Shuaib A, et al. A comparative trial of three agents in the treatment of acute migraine headache. Ann Emerg Med 1990;19:1079.

100. Colman I, Brown MD, Innes GD, et al. Parenteral metoclopramide for acute migraine: meta-analysis of randomised controlled trials. BMJ 2004;329:1369.

101. Weaver CS, Jones JB, Chisholm CD, et al. Droperidol vs prochlorperazine for the treatment of acute headache. J Emerg Med 2004;26:145.

102. Miner JR, Fish SJ, Smith SW, et al. Droperidol vs. prochlorperazine for benign headaches in the emergency department. Acad Emerg Med 2001;8:873.

103. Coppola M, Yealy DM, Leibold RA. Randomized, placebo-controlled evaluation of prochlorperazine versus metoclopramide for emergency department treatment of migraine headache. Ann Emerg Med 1995;26:541.

104. Jones J, Pack S, Chun E. Intramuscular prochlorperazine versus metoclopramide as single-agent therapy for the treatment of acute migraine headache. Am J Emerg Med 1996;14:262.

105. Richman PB, Reischel U, Ostrow A, et al. Droperidol for acute migraine headache. Am J Emerg Med 1999;17:398.

106. Vinson DR. Treatment patterns of isolated benign headache in US emergency departments. Ann Emerg Med 2002;39:215.

107. Hurtado TR, Vinson DR, Vandenberg JT. ED treatment of migraine headache: factors influencing pharmacotherapeutic choices. Headache 2007;47:1134.

108. Gupta A, Lawrence AT, Krishnan K, et al. Current concepts in the mechanisms and management of drug-induced QT prolongation and torsade de pointes. Am Heart J 2007;153:891.

109. Vinson DR. Diphenhydramine in the treatment of akathisia induced by prochlorperazine. J Emerg Med 2004;26:265.

110. Vinson DR, Migala AF, Quesenberry CP Jr. Slow infusion for the prevention of akathisia induced by prochlorperazine: a randomized controlled trial. J Emerg Med 2001;20:113.

111. Vinson DR, Drotts DL. Diphenhydramine for the prevention of akathisia induced by prochlorperazine: a randomized, controlled trial. Ann Emerg Med 2001;37:125.

112. Friedman BW, Grosberg BM. Diagnosis and management of the primary headache disorders in the emergency department setting. Emerg Med Clin North Am 2009;27:71.

113. Colman I, Brown MD, Innes GD, et al. Parenteral dihydroergotamine for acute migraine headache: a systematic review of the literature. Ann Emerg Med 2005;45:393.

114. Tomita M, Suzuki N, Igarashi H, et al. Evidence against strong correlation between chest symptoms and ischemic coronary changes after subcutaneous sumatriptan injection. Intern Med 2002;41:622.

115. Dodick D, Lipton RB, Martin V, et al. Consensus statement: cardiovascular safety profile of triptans (5-HT agonists) in the acute treatment of migraine. Headache 2004;44:414.

116. Proulx N, Frechette D, Toye B, et al. Delays in the administration of antibiotics are associated with mortality from adult acute bacterial meningitis. QJM 2005; 98:291.

117. Miner JR, Heegaard W, Mapes A, et al. Presentation, time to antibiotics, and mortality of patients with bacterial meningitis at an urban county medical center. J Emerg Med 2001;21:387.

118. Radetsky M. Duration of symptoms and outcome in bacterial meningitis: an analysis of causation and the implications of a delay in diagnosis. Pediatr Infect Dis J 1992;11:694.

119. Talan DA, Hoffman JR, Yoshikawa TT, et al. Role of empiric parenteral antibiotics prior to lumbar puncture in suspected bacterial meningitis: state of the art. Rev Infect Dis 1988;10:365.
120. de Gans J, van de Beek D. Dexamethasone in adults with bacterial meningitis. N Engl J Med 2002;347:1549.
121. van de Beek D, de Gans J, McIntyre P, et-al: Corticosteroids for acute bacterial meningitis. Cochrane Database Syst Rev, 2007;(1):CD004405.
122. Fitch MT, van de Beek D. Emergency diagnosis and treatment of adult meningitis. Lancet Infect Dis 2007;7:191.
123. Tunkel AR, Hartman BJ, Kaplan SL, et al. Practice guidelines for the management of bacterial meningitis. Clin Infect Dis 2004;39:1267.
124. Ducharme J, Beveridge RC, Lee JS, et al. Emergency management of migraine: is the headache really over? Acad Emerg Med 1998;5:899.
125. Friedman BW, Hochberg ML, Esses D, et al. Recurrence of primary headache disorders after emergency department discharge: frequency and predictors of poor pain and functional outcomes. Ann Emerg Med 2008;52:696.
126. Rowe BH, Colman I, Edmonds ML, et al. Randomized controlled trial of intravenous dexamethasone to prevent relapse in acute migraine headache. Headache 2008;48:333.
127. Akpunonu BE, Mutgi AB, Federman DJ, et al. Subcutaneous sumatriptan for treatment of acute migraine in patients admitted to the emergency department: a multicenter study. Ann Emerg Med 1995;25:464.
128. Donaldson D, Sundermann R, Jackson R, et al. Intravenous dexamethasone vs placebo as adjunctive therapy to reduce the recurrence rate of acute migraine headaches: a multicenter, double-blinded, placebo-controlled randomized clinical trial. Am J Emerg Med 2008;26:124.
129. Kelly AM, Kerr D, Clooney M. Impact of oral dexamethasone versus placebo after ED treatment of migraine with phenothiazines on the rate of recurrent headache: a randomised controlled trial. Emerg Med J 2008;25:26.
130. Friedman BW, Greenwald P, Bania TC, et al. Randomized trial of IV dexamethasone for acute migraine in the emergency department. Neurology 2007;69:2038.
131. Colman I, Friedman BW, Brown MD, et al. Parenteral dexamethasone for acute severe migraine headache: meta-analysis of randomised controlled trials for preventing recurrence. BMJ 2008;336:1359.

Toxicology: Pearls and Pitfalls in the Use of Antidotes

Craig G. Smollin, MD[a,b,c]

KEYWORDS

• Toxicology • Antidotes • Acute poisoning • Toxin therapy

The management of the acutely poisoned patient first and foremost requires careful attention to the basic principles of emergency medicine. The patient's airway, breathing, and circulation must be evaluated and addressed systematically, and supportive care instituted expeditiously. With few exceptions, supportive care alone will effectively treat the majority of patients who present with acute poisoning. In 2008, according to the American Association of Poison Control Centers Toxic Exposure Surveillance System (TESS), besides decontamination, the most commonly instituted specific therapy in acute poisoning was the administration of intravenous fluids followed by the administration of oxygen.[1] In certain circumstances, however, prompt administration of a specific antidote may be required, and failure to identify these circumstances may lead to significant morbidity or mortality. This article aims to describe select antidotes, and to discuss their indications and the potential pitfalls with their use.

HIGH-DOSE INSULIN EUGLYCEMIC THERAPY FOR THE TREATMENT OF CALCIUM CHANNEL BLOCKER OVERDOSE

Acute calcium channel blocker (CCB) overdose is associated with significant morbidity and mortality. In 2008, the American Association of Poison Control Centers TESS reported 10,084 CCB exposures, of which 2232 were treated in health care facilities. Outcomes were defined as moderate in 361 cases and major in 74 cases, and there were 17 deaths.[1] The clinical features of severe CCB toxicity are the result of excessive blockade at L-type calcium channels located in myocardial cells, smooth muscle cells of the peripheral vasculature, and β cells in the pancreas. Antagonism of these channels produces decreased inotropy, bradycardia, myocardial conduction disturbances, peripheral vasodilation, and hypoinsulinemia, resulting in hyperglycemia. The combination of these effects can result in metabolic acidosis and refractory hypotension and shock.

[a] University of California San Francisco, Department of Emergency Medicine, 505 Parnassus Avenue, Rm. L-126, Box 0208, San Francisco, CA 94143-0208, USA
[b] California Poison Control System, San Francisco Division, University of California San Francisco, UCSF Box 1369, San Francisco, CA 94143-1369
[c] San Francisco General Hospital, Emergency Services, 1001 Potrero Avenue, Suite 1E21, San Francisco, CA 94110, USA
E-mail address: craig.smollin@emergency.ucsf.edu

Emerg Med Clin N Am 28 (2010) 149–161
doi:10.1016/j.emc.2009.09.009
0733-8627/09/$ – see front matter © 2010 Published by Elsevier Inc.

emed.theclinics.com

Significant CCB ingestions can pose a particular challenge to the emergency physician, because although the patient may initially appear well, hemodynamic decompensation can rapidly ensue.[2] In addition, conventional treatments produce variable responses, and often fail to restore hemodynamic stability.[3,4] These treatments include the administration of intravenous fluids to increase intravascular volume, calcium salts such as calcium gluconate or calcium chloride to increase transmembrane calcium flow, atropine to decrease vagal tone and increase heart rate, and the administration of vasoactive agents or glucagon. In some cases, intravenous pacing or an intra-aortic balloon pump may be necessary.[5]

High-dose insulin euglycemic therapy (HIET) consists of the infusion of high-dose regular insulin, most commonly as a bolus of 1 IU/kg followed by an infusion of 0.5 IU/kg per hour, along with the administration of supplemental glucose to maintain euglycemia (**Table 1**). HIET requires frequent blood glucose monitoring (every 30 minutes), and serum potassium should also be monitored and repleted as needed. The duration of therapy should be tailored to clinical response, in particular to hemodynamic parameters.[2]

The proposed mechanism by which HIET reverses hemodynamic collapse is through direct metabolic effects on myocardial cells.[6–8] It is hypothesized that in a state of shock, myocytes switch from the utilization of free fatty acids to glucose in order to meet metabolic demands. CCBs induce a state of hypoinsulinemia, preventing the uptake of glucose by myocytes and causing a loss of inotropy, decreased peripheral vascular resistance, and shock.[6–8] High doses of insulin might therefore be able to reverse these metabolic derangements.

Animal studies suggest that the administration of HIET may be more effective than conventional therapies. In a series of studies of verapamil-poisoned canines performed by Kline and colleagues,[6–8] HIET outperformed epinephrine, glucagon, and calcium chloride in increasing myocardial contractility, and resulted in improved survival. Although there are no randomized controlled trials in humans, there are numerous human case reports in the literature demonstrating the efficacy of HIET in improving blood pressure and hemodynamic collapse in patients refractory to other interventions including atropine, calcium chloride, glucagon, and vasoactive agents.[4–15]

It should not be overlooked, however, that there are many published case reports demonstrating the failure of HIET to reverse CCB-induced hemodynamic collapse. Some of these reports have in common the late initiation of HIET, after the development of severe symptoms,[16–18] and may indicate that HIET should be considered early in severe CCB toxicity rather than as a therapy of "last resort."

Given the small numbers of patients presenting to any given institution with CCB overdose and the variability of individual ingestion, it is unlikely that randomized prospective data on the efficacy of HIET will ever become available. However, this limitation is shared by all of the conventional therapies currently used in the treatment of CCB overdose. Both the animal data and human case reports provide some evidence that early treatment with HIET in conjunction with conventional measures may be of benefit. Given the significant potential for precipitous hemodynamic decline in patients who overdose on CCBs, emergency physicians should likely be prepared to initiate early and aggressive therapy that includes HIET.

INTRAVENOUS LIPID EMULSION

The administration of intravenous lipid emulsion (ILE) has rapidly emerged as a possible antidote for a variety of lipophilic cardiotoxic drugs. ILE conventionally provides calories in the form of free fatty acids to patients requiring total parenteral

Table 1
Antidotes discussed and their usage

Antidote	Primary Indication by Substance	Dose and Administration
High dose insulin euglycemic therapy (HIE)	Severe calcium channel blocker poisoning	• Bolus of Regular Insulin 1U/kg followed by infusion at 0.5–1.0 U/kg/h. Give 25 gm (50 cc of D50W) initially and monitor glucose frequently to prevent hypoglycemia. Monitor serum potassium and replace as needed to avoid hypokalemia.
Intravenous lipid emulsion (Intralipid)	Lipophillic cardiotoxic agents	• 1.5 mL/kg of 20% intralipid as an initial bolus followed by 0.25 mL/kg/min for 30–60 min. • Depending upon response, bolus could be repeated 1-2 times and infusion rate increased.
Hydroxocobalamin (Cyanokit, 5 g per kit)	Cyanide	• 5 grams as intravenous infusion over 15 min. • Depending on severity of poisoning, a second dose of 5 grams may be administered.
Oral N-Acetylcysteine(NAC) Mucomyst (Apothecon; Plainsboro, NJ) or equivalent, 10% or 20%	Acetaminophen	• **Loading dose**: 140 mg/kg diluted in juice or soda to produce a 5% solution • **Maintenance dose**: 70 mg/kg every 4 hours for 4 doses (uncomplicated cases)
Intravenous N-Acetylcysteine (NAC) Acetadote, 20%	Acetaminophen	• **Loading dose**: 150 mg/kg in 200 mL of 5% dextrose in water (D5W) over one hour • **Maintenance dose**: 50 mg/kg in 500 mL of D5W over four hours then 100 mg/kg in 1000 mL of D5W over 16 hours • Note: dosing based on ideal body weight; and, use smaller diluents doses of D5W in children
Crotalid Antivenom CroFab [Crotalidae polyvalent immune Fab (ovine)]; Protherics PLC; Cheshire UK	Rattlesnake envenomation	• Depending on severity of bite, initial dose ranges from 4-8 vials. • Repeat until there is a halt in progression of symptoms • Additional 2-vial doses every 6 hours for up to 18 hours, if needed

nutrition.[19] In addition, animal studies have suggested its effectiveness in resuscitation from the cardiotoxic effects of bupivacaine,[20,21] chlorpromazine,[22] clomipramine,[23] propranolol,[24] and verapamil.[19] The first case report of the use of ILE in humans appeared in the anesthesia literature in relation to the rare occurrence of cardiovascular collapse in the setting of regional anesthesia with ropivacaine.[25] Since then, numerous case reports have emerged demonstrating its efficacy in bupivacaine-induced cardiovascular collapse.[26–28]

In the last several years, the use of ILE in humans has been reported for overdoses of other lipid-soluble cardiac toxins. In a case report of a combined buproprion and lamotrigine overdose in which cardiac arrest had proved refractory to conventional treatment, ILE infusion was associated with the return of spontaneous circulation and a good patient outcome.[29] In a report of a combined quetiapine and sertraline overdose it was demonstrated to reverse coma, allowing the treating physicians to avoid intubation.[30] Finally, in a case of sustained-release verapamil overdose resulting in shock, its administration was temporally associated with a dramatic improvement in blood pressure and cessation of vasopressors and glucagon.[31] Although there is no standard protocol for ILE, a 1.5 mL/kg bolus of Intralipid 20% followed by an infusion of 0.25 mL/kg/min for 30 to 60 minutes has been described (see **Table 1**).[32]

Several mechanisms of action have been suggested. One theory is that ILE acts as a "lipid sink," expanding the lipid compartment within the intravascular space, and sequestering lipid-soluble drugs from the tissues. The success of ILE in the treatment of poisoning by lipid-soluble drugs such as bupivacaine, propranolol, and verapamil supports this theory. Another explanation suggests that its efficacy is related to metabolic effects in the myocardium, specifically its ability to enhance fatty acid intracellular transport in myocardial cells.[19]

Many questions remain, including the identification of potential safety hazards. ILE is contraindicated in patients with known egg allergies, disorders of fat metabolism, and liver disease.[19] In patients receiving total parenteral nutrition (TPN), high triglycerides resulting from ILE infusion may alter immunity, lung function, and hemodynamics.[19] Yet TPN patients receive intravenous lipid emulsion for an extended period of time, rather than as short-term rescue dosing. With bolus dosing and at high doses, ILE can potentially result in pulmonary and fat emboli.[19] Finally, there is also evidence to suggest that ILE is contraindicated in acute myocardial infarction, because free fatty acids administered during ischemia may increase myocardial damage through lipid peroxidation.[19]

For now, ILE is an intriguing antidote that holds the promise of a potential "intravascular decontamination" method for lipophilic drugs. The use of ILE as an adjunctive therapy to standard Advanced Cardiac Life Support protocols in the rare setting of cardiac arrest due to the administration of regional anesthesia with bupivacaine seems justified. Case reports of its use in the setting of lipophilic drug overdose are compelling, but more research is needed. Although it is too early to consider ILE a stand-alone therapy in the setting of lipophilic drug overdose, it should be considered when conventional therapies fail.

THE USE OF HYDROXOCOBALAMIN IN SMOKE INHALATION VICTIMS

Inhalation of smoke accounts for more fire-related morbidity and mortality than burns.[33] Fire smoke contains a complex mixture of gases released from the combustion of natural and synthetic materials, which contribute to smoke inhalation-associated death. Among these are carbon monoxide (CO) and hydrogen cyanide (HCN).

CO binds to hemoglobin with 250 times the affinity of oxygen and shifts the oxygen hemoglobin dissociation curve to the left.[34] This results in decreased carrying capacity of hemoglobin for oxygen (functional anemia) and impaired delivery of oxygen to vital tissues, resulting in cellular hypoxia, cardiovascular collapse, and death. HCN inhibits oxidative phosphorylation by binding to cytochrome oxidase in the electron transport chain. The end result is similar to CO, in that cellular hypoxia ensues, causing lactic acidosis, cardiovascular collapse and death.

Studies on smoke exposure victims indicate that CO and HCN are often both present.[33] Whereas CO can be quickly detected in venous or arterial blood with the use of cooximetry, cyanide levels cannot be obtained rapidly in most hospitals. A surrogate marker, lactic acidosis, may be elevated in cyanide exposure, but can also be present in CO poisoning.

Management of smoke inhalation involves removal of the victim from further exposure, airway support, and the administration of supplement oxygen. CO poisoning is usually treated with high-flow oxygen, and sometimes hyperbaric oxygen, whereas HCN poisoning requires the administration of a specific antidote.

The conventional cyanide antidote kit (consisting of amyl nitrite, sodium nitrite, and sodium thiosulfate) may be unsuitable for the empiric treatment of the undifferentiated smoke inhalation victim. Amyl nitrite and sodium nitrite work through the induction of methemoglobinemia. Cyanide preferentially binds to methemoglobin, preventing or delaying its binding to the cytochrome oxidase in the electron transport chain. However, methemoglobinemia also reduces the oxygen-carrying capacity of blood, and can therefore exacerbate CO toxicity and hypoxemia from lung injury due to smoke inhalation. Furthermore, both amyl nitrite and sodium nitrite can cause vasodilation and exacerbate hypotension.[35] Therefore, empiric use of these agents is not recommended in smoke inhalation victims. The third component of the kit, sodium thiosulfate, does not induce methemoglobinemia, but enhances the elimination of cyanide by acting as a sulfhydryl donor in the conversion of cyanide to thiocyanate. Although sodium thiosulfate can be given alone, it has been suggested that its delayed onset of action, and limited penetration into the brain and mitochondria, may make it a less effective antidote.[35]

An alternative antidote, hydroxocobalamin, has been used in France since the 1980s. Hydroxocobalamin is the natural form of vitamin B_{12a}, which directly binds to cyanide to form nontoxic cyanocobalamin (vitamin B_{12}). In multiple animal models, hydroxocobalamin was an effective antidote even when given after cyanide exposure rather than as prophylaxis.[36–38] Hydroxocobalamin's efficacy was compared with saline in dogs administered intravenous potassium cyanide.[38] In the saline-treated dogs, the overall mortality rate was 82% (14/17), whereas 79% (15/19) and 100% (18/18) of the dogs treated with 75 mg/kg or 150 mg/kg, respectively, survived. Although no efficacy data are available in humans (due to the ethical issues of a placebo controlled trial), a prospective noncomparative trial in victims of fire-smoke inhalation and documented cyanide exposure demonstrated a survival rate of 72% (50/69) in patients treated with 5 to 15 g intravenously.[33] In addition, 82% (41/50) of the survivors showed no neuropsychiatric sequelae. Many of the patients in this study were also shown to have concomitant CO exposure, suggesting that the antidote is safe for administration in the setting of concomitant CO exposure. A retrospective review of 101 smoke inhalation victims treated with hydroxocobalamin showed a survival rate of 41.7%, and of 38 patients found in cardiac arrest, 21 had return of spontaneous circulation.[39]

The recommended dosing for hydroxocobalamin (Cyanokit) is an intravenous initial infusion of 5 g over 15 minutes (see **Table 1**). Depending on the severity of the poisoning and the clinical response, a second dose of 5 g may be administered.[40] The most frequently reported adverse effect of hydroxycobalamin is a red discoloration of the urine and skin that does not appear to be of any clinical significance, but can last for several days.[39] This red discoloration may also affect some laboratory tests that depend on colorimetric assays. Temporary increases in blood pressure, headache, nausea, and injection site reactions have also been reported.[40] Allergic reactions have been observed in a small number of individuals, but are relatively mild and have responded quickly to standard treatment.[36]

Hydroxocobalamin seems to be a safe and effective therapy in the undifferentiated smoke inhalation victim, and has a limited side effect profile. Of importance is that the use of sodium thiosulfate alone may also be an effective and cheaper option, but no trials directly comparing the 2 antidotes have been carried out. Until then, both drugs should be considered options for the treatment of this patient population.

INTRAVENOUS *N*-ACETYLCYSTEINE FOR THE TREATMENT OF ACETAMINOPHEN POISONING AND SHORT-COURSE THERAPY

Acetaminophen is one of the most common causes of poisoning worldwide.[41] According to the American Association of Poison Control Centers TESS, in the United States in 2008 alone, acetaminophen was responsible for more than 26,000 visits to health care facilities and approximately 74 deaths.[1] In overdose, acetaminophen is metabolized by the P450 system of the liver to the toxic metabolite, *N*-acetyl-*p*-benzoquinone imine (NAPQI), resulting in the destruction of liver cells.[42] *N*-Acetylcysteine (NAC) prevents hepatic injury primarily by restoring hepatic glutathione, which binds to NAPQI to form nontoxic metabolites.[42]

Intravenous NAC was first suggested as an antidote for acetaminophen toxicity in 1974, and NAC was first introduced to the United States as an oral preparation with a 72-hour treatment protocol.[41] Following its introduction, a multicenter study involving 2540 patients over 9 years showed that 6.1% of patients who received oral NAC within 10 hours of their ingestion developed hepatotoxicity.[43] This result was a marked improvement when compared with historical controls, and contributed to the widespread acceptance of NAC for the treatment of acetaminophen overdose.

Over the years, emergency physicians have become familiar with the use of NAC. When no approved intravenous formulation was available, physicians could administer the oral form intravenously after running it through a micropore filter. In 2004, the Food and Drug Administration (FDA) approved an intravenous formulation of NAC (Acetadote). The approved 20-hour dosing regimen for Acetadote is identical to that used for many years in Canada and Europe, and is considerably shorter than the conventional 72-hour oral NAC regimen. Acetadote's ease of use and shorter course have made intravenous NAC a popular choice for treatment of acetaminophen overdose. According to data collected by the American Association of Poison Control Centers in the 4 years from 2004 to 2008, the use of intravenous NAC jumped from 3807 to 11,895 instances and exceeded the use of oral NAC by approximately 150.[1,44] That same time period saw the use of oral NAC decrease from 15,333 to 11,764 uses.[1,44]

The dosing regimens of the oral and intravenous formulations of NAC are listed in **Table 1**. There are no formal studies comparing the use of intravenous versus oral NAC, but experience suggests that they are equally efficacious. Intravenous NAC may be advantageous in the patient with an altered level of consciousness, or when there is significant nausea and vomiting precluding the use of oral medications. It should be noted, however, that oral NAC is generally well tolerated, especially when given in conjunction with an antiemetic. While both therapies are relatively inexpensive, intravenous NAC costs approximately $470 for a 20-hour course compared with $50 for a 72-hour course of oral NAC,[41] and there may be additional administration costs for intravenous use.

The most commonly reported adverse side effect of intravenous NAC is anaphylactoid reactions, which may occur in up to 15% of patients.[45] Most symptoms are mild and include rash and pruritus; however, 1% are severe and may include bronchospasm, tachycardia, and hypotension.[42] Depending on the severity of the reaction, treatment includes the administration of diphenhydramine, corticosteroids, and bronchodilators. Although a decrease in the infusion rate of intravenous NAC may result in a decreased incidence of anaphylactoid reactions, studies have produced conflicting results.[45,46] Nonetheless, the manufacturer has changed the recommended initial infusion rate from 15 minutes to 60 minutes.

Studies have shown that patients with a family history of allergy and asthmatics are at increased risk of anaphylactoid reactions to NAC.[47] Death has been reported in a patient with a history of asthma,[48] and physicians should be particularly cautious with the administration of intravenous NAC in this patient population. In addition, an inverse correlation has been observed between serum N-acetyl-para-aminophenol concentrations and anaphylactoid reactions,[47,49–52] suggesting that acetaminophen itself has protective properties against the adverse effects of NAC. This unexpected finding suggests that physicians should use the oral formulation in patients with low or borderline acetaminophen concentration. Finally, dosing errors with the intravenous infusion have also led to deaths.[53,54] Dilutional hyponatremia and seizures developed in a child receiving the adult volume of intravenous NAC.[55] For pediatric patients, volumes should be adjusted to body weight, and normal saline solution should be used as the diluent.

The conventional oral NAC regimen has a recommended duration of therapy of 72 hours, whereas the intravenous preparation has a recommended 20-hour protocol. This discrepancy can often lead to confusion over when to stop treatment. Evidence supports the use of a shortened protocol in patients with acute acetaminophen overdose, who receive their first dose of NAC (either intravenously or orally) within 8 hours of arrival in the emergency department.[56,57] Patients should have repeat acetaminophen measurements and liver function test performed at the end of the 20-hour protocol to ensure the absence of liver damage and nondetectable acetaminophen levels. A critical mistake is the use of the 20-hour regimen in the setting of delayed presentations, and large or chronic acetaminophen ingestions. Premature cessation of therapy in this setting has resulted in hepatotoxicity.[58]

In summary, NAC is a safe and effective therapy for the treatment of acetaminophen overdose, and has been used by emergency physicians for several decades. The introduction of an FDA-approved intravenous formulation has greatly increased this route of administration. Physicians must be aware of the risk of anaphylactoid reactions, especially among asthmatics and those with low serum acetaminophen levels. Dosing errors, in particular among pediatric patients, have led to deaths. The shortened (20-hour) protocol is appropriate for patients with acute ingestions, who receive NAC within 8 hours of ingestion, and have normal liver function tests and undetectable acetaminophen levels at the end of treatment.

CROTALIDAE POLYVALENT IMMUNE FAB (OVINE; FabAV) and thrombocytopenia

Each year, there are approximately 8000 venomous snakebites in the United States, most of which are caused by the Crotalidae (pit viper) family.[59] Snake venoms are complex mixtures of substances that function to immobilize, kill, and predigest prey.[34] In humans these substances precipitate tissue destruction at the bite site, and have hemotoxic, neurotoxic, and other systemic effects. The relative predominance of these effects is variable and depends on the species of snake, as well as geographic and seasonal factors.[34]

The clinical presentation after a significant rattlesnake bite includes stinging and burning pain at the site of the bite, accompanied by progressive swelling and erythema. Petechiae, ecchymosis, and hemorrhagic blebs may develop over several hours. Hypovolemic shock and local compartment syndrome may occur secondary to fluid and blood sequestration in the affected area.[34] Neurotoxic effects may result in nausea, vomiting, weakness, muscle fasciculations, a metallic taste in the mouth, and perioral and peripheral paresthesias. Venom-induced hematologic effects can include thrombocytopenia and coagulopathy.

The evaluation of the snakebite victim begins with an assessment of the bite site and identification of systemic toxicity. The affected area should be measured, and the leading edge of swelling demarcated and frequently reassessed. Complete blood cell count, coagulation studies, chemistry panel, and creatine phosphokinase along with fibrinogen and D-dimer levels should be obtained. It should be noted that approximately 25% of rattlesnake bites are "dry" bites, in which no envenomation has occurred.[59] In such cases there will be minimal to no swelling at the bite site, with no progression of symptoms over time and no systemic symptoms. Patients with apparent dry bites should be observed for at least 12 hours to ensure that no delayed symptoms develop before being sent home. Patients with signs or symptoms of envenomation should be given antivenom.

For many years, the only available antivenom was the equine-derived Antivenin Crotalidae polyvalent (ACP), and a significant proportion of patients receiving this antidote developed both immediate and delayed-onset hypersensitivity reactions. In retrospective studies, the incidence of acute allergic reactions from ACP (including hypotension and anaphylaxis) ranged between 23% and 56%, and virtually all patients who received more than 12 vials developed serum sickness.[34]

In 2000, Crotalidae polyvalent immune fab (ovine; FabAV) became available as an alternative to ACP. FabAV is derived from sheep immunized with the venom of 1 of 4 species of rattlesnake (*Crotalus atox*, *Crotalus adamantus*, *Crotalus scutulatus*, and *Agkistrodon piscivorus*). Papain is used to cleave the immunogenic Fc fragment from the IgG antibody, producing a purified Fab fragment antivenom. Experience using Crofab compared with ACP indicates a substantially reduced incidence of allergic reactions and serum sickness with apparently equal efficacy.[60] Because of its improved safety profile, FabAV has essentially replaced ACP for the treatment of rattlesnake bites in the United States (see **Table 1** for a description of dosing regimens).

The adoption of FabAV as the treatment of choice in snakebite victims has coincided with the documentation of recurrent thrombocytopenia and thrombocytopenia refractory to additional doses of antivenom. Published case reports and postmarketing surveillance describe patients with thrombocytopenia that is initially responsive to antivenom, but refractory to additional doses of FabAV when it recurs.[61–65] Boyer and colleagues[66] conducted a multicenter, prospective clinical trial designed to detect recurrent and persistent coagulation abnormalities after FabAV administration. These investigators showed that 53% (20 of 38 patients) had recurrent, persistent or late coagulopathy from 2 to 14 days after envenomation. Even more concerning are reports of clinically significant bleeding in association with thrombocytopenia.[61]

These findings were not previously reported following the administration of the ACP antivenom. Some investigators have hypothesized that the smaller molecular weight of FabAV compared with ACP allows for more rapid renal clearance, resulting in recurrent symptoms. This theory, however, does not explain why some patients' recurrent thrombocytopenia is resistant to further FabAV administration. Others suggest that delayed coagulation abnormalities were simply not recognized with the use of the ACP, because clinicians did not repeat coagulation studies after discharge. In a retrospective review, Bogdan and colleagues[67] tried to reevaluate patients treated with ACP for recurrent coagulopathy. Unfortunately, in a review of 354 consecutive cases, they found only 31 with adequate follow-up testing, but 14 of these 31 cases (45%) did reveal recurrent coagulopathy.

Whether recurrent and refractory thrombocytopenia is a function of the new FabAV antivenom or just a newly recognized phenomenon, it may result in a real risk of clinically significant bleeding. Clinicians must be aware of this risk, and should follow coagulation parameters closely after the discontinuation of antivenom therapy. Recurrent thrombocytopenia should be treated with additional antivenom in consultation with a poison control center or a medical toxicologist.

SUMMARY

Although the majority of poisonings require only supportive care, the emergency physician must recognize when the use of an antidote is required, and understand the risks and benefits of the treatment rendered. This article focuses on several selected antidotes, their indications, and potential pitfalls in their use. Both HIE therapy for the treatment of CCB overdose and the use of ILEs for the treatment of lipophilic cardiotoxic drug overdoses represent cutting-edge therapies that hold promise for poisonings that currently have limited treatment options. Further study may shed light on their effectiveness and continue to define their side effect profiles. Hydroxycobalamin is an antidote that has the potential to replace the cyanide antidote kit for the treatment of cyanide exposure in the undifferentiated smoke inhalation victim. Preliminary evidence suggests that it is effective and has minimal side effects. Further study comparing it with sodium thiosulfate alone (a cheaper and potentially equally efficacious option) should be conducted. NAC is a well-established antidote with a newly FDA-approved intravenous formulation and shortened protocols for administration. With its increasing use, physicians must be aware of the risks associated with anaphylactoid reactions and dosing errors. Physicians must also understand the limited indications for the shortened protocol, as premature cessation of therapy can result in irreversible hepatotoxicity. Finally, several years into use of the new rattlesnake antivenom, FabAV, delayed and refractory thrombocytopenia and bleeding complications have been documented in snakebite victims. It remains to be seen whether these complications result from the new therapy or represent greater detection from improved follow-up.

REFERENCES

1. Bronstein AC, Spyker DA, Cantilena LR Jr, et al. 2007 Annual report of the American Association of Poison Control Centers' National Poison Data System (NPDS): 25th annual report. Clin Toxicol (Phila) 2008;46(10):927–1057.
2. Lheureux PE, Zahir S, Gris M, et al. Bench-to-bedside review: hyperinsulinaemia/euglycaemia therapy in the management of overdose of calcium-channel blockers. Crit Care 2006;10(3):212.
3. Enyeart JJ, Price WA, Hoffman DA, et al. Profound hyperglycemia and metabolic acidosis after verapamil overdose. J Am Coll Cardiol 1983;2(6):1228–31.

4. Shepherd G, Klein-Schwartz W. High-dose insulin therapy for calcium-channel blocker overdose. Ann Pharmacother 2005;39(5):923–30.
5. Salhanick SD, Shannon MW. Management of calcium channel antagonist overdose. Drug Saf 2003;26(2):65–79.
6. Kline JA, Tomaszewski CA, Schroeder JD, et al. Insulin is a superior antidote for cardiovascular toxicity induced by verapamil in the anesthetized canine. J Pharmacol Exp Ther 1993;267(2):744–50.
7. Kline JA, Leonova E, Raymond RM. Beneficial myocardial metabolic effects of insulin during verapamil toxicity in the anesthetized canine. Crit Care Med 1995;23(7):1251–63.
8. Kline JA, Raymond RM, Leonova ED, et al. Insulin improves heart function and metabolism during non-ischemic cardiogenic shock in awake canines. Cardiovasc Res 1997;34(2):289–98.
9. Yuan TH, Kerns WP 2nd, Tomaszewski CA, et al. Insulin-glucose as adjunctive therapy for severe calcium channel antagonist poisoning. J Toxicol Clin Toxicol 1999;37(4):463–74.
10. Boyer EW, Shannon M. Treatment of calcium-channel-blocker intoxication with insulin infusion. N Engl J Med 2001;344(22):1721–2.
11. Rasmussen L, Husted SE, Johnsen SP. Severe intoxication after an intentional overdose of amlodipine. Acta Anaesthesiol Scand 2003;47(8):1038–40.
12. Marques M, Gomes E, de Oliveira J. Treatment of calcium channel blocker intoxication with insulin infusion: case report and literature review. Resuscitation 2003; 57(2):211–3.
13. Ortiz-Munoz L, Rodriguez-Ospina LF, Figueroa-Gonzalez M. Hyperinsulinemic-euglycemic therapy for intoxication with calcium channel blockers. Bol Asoc Med P R 2005;97(3 Pt 2):182–9.
14. Megarbane B, Karyo S, Baud FJ. The role of insulin and glucose (hyperinsulinaemia/euglycaemia) therapy in acute calcium channel antagonist and beta-blocker poisoning. Toxicol Rev 2004;23(4):215–22.
15. Min L, Deshpande K. Diltiazem overdose haemodynamic response to hyperinsulinaemia-euglycaemia therapy: a case report. Crit Care Resusc 2004;6(1):28–30.
16. Herbert J, O'Malley C, Tracey J, et al. Verapamil overdosage unresponsive to dextrose/insulin therapy [abstract]. J Toxicol Clin Toxicol 2001;39:293–4.
17. Cumpston K, Mycyk M, Pallash E, et al. Failure of hyperinsulinemia/euglycemia therapy in severe diltiazem overdose [abstract]. J Toxicol Clin Toxicol 2002;40:618.
18. Pizon AF, Lovecchio F, Matesick LF. Calcium channel blocker overdose: one center's experience. Clin Toxicol 2005;43:679–80.
19. Bania TC, Chu J, Perez E, et al. Hemodynamic effects of intravenous fat emulsion in an animal model of severe verapamil toxicity resuscitated with atropine, calcium, and saline. Acad Emerg Med 2007;14(2):105–11.
20. Weinberg GL, VadeBoncouer T, Ramaraju GA, et al. Pretreatment or resuscitation with a lipid infusion shifts the dose-response to bupivacaine-induced asystole in rats. Anesthesiology 1998;88(4):1071–5.
21. Weinberg G, Ripper R, Feinstein DL, et al. Lipid emulsion infusion rescues dogs from bupivacaine-induced cardiac toxicity. Reg Anesth Pain Med 2003;28(3): 198–202.
22. Krieglstein J, Meffert A, Niemeyer DH. Influence of emulsified fat on chlorpromazine availability in rabbit blood. Experientia 1974;30(8):924–6.
23. Yoav G, Odelia G, Shaltiel C. A lipid emulsion reduces mortality from clomipramine overdose in rats. Vet Hum Toxicol 2002;44(1):30.

24. Cave G, Harvey MG, Castle CD. The role of fat emulsion therapy in a rodent model of propranolol toxicity: a preliminary study. J Med Toxicol 2006;2(1):4–7.
25. Litz RJ, Popp M, Stehr SN, et al. Successful resuscitation of a patient with ropivacaine-induced asystole after axillary plexus block using lipid infusion. Anaesthesia 2006;61(8):800–1.
26. Rosenblatt MA, Abel M, Fischer GW, et al. Successful use of a 20% lipid emulsion to resuscitate a patient after a presumed bupivacaine-related cardiac arrest. Anesthesiology 2006;105(1):217–8.
27. Warren JA, Thoma RB, Georgescu A, et al. Intravenous lipid infusion in the successful resuscitation of local anesthetic-induced cardiovascular collapse after supraclavicular brachial plexus block. Anesth Analg 2008;106(5):1578–80.
28. Zimmer C, Piepenbrink K, Riest G, et al. [Cardiotoxic and neurotoxic effects after accidental intravascular bupivacaine administration. Therapy with lidocaine propofol and lipid emulsion]. Anaesthesist 2007;56(5):449–53 [in German].
29. Sirianni AJ, Osterhoudt KC, Calello DP, et al. Use of lipid emulsion in the resuscitation of a patient with prolonged cardiovascular collapse after overdose of bupropion and lamotrigine. Ann Emerg Med 2008;51(4):412–5, 415, e411.
30. Finn SD, Uncles DR, Willers J, et al. Early treatment of a quetiapine and sertraline overdose with Intralipid. Anaesthesia 2009;64(2):191–4.
31. Young AC, Velez LI, Kleinschmidt KC. Intravenous fat emulsion therapy for intentional sustained-release verapamil overdose. Resuscitation 2009;80(5):591–3.
32. Intralipid 20%. Baxter Healthcare Corporation, Deerfield, IL [package insert].
33. Borron SW, Baud FJ, Barriot P, et al. Prospective study of hydroxocobalamin for acute cyanide poisoning in smoke inhalation. Ann Emerg Med 2007;49(6):794–801, 801, e791–2.
34. Olson K. Poisoning and drug overdose. 5th edition. New York: McGraw-Hill Professional; 2006.
35. Gracia R, Shepherd G. Cyanide poisoning and its treatment. Pharmacotherapy 2004;24(10):1358–65.
36. Borron SW, Stonerook M, Reid F. Efficacy of hydroxocobalamin for the treatment of acute cyanide poisoning in adult beagle dogs. Clin Toxicol (Phila) 2006;44(Suppl 1):5–15.
37. Krapez JR, Vesey CJ, Adams L, et al. Effects of cyanide antidotes used with sodium nitroprusside infusions: sodium thiosulphate and hydroxocobalamin given prophylactically to dogs. Br J Anaesth 1981;53(8):793–804.
38. Ivankovich AD, Braverman B, Kanuru RP, et al. Cyanide antidotes and methods of their administration in dogs: a comparative study. Anesthesiology 1980;52(3):210–6.
39. Fortin JL, Giocanti JP, Ruttimann M, et al. Prehospital administration of hydroxocobalamin for smoke inhalation-associated cyanide poisoning: 8 years of experience in the Paris fire brigade. Clin Toxicol (Phila) 2006;44(Suppl 1):37–44.
40. Cyanokit, Dey, LP, Napa, CA [package insert].
41. Heard KJ. Acetylcysteine for acetaminophen poisoning. N Engl J Med 2008;359(3):285–92.
42. Goldfrank L, Flomenbaum N, Howland MA, et al. Goldfrank's toxicologic emergencies. 8th edition. New York: McGraw-Hill Professional; 2006.
43. Smilkstein MJ, Knapp GL, Kulig KW, et al. Efficacy of oral N-acetylcysteine in the treatment of acetaminophen overdose. Analysis of the national multicenter study (1976 to 1985). N Engl J Med 1988;319(24):1557–62.

44. Watson WA, Litovitz TL, Rodgers GC Jr, et al. 2004 Annual report of the American Association of Poison Control Centers Toxic Exposure Surveillance System. Am J Emerg Med 2005;23(5):589–666.
45. Kerr F, Dawson A, Whyte IM, et al. The Australasian clinical toxicology investigators collaboration randomized trial of different loading infusion rates of N-acetylcysteine. Ann Emerg Med 2005;45(4):402–8.
46. Whyte AJ, Kehrl T, Brooks DE, et al. Safety and effectiveness of Acetadote for acetaminophen toxicity. J Emerg Med 2008, in press.
47. Pakravan N, Waring WS, Sharma S, et al. Risk factors and mechanisms of anaphylactoid reactions to acetylcysteine in acetaminophen overdose. Clin Toxicol (Phila) 2008;46(8):697–702.
48. Appelboam AV, Dargan PI, Knighton J. Fatal anaphylactoid reaction to N-acetylcysteine: caution in patients with asthma. Emerg Med J 2002;19(6):594–5.
49. Dawson AH, Henry DA, McEwen J. Adverse reactions to N-acetylcysteine during treatment for paracetamol poisoning. Med J Aust 1989;150(6):329–31.
50. Lynch RM, Robertson R. Anaphylactoid reactions to intravenous N-acetylcysteine: a prospective case controlled study. Accid Emerg Nurs 2004;12(1):10–5.
51. Waring WS, Stephen AF, Robinson OD, et al. Lower incidence of anaphylactoid reactions to N-acetylcysteine in patients with high acetaminophen concentrations after overdose. Clin Toxicol (Phila) 2008;46(6):496–500.
52. Schmidt LE, Dalhoff K. Risk factors in the development of adverse reactions to N-acetylcysteine in patients with paracetamol poisoning. Br J Clin Pharmacol 2001;51(1):87–91.
53. Bailey B, Blais R, Letarte A. Status epilepticus after a massive intravenous N-acetylcysteine overdose leading to intracranial hypertension and death. Ann Emerg Med 2004;44(4):401–6.
54. Hershkovitz E, Shorer Z, Levitas A, et al. Status epilepticus following intravenous N-acetylcysteine therapy. Isr J Med Sci 1996;32(11):1102–4.
55. Sung L, Simons JA, Dayneka NL. Dilution of intravenous N-acetylcysteine as a cause of hyponatremia. Pediatrics 1997;100(3 Pt 1):389–91.
56. Woo OF, Mueller PD, Olson KR, et al. Shorter duration of oral N-acetylcysteine therapy for acute acetaminophen overdose. Ann Emerg Med 2000;35(4):363–8.
57. Tsai CL, Chang WT, Weng TI, et al. A patient-tailored N-acetylcysteine protocol for acute acetaminophen intoxication. Clin Ther 2005;27(3):336–41.
58. Smith SW, Howland MA, Hoffman RS, et al. Acetaminophen overdose with altered acetaminophen pharmacokinetics and hepatotoxicity associated with premature cessation of intravenous N-acetylcysteine therapy. Ann Pharmacother 2008;42(9):1333–9.
59. Gold BS, Barish RA, Dart RC. North American snake envenomation: diagnosis, treatment, and management. Emerg Med Clin North Am 2004;22(2):423–43, ix.
60. Cannon R, Ruha AM, Kashani J. Acute hypersensitivity reactions associated with administration of crotalidae polyvalent immune Fab antivenom. Ann Emerg Med 2008;51(4):407–11.
61. Fazelat J, Teperman SH, Touger M. Recurrent hemorrhage after western diamondback rattlesnake envenomation treated with crotalidae polyvalent immune fab (ovine). Clin Toxicol (Phila) 2008;46(9):823–6.
62. Offerman SR, Barry JD, Schneir A, et al. Biphasic rattlesnake venom-induced thrombocytopenia. J Emerg Med 2003;24(3):289–93.
63. Wasserberger J, Ordog G, Merkin TE. Southern Pacific Rattlesnake bite: a unique clinical challenge. J Emerg Med 2006;31(3):263–6.

64. Odeleye AA, Presley AE, Passwater ME, et al. Report of two cases: rattlesnake venom-induced thrombocytopenia. Ann Clin Lab Sci 2004;34(4):467–70.
65. Gold BS, Barish RA, Rudman MS. Refractory thrombocytopenia despite treatment for rattlesnake envenomation. N Engl J Med 2004;350(18):1912–3 [discussion: 1912–3].
66. Boyer LV, Seifert SA, Clark RF, et al. Recurrent and persistent coagulopathy following pit viper envenomation. Arch Intern Med 1999;159(7):706–10.
67. Bogdan GM, Dart RC, Falbo SC, et al. Recurrent coagulopathy after antivenom treatment of crotalid snakebite. South Med J 2000;93(6):562–6.

Pitfalls in the Evaluation of Shortness of Breath

Charlotte Page Wills, MD*, Megann Young, MD,
Douglas W. White, MD

KEYWORDS

• Shortness of breath • Pneumothorax • Asthma
• Pericardial effusion • Pulmonary embolism • Anemia

Shortness of breath is frequently the chief complaint in the emergency department (ED) and is commonly associated with hospital admission.[1] Dyspnea can be caused by disease in almost any organ system, and the emergency physician (EP) must maintain a high index of suspicion for causes besides the most common, such as pneumonia, congestive heart failure, reactive airway disease, and cardiac disease. "Premature closing" or early narrowing of the differential diagnosis[2] is particularly hazardous in emergency medicine, where undifferentiated patients are frequently treated in the setting of limited clinical information. Delayed diagnosis and treatment of underlying conditions can lead to substantial morbidity and mortality. The following cases illustrate some of the pitfalls that may accompany the diagnoses associated with dyspnea in the ED setting.

CASE 1

A 50-year-old homeless man is brought to the ED after he wandered into a store and sat down refusing to move. He tells paramedics that he cannot breathe but appears in no distress and refuses to give any history. He has a history of severe schizophrenia and catatonia. He has a normal blood pressure, a heart rate of 160, is afebrile, and his oxygen saturation by pulse oximetry is 92%. His lungs are clear and the remainder of his examination is notable only for cachexia. His electrocardiogram (ECG) shows atrial fibrillation at a rate of 160 beats per minute (bpm), and his chest radiograph (CXR) shows mild cardiomegaly with no evidence of edema or pneumonia. Heart

Disclosure: No funding or financial support of any type was received by any of the authors in the preparation of this article. CPW is an employee of the Oakcare Medical Group. MY and DWW are both employees of Alameda County Medical Center.
Department of Emergency Medicine, Alameda County Medical Center-Highland Hospital, 6th Floor, 1411 East 31st Street, Oakland, CA 94602, USA
* Corresponding author.
E-mail address: cwills@acmedctr.org (C.P. Wills).

rate control is attempted with intravenous atrioventricular nodal blocking agents with mild resulting hypotension. Bedside ultrasonography performed several hours after presentation reveals a 3-cm pericardial effusion with tamponade physiology.

Although cardiac dysrhythmia is an important cause of dyspnea, the providers in this case assumed atrial fibrillation was the primary cause of this patient's dyspnea and delayed evaluation of contributing causes of dyspnea. In addition, these providers did not initially consider effusion in the differential diagnosis of the cardiomegaly seen on CXR. Cardiac tamponade may be easily recognized in extreme cases when accompanied by hypotension, jugular venous distension, and muffled heart tones, but can be overlooked in the absence of hemodynamic instability. Pericardial effusion and tamponade should always be considered in the differential diagnosis of dyspnea; in one study of 103 patients with unexplained dyspnea, 14 were found to have pericardial effusions, 4 of which were clinically significant.[3]

Cardiac Tamponade in Medical Patients

The term "cardiac tamponade" was first described in the late nineteenth century as the compression of the heart and impaired diastolic filling caused by fluid within the pericardial sac.[4] Rephrased over a hundred years later, cardiac tamponade is a state of hemodynamic compromise caused by cardiac compression from confined fluid in the pericardial space.[5]

Although the symptoms of rapidly progressive traumatic effusion are dramatic and ultrasound evaluation for pericardial effusion has become a standard part of trauma evaluation, tamponade resulting from an underlying medical condition can be far more insidious. The incidence of tamponade from medical pericardial effusion has been estimated at approximately 3 cases per year per 100,000 population.[6] The causes of cardiac effusion are numerous and include infectious, rheumatologic, and inflammatory conditions. Malignancy is a common cause of effusion, found in 65% of cases in one study,[6–8] as are viral infections and anticoagulant therapy.[6] Tuberculous and uremic effusions, once common, have been declining in incidence in the United States. Even with intervention and treatment, overall in-hospital mortality for medical cardiac tamponade ranges from 10% to 15%.[6]

The stiffness of the pericardium determines the rate at which cardiac filling is compromised by accumulating fluid. Processes causing a slow accumulation over time allow the pericardium to "stretch". It is this gradual accommodation in the setting of increasing fluid that makes medical pericardial effusion and tamponade a diagnostic challenge.

Clinical Presentation and Diagnosis

Dyspnea, tachycardia, elevated jugular venous pressure, and pulsus paradoxus are evident in more than 70% of patients with cardiac tamponade. Cardiomegaly on CXR is also common.[5] However, fewer than 50% of patients will have the classic findings of diminished heart tones, hypotension, and low-voltage (ECG).[5] Pulsus paradoxus is the hallmark finding defined as a 10-mm Hg or greater drop in systolic arterial pressure during inspiration, and the degree of pulsus paradoxus has been shown to correlate with the severity of tamponade.[9]

Other presenting symptoms may be vague, including fullness, fatigue, loss of appetite, and difficulty swallowing.[9] Additionally, depending on the underlying cause of the pericardial effusion, patients may report fever, weight loss, rales, lower extremity edema, ascites, and myalgias. Late-presenting symptoms of poor cardiac output may include dysphoria,[10] syncope, respiratory distress, altered mental status, and ultimately, cardiac arrhythmia, or arrest. Atrial arrhythmias, as in this patient, are less common but have been reported.[11]

Finally, this case illustrates the pitfalls of medical evaluation in the setting of psychiatric disease. In one study, an estimated 4% of patients presenting with psychiatric disease had significant underlying medical disease requiring treatment. These patients are more likely to provide inadequate history and have inadequate physical examinations.[12] Another study found that 64% of patients with psychiatric disease who presented to the ED with altered mental status required hospital admission and had hospital stays of more than a week.[13]

Cardiac Ultrasonography

Doppler echocardiography is the gold standard for diagnosing cardiac tamponade, but is not always readily available. EPs have been shown to do well identifying pericardial effusion by bedside ultrasonography, with an overall sensitivity of 96% in one study.[14] Even in patients in pulseless electrical activity or with cardiac standstill, EPs perform well, correctly identifying effusion.[15] Distinguishing cardiac tamponade physiology by diastolic collapse of one or more chambers may be more challenging. The right ventricular wall is usually the first site where diastolic collapse is seen on ultrasound scan.[16] Once pericardial effusion is identified, cardiac tamponade should be suspected in any symptomatic or hemodynamically unstable patient.

CASE 2

A 35-year-old woman presents to the ED requesting refills of her asthma inhalers. She was recently discharged from the hospital after a 1-week admission for severe asthma and lost her medications on the bus. She reports that she is currently taking prednisone as directed, in addition to an inhaled steroid, a long-acting beta agonist, and a leukotriene receptor antagonist. She reports dyspnea similar to her usual asthma symptoms. Review of her medical record shows multiple prior hospital admissions for asthma, but no history of intubation. Her vital signs are notable for a heart rate of 100 bpm and an oxygen saturation of 91% on room air. Physical examination reveals diffuse wheezing throughout all lung fields, poor air movement, but no accessory muscle use. Her best peak expiratory flow (PEF) is 150. She is treated with nebulized albuterol and requests to be discharged after the third treatment, stating that she "feels fine." She is discharged with prescriptions for the lost medications and 2 hours later develops severe wheezing at home. On paramedic arrival she is in acute respiratory distress. She is intubated and transported to the ED but experiences cardiac arrest en route and does not survive the hospitalization.

Severe and Fatal Asthma

Asthma affects 6% to 8% of the population[17] and is one of the most commonly encountered chronic diseases in the ED. Patients with severe asthma, however, represent less than 10%[18] of more than 22 million Americans afflicted by asthma, and these patients suffer markedly higher rates of ED visits, hospital admissions, and death.[19] The in-hospital mortality approaches 17% for patients who require intubation, and a further 14% of patients die subsequently.[19,20] Severe asthma kills between 3000 and 5000 people each year in the United States alone.[21]

Though it is more common in patients with severe asthma, fatal asthma may result from any asthma attack that remains untreated. Deciding which patients fall into this high-risk category among the hundreds of thousands who present annually to the ED for asthma can be challenging. However, identifying patients at risk is crucial, because at least some asthma-related deaths may be preventable.

Identifying Asthmatics at Risk

Every asthmatic patient should be screened for severe asthma. Clinical assessment of asthma severity should include a patient's use of medication and consumption of health care resources for asthma exacerbations.[22] Certain populations are particularly vulnerable. African Americans with asthma who suffer severe disease are disproportionate, with prevalence rates reported at 12.5% compared with approximately 7% in whites and Hispanics.[23] Hospital admissions rates in one study of patients in a predominantly African American community in New York City were 3 times higher and rates of ED visits 5 times higher than the national average.[24]

Assessment of risk for fatal asthma should also include a psychosocial screening. Noncompliance with treatments, missed appointments, self-discharge from the hospital, psychiatric issues, drug or alcohol abuse, learning difficulties, job and income problems, and domestic stressors have all been implicated as risk factors of severe and fatal asthma.[25,26] The nonmedical obstacles that asthmatic patients face in complying with their care can be enormous, and added stress is a significant factor in worsening of their disease. Identifying these issues at the time of treatment and mobilizing appropriate resources in the ED is crucial.

Assessing Asthma Severity

Severe asthma requires high intensity treatment.[27] The National Institutes of Health defines severe asthma as persistent or continual symptoms that cause a limitation in physical activity, frequent exacerbations, a PEF of less than 60% of that predicted, or a diurnal variation in the PEF of greater than 30%. The American Thoracic Society Workshop generated a definition that includes major and minor criteria. The major criteria are treatment with oral corticosteroids for more than 50% of the year and with high-dose inhaled steroids. Minor criteria include the following: use of a daily controller medication, such as a long-acting beta agonist, theophylline, or leukotriene receptor antagonist, daily use of a short-acting beta agonist, forced expiratory volume in one second less than 80%, one or more ED visits per year, 3 or more oral steroid bursts per year, intolerance of decrease in oral or inhaled steroid dosing, or any history of near-fatal asthma exacerbation.[17] Only one major or 2 minor criteria are needed for classification as a severe asthmatic. Of 800 patients meeting these criteria and enrolled in the Severe Asthma Research Program database, 12% had an ICU admission in the preceding year.[17]

Clinical Presentation

Severe asthma exacerbations may be slow or rapid in onset.[28,29] Slow-onset asthma attacks evolve over a period of time, usually greater than 3 hours,[29] and have a slower response to therapy. Patients suffering slow-onset attacks have a higher degree of eosinophilic inflammation, mucous plugging, epithelial sloughing, and resultant airway obstruction. Because the onset of symptoms is more gradual, patients have a longer lead time to start therapy and seek treatment.

In contrast, rapid-onset attacks can manifest symptoms in less than an hour[30] and usually less than 3 hours.[31] In one study, patients with sudden-onset symptoms were more likely to present to the ED between midnight and 8:00 AM, to require intubation, and to be admitted to the intensive care unit. However, they also had more rapid response to treatment[29] and shorter hospital stays.[31] Rapid-onset attacks may follow a long history of the disease in young to middle-aged patients, previous life-threatening attacks or hospitalizations, or delay in obtaining medical aid.[32] In contrast to patients with slow-onset asthma attacks, patients with rapid-onset attacks have more smooth muscle bronchospasm and a neutrophil-predominant inflammatory process.[28,33] Patients with sudden-onset asthma are less likely to report an upper respiratory tract infection or clear trigger,[28,29] making the identification of patients at risk even more challenging.

Perception of Dyspnea

The unstable asthmatic is usually not a diagnostic dilemma. However, the stable severe asthmatic may be more challenging, as in our introductory case. Indeed the stable patient with near-fatal asthma may initially be difficult to distinguish from the mild asthmatic.[34] Dyspnea is subjective, but severe asthmatics, in particular, suffer from decreased or blunted perception of dyspnea.[35] Blunted perception of dyspnea results in an inadequate sense of the onset or severity of bronchoconstriction and leads to underreporting of duration and severity of symptoms, delay in seeking treatment,[36] and lack of recognition of severity of disease by physicians.[37] Patients with low perception of dyspnea have more ED visits, hospitalizations, near-fatal asthma attacks, and deaths.[19]

Smoking further affects the perception of dyspnea even in mild asthmatics.[37] Smoking in patients with severe asthma is associated with a higher in-hospital mortality and with a higher posthospitalization mortality.[20] Further, smoking decreases the efficacy of corticosteroids. Drugs and alcohol may also suppress awareness of symptoms and result in poor compliance and delay to appropriate medical treatment.[38] Standard antiasthma therapies have been shown to improve the perception of dyspnea,[37] although studies conflict as to whether corticosteroids directly improve perception of dyspnea.[39]

Predictors of Complications in the ED

Failure of initial therapy to improve expiratory flow predicts a more severe course and need for hospitalization.[40] Recent severe asthma exacerbations, such as the hospital admission in case 2, is a strong independent risk factor of future exacerbations and must be part of the clinical assessment of patients with severe or difficult-to-treat asthma.[22] Any patient who suffers an exacerbation in the setting of oral steroid use and multidrug therapy, like the patient in case 2, requires serious consideration for inpatient admission.

After discharge from the ED, many patients have persistent respiratory symptoms and impairment of activities of daily living. One study found that 17% of patients seen in the ED relapse within 2 weeks, requiring urgent medical treatment. The factors associated with asthma relapse were a history of frequent ED visits over the previous year, use of a home nebulizer, multiple asthma triggers, and symptoms lasting for more than a day. Lack of a regular primary-care physician was also associated with a higher incidence of relapse.[41]

In the treatment and assessment of the asthmatic, it is crucial to be aware of the criteria for severe asthma, and screening patients for predictors of near-fatal and fatal asthma attacks should be part of the discharge planning for every patient who presents to the ED with asthma.

CASE 3

A 48-year-old woman presents to the ED after several days of severe dyspnea and some wheezing. She describes a remote history of asthma, but has not been on medications recently and has never required intubation or hospitalization. On examination, she has mild expiratory wheezing and her oxygen saturation is 93% on room air by pulse oximetry. The CXR is remarkable for mildly increased interstitial markings with no infiltrates. She is started on nebulized albuterol, given prednisone, and signed out to the next shift of providers. Her wheezing resolves after the first nebulizer and her oxygen saturation remains stable, but over the course of the next 4 hours, her subjective dyspnea does not improve, and she is admitted to the hospital for status asthmaticus. Routine admission laboratory tests show severe anemia with a hemoglobin level of 4. On further review of systems, the patient reports vaginal bleeding, and her inpatient evaluation ultimately reveals invasive cervical cancer.

Even at the time of presentation, this patient reported severe dyspnea out of proportion to her mild wheezing and her borderline oxygen saturation. Although a trial of nebulized therapy was probably appropriate, given her history and wheezing on examination, asthma was unlikely to be the complete explanation for her severe symptoms. In addition, in a patient with wheezing and increased interstitial markings on CXR, heart failure, including high-output failure, must be considered. In general, a history of dyspnea that is out of proportion to clinical findings, or that does not resolve with initial therapy, will always require a broad differential diagnosis and complete workup.

Symptomatic Anemia

Anemia is a pervasive health problem, particularly among elderly patients. In one UK study of developed nations, the overall prevalence of anemia was 17% in patients older than 65 years.[42] In the United States, it is estimated that 10% to 11% of all adults older than 65 years and up to 28% of African Americans have anemia.[43] Risk factors for anemia include chronic kidney disease, dialysis, inherited disorders of red blood cell structure and function, certain medications, and poor diet.[44] Worldwide, up to one-third of cases of anemia are due to dietary deficiency (insufficiency of iron, vitamin B12, and/or folate); an additional one-third are due to chronic disease.[43]

There is no single hemoglobin level at which most patients begin to have symptoms. One study found that in otherwise healthy patients, oxygen delivery to tissues could be maintained at rest at a hemoglobin level of 5g/dL as long as intravascular volume was maintained.[45] Symptoms may occur at a higher hemoglobin level with exertion or in patients with heart disease that impairs cardiac output.[45]

Clinical Presentation

The clinical signs of anemia vary and depend on several factors: the absolute hemoglobin level, the rate of development of the anemia, comorbid conditions, and the underlying cause. When anemia develops gradually, patients are often able to tolerate strikingly low hemoglobin levels that might not be tolerated in acute cases. In addition, patients with normal cardiac function are more likely to be able to compensate for lower oxygen-carrying capacity by increasing cardiac output, thus maintaining oxygen delivery to tissues.[45] The earliest symptoms of mild-to-moderate anemia are generally exertional dyspnea, fatigue, weakness, and tachycardia.[46] In patients who develop anemia rapidly due to acute blood loss, symptoms of hypovolemia, such as orthostasis, hypotension, syncope, tachycardia, and palpitations are likely to predominate. However, in a patient with a slowly progressive chronic anemia, symptoms may be limited to fatigue and exertional dyspnea, and they may not occur until patients reach a hemoglobin level of 5 or 6.[45,46]

Anemia-associated high-output heart failure is caused by a supraphysiologic increase in cardiac output that attempts to compensate for decreased oxygen-carrying capacity. It is characterized by dyspnea, wide pulse pressure, midsystolic flow murmur, and wheezing; is defined as a resting cardiac index more than the normal range (>4 L/min/m^2); and typically occurs at a hemoglobin level less than 5 g/dL.[47]

Diagnostic Evaluation

History and physical

Important historical findings in a patient with chronic anemia include past medical history, medication use, occupational history of toxic exposures, social history of alcohol or drug use, dietary history, and family history.[44] Physical findings may include pallor of the skin and mucosa; conjunctival pallor seems to be the most predictive of low hemoglobin levels.[48,49] Other physical findings may be related to the cause of anemia: angular cheilitis and koilonychia are found in iron deficiency, whereas jaundice and splenomegaly are noted in hemolytic anemias.[44] Evaluation should include fecal occult blood testing for gastrointestinal bleeding.

Diagnostic testing

Ultimately, the diagnosis of anemia is made by a complete blood count demonstrating low hemoglobin or hematocrit. Anemias are generally categorized morphologically as macrocytic, microcytic, or normocytic[50]; or etiologically due to increased destruction, sequestration, or decreased production of red blood cells.[46] Critical adjunctive blood tests include reticulocyte count and peripheral blood smear. Other specific etiologic tests include iron, transferrin saturation, ferritin, total iron-binding capacity for iron deficiency, and haptoglobin for suspected hemolysis. If a patient is noted to be pancytopenic, a bone marrow biopsy may be required. Although much of this workup is completed after a patient has left the ED, iron studies and reticulocyte count should be done before any transfusion.

In most cases, patients with symptomatic anemia of unknown cause will be transfused and admitted to the hospital to determine its cause. Although the onus of determining the cause of anemia falls on the inpatient service, it is important for the EP not to close the differential diagnosis too early, and to consider anemia as a cause of dyspnea.

CASE 4

A 52-year-old man presents to the ED after 2 weeks of cough and dyspnea. He is well-appearing with normal vital signs and oxygen saturation and is triaged to the fast-track area of the ED. The patient describes his cough as dry and nonproductive. He denies any fever, fatigue, hemoptysis, or chest pain. He does admit to smoking tobacco and marijuana and has had multiple episodes of bronchitis, although he has never been diagnosed with chronic obstructive pulmonary disease (COPD). On physical examination, he has diminished breath sounds over the right lung field. CXR reveals a 90% right pneumothorax, which is treated with a 22-French tube thoracostomy. Shortly after chest tube placement, he develops dyspnea, a severe constant cough productive of clear frothy sputum, and profound hypoxia. His CXR is consistent with pulmonary edema. The patient's respiratory distress worsens, ultimately requiring intubation and mechanical ventilation.

Spontaneous Pneumothorax

Pneumothorax is the presence of air in the pleural space,[51] a finding which is always abnormal. A pneumothorax may be classified as spontaneous, traumatic, or iatrogenic when it results from any medical procedure, including mechanical ventilation.[51,52] Spontaneous pneumothorax is further described as primary if there is no identifiable cause or secondary if there is clinically apparent underlying lung disease, such as COPD.[53]

Epidemiology and Risk Factors of Spontaneous Pneumothorax

In a population study in Olmsted County, Minnesota, the incidence of pneumothorax (all types) ranged from 7.4 to 18 cases per 100,000 population.[54] Risk factors of primary spontaneous pneumothorax include being male, younger,[51] and thin/underweight or tall.[55,56] Secondary pneumothorax is most commonly associated with blebs or bullae in the pulmonary parenchyma.[51] In primary and secondary spontaneous pneumothorax, smoking confers a 9-fold relative risk of developing spontaneous pneumothorax in women and a 22-fold relative risk in men.[55] In fact, smoking cessation is included in the British Thoracic Society guidelines for the management of spontaneous pneumothorax.[57] Although COPD is the disease most commonly associated[52,56] with secondary spontaneous pneumothorax,[58] infectious pathogens, such as pneumocystis carinii,[56] interstitial lung disease, connective tissue disease, pleural-based cancers, and rarely, thoracic endometrial implants, can also cause spontaneous pneumothorax.[51] Secondary spontaneous pneumothorax in the setting of COPD is associated with a 4-fold increased risk of dying,[59,60] and in one study, 5% of patients with a pneumothorax related to COPD died before intervention.[61] It is critical to recognize diminished pulmonary reserve in any patient with a pneumothorax, including those related to trauma or iatrogenic causes.

Clinical Presentation

Dyspnea is the most common complaint in patients with spontaneous pneumothorax. Patients also frequently complain of pleuritic chest pain. Approximately 60% of patients complain of dyspnea and chest pain.[58,62] Tachycardia is the most common physical finding,[52] and diminished breath sounds are notoriously unreliable, especially in the ED setting. Furthermore, diminished breath sounds may be difficult to identify in the COPD patient who already has significantly decreased air movement with respiration. Other physical findings include decreased movement of the chest wall, diminished tactile fremitus, and hyperresonance.[52,56] Tension pneumothorax should be suspected in any patient with severe respiratory distress, tachycardia, hypotension, hypoxia, or deviated trachea, and it requires immediate needle or tube thoracostomy with no delay for imaging studies.

Diagnostic Evaluation

Although chest computed tomography (CT) is the most sensitive screening modality and able to detect even a very small pneumothorax, CXR is still the preferred initial study. The classic finding in an upright film is visualization of the visceral pleural line without distal lung markings.[63] A pneumothorax is considered large when the distance from the pleural surface to the lung is greater than 2 cm[57,63] or the distance from apex to cupola is greater than 3 cm.[53] End-expiratory views are no longer recommended as they have been shown to add little value in diagnosing a pneumothorax.[64] Bedside ultrasonography can be used in trauma and medical patients to detect pneumothorax, with sensitivities of up to 98%[65,66] and has recently been shown to outperform supine CXR, which has a false-negative rate that approaches 50% in some studies.[67,68]

Ultrasonography and CXR provide limited ability to differentiate bullous disease from pneumothorax, although there are case reports of using the presence of "comet tailing" on ultrasound scan to distinguish bullae from pneumothorax. Comet tailing confirms pleural sliding and indicates the absence of pneumothorax, although accuracy is limited by the number of locations on the chest wall that are scanned.[69] Chest CT scan is the definitive study for bullous disease and should be obtained in most patients in whom bullous disease is suspected.[52] Chest CT scan is recommended for all patients with recurrent pneumothorax, persistent air leaks, or planned surgical interventions.[53]

Treatment Alternatives

Determining whether a spontaneous pneumothorax is primary or secondary is crucial. Clinically stable patients with small pneumothoraces, defined as less than 2 cm from the pleural surface to lung edge, may be observed without intervention for up to 6 hours in the ED and discharged if there is no expansion.[63] Needle aspiration of the pleural space, placement of small bore catheters, and traditional tube thoracostomy are other alternatives. In a study comparing these treatment modalities in patients with primary spontaneous pneumothoraces ranging in size from 5% to 60%, 79% of patients treated with observation alone required no further intervention.[70] Although not part of the consensus recommendations of the American College of Chest Physicians,[53] needle aspiration of small primary spontaneous pneumothoraces may be a reasonable first-line treatment option in the otherwise stable patient. The British Thoracic Society recommends needle aspiration as first-line treatment for all patients with primary spontaneous pneumothoraces measuring less than 2 cm that require intervention.[57] Several studies have demonstrated that needle aspiration is as safe and effective as tube thoracostomy,[71–73] although it is less likely to succeed in patients older than 50 years and those who have moderate-to-large pneumothoraces.[74,75] Patients with large pneumothoraces, whether primary or secondary, should undergo lung re-expansion with small-bore catheter or tube thoracostomy.[53] Patients with underlying lung disease always require hospitalization,[53] because they are at much higher risk of complications.

Re-expansion Pulmonary Edema

Re-expansion pulmonary edema (REPE) occurs in a small number of patients who undergo rapid inflation of the lung after a prolonged period of collapse from either pneumothorax or pleural effusion.[58] REPE is a rare complication with an estimated incidence of 0% to 1%.[76] However, mortality rates are reported as high as 20%.[77] Symptoms include coughing,[78] hypoxia, and in severe cases, hypotension. Onset of symptoms occurs soon after lung reinflation, with most cases developing within 1 hour.[77] REPE results from increased vascular permeability in the collapsed lung and the mechanical stress of re-expansion.[79] REPE tends to occur in patients with a period of collapse greater than 3 days, and those who undergo evacuation of a volume greater than 2.0 L.[79] Rates of REPE are highest in patients aged 20 to 39 years,[80] and other risk factors include negative pleural suction pressures of greater than 20 cm H_2O[77] and rapid re-expansion.[78] Gradually reinflating the lung by using either water seal[58] or negative pleural pressures of 10 to 12 cm H_2O[78,80,81] may reduce the occurrence of REPE. Identifying patients at risk of REPE and recognizing symptoms quickly is imperative. Treatment is supportive and may include supplemental oxygen, mechanical ventilation, and diuretics.

CASE 5

A 65-year-old man presents to the ED with dyspnea. He has a long history of COPD and suffers exacerbations every several months. His physical examination reveals end-expiratory wheezing and diminished air movement throughout. His vital signs are remarkable only for a pulse oximetry reading of 92%, which he reports as his baseline. He is treated with nebulized albuterol and ipratropium bromide, but his dyspnea and wheezing persist. No evidence of pneumonia is found on CXR, and he is admitted for continuous nebulizer therapy and observation. On day 2 at the hospital, the patient suffers a cardiopulmonary arrest and dies. Postmortem examination reveals a massive pulmonary embolism (PE).

Providers in this case failed to consider PE as a possible cause of this man's dyspnea and wheezing, despite data showing that the rates of PE in admitted COPD patients approach 25%.[82] The differential diagnosis was narrowed prematurely based on this patient's prior presentations and was not reassessed when he failed to respond to COPD therapy. In particular, these providers stopped at the first explanation (bronchospasm) for this patient's dyspnea, attributed it to a known prior diagnosis (COPD), and did not evaluate other possible underlying causes of bronchospasm and dyspnea.

PE

The wide variation in the clinical presentation of PE makes it a diagnostic challenge, and the incidence and prevalence of PE are poorly defined. One retrospective study of all-cause mortality estimated that 1.3% of patients had PE at the time of death; among these, PE was deemed the actual cause of death in 34%.[83] If untreated, PE has a mortality rate as high as 30%; when treated with anticoagulation, the mortality rate decreases to approximately 2%.[84,85] Risk factors for PE include immobilization, recent travel longer than 4 hours, surgery within the previous 3 months, paresis/paralysis, malignancy, history of venous thromboembolism or PE, and central venous instrumentation within the previous 3 months.[86] Additional factors that may increase risk in women include cigarette smoking, obesity, and hypertension.[85]

Clinical Presentation

The clinical presentation of PE varies widely. In the Prospective Investigation of Pulmonary Embolism Diagnosis (PIOPED) II study, the most common presenting symptoms in patients ultimately diagnosed with PE were dyspnea (79%), pleuritic chest pain (47%), cough (43%), calf or thigh pain (42%), and calf or thigh swelling (39%). The most common signs were tachypnea greater than 20 breaths per minute (57% of all patients with PE), deep vein thrombosis (DVT) signs (edema, erythema, tenderness, or palpable cord) in the calf or thigh (47%), tachycardia greater than100 bpm (26%), and decreased lung sounds (21%).[86] Given the wide variation in clinical presentation, a high index of suspicion for PE is required to initiate appropriate and timely diagnostic testing.

Diagnostic Evaluation

History and physical

The history and physical examination are rarely diagnostic of PE but can suggest the need for further evaluation. The history should focus on the timing and onset of symptoms, and any risk factors of PE should be explored; 67% of all patients with PE describe a rapid onset of dyspnea over seconds to minutes.[86] On physical examination, tachycardia and tachypnea are the classically taught findings, but occur in only half to three-quarters of patients with proven PE.[86] In massive PE, cardiopulmonary examination may show evidence of acute right heart strain, such as increased jugular venous pressure or right ventricular lift.

Adjunctive Methods

Scoring systems

Clinical prediction rules provide a standardized method for estimating disease likelihood and can guide the use of diagnostic tests (such as contrast CT) and medications (such as anticoagulants) that carry their own risk.[87] Numerous clinical decision rules and scoring systems exist for the evaluation of pretest probability or likelihood of PE.[88] The Wells criteria[89] have been extensively studied and have performed well in prospective validation studies; a low-risk Wells score combined with negative D-dimer test result has a negative predictive value of 96% to 100%.[87,90] The PE rule-out criteria (PERC) is another widely-used, prospectively validated clinical decision rule for the evaluation of possible PE. PERC variables are shown in **Table 1**. The PERC criteria have similar test characteristics to the D-dimer test. Therefore, PE can be excluded in a patient with low pretest probability if the PERC criteria are met, without additional diagnostic testing.[91,92]

CXR

Although CXR is a poor diagnostic tool for PE, in the PIOPED cohort of patients ultimately diagnosed with PE and with no preexisting cardiac or pulmonary disease, the most common CXR findings included atelectasis (seen in 68% of patients with PE vs 48% without) and pleural effusion (seen in 48% with PE vs 31% without).[93]

ECG

Many patients with acute PE have abnormalities on ECG. The classically taught S1Q3T3 (wide S wave in lead I and Q wave and inverted T wave in lead III) pattern for PE was first described in 1935,[94] probably in a sample of patients who had acute right heart strain from massive PE. Several more recent studies have demonstrated that these findings are neither sensitive nor specific for PE.[95] Other commonly reported ECG findings include sinus tachycardia, atrial tachyarrhythmias, and complete or incomplete right bundle branch block.[95] Sinha and colleagues[96] found the most common PE-associated ECG patterns to be sinus tachycardia, S1Q3T3 pattern, and atrial tachyarrhythmias; Ferrari and colleagues[97] found that negative T waves in the precordial leads (occurring in 68% of patients with proven PE) were most predictive of PE; Stein and colleagues[86] found that the most common and most predictive findings were nonspecific ST-T–wave changes; and Richman and colleagues[98] found

Table 1 Wells and PERC criteria	
Wells Criteria for PE	**PERC**
Signs or symptoms of DVT–3 points	Age<50
Heart Rate >100–1.5 points	Heart Rate<100
Surgery/immobilization within 4 weeks–1.5 points	Oxygen saturation>95%
	No unilateral leg swelling
Previous DVT or PE–1.5 points	No hemoptysis
Hemoptysis–1 point	No recent surgery
Malignancy–1 point	No history of venous thromboembolism
Other diagnosis less likely than PE–3 points	No oral hormone use
>6 points: high risk (>78% probability of PE)	
2-6 points: moderate risk (28% probability of PE)	
<2 points: low risk (3.4% probability of PE)	

Data from Wells PS, Ginsberg JS, Anderson DR, et al. Use of a clinical model for safe management of patients with suspected PE. Ann Intern Med 1998;129(12):997-1005; and Kline JA, Courtney DM, Kabrhel C, et al. Prospective multicenter evaluation of the PE rule-out criteria. J Thromb Haemost 2008;6(5):772–80.

that normal sinus rhythm was the most common (occurring in more than two-thirds of patients with PE). Given this heterogeneity of findings, it is difficult to draw conclusions about typical ECG findings in patients with PE, and it is clear that none of these ECG findings is sensitive to or specific for PE. Therefore, the primary utility of the ECG in patients with suspected PE is in excluding other causes of dyspnea or chest pain, such as acute coronary syndrome.

D-dimer

The D-dimer is a breakdown product of cross-linked fibrin and, as such, is a marker of thrombus. D-dimer testing has poor positive predictive value because many different disease processes can cause a positive test result. However, the negative predictive value for D-dimer testing in low-risk patients is good. Combined with clinical decision rules indicating that a patient has a low pretest probability of thromboembolic disease, a negative D-dimer level is adequate to withhold anticoagulation and further diagnostic testing.[99] In high-probability patients, however, D-dimer testing does not confer the same benefits, and further testing should be pursued regardless of D-Dimer test results.[99] In one study, patients with a normal D-dimer level had a 95% likelihood of not having a PE, leading the investigators to conclude that "for excluding PE or DVT, a negative test result on a quantitative rapid ELISA (enzyme-linked immunosorbent assay) is as diagnostically useful as a normal lung scan or negative duplex ultrasonography finding.[100]"

CT Angiography of the Chest

CT angiography is one of the most frequently used diagnostic modalities for PE because of its availability in the ED and the possibility that it may also diagnose other causes of a patient's symptoms. Some debate exists about the accuracy of chest CT scan for the diagnosis of PE, with initial reported sensitivities as low as 53% to 70%.[101,102] However, in the setting of improving CT technology and in combination with a clinical scoring system to determine pretest probability, sensitivities of 83% and specificities of 96% have been reported. The addition of venous phase imaging of the pelvis and lower extremities also improves sensitivity.[103] Anderson and colleagues[104] conducted a randomized controlled trial of noninferiority between chest CT scan and ventilation/perfusion (V/Q) scan, which reported essentially equal rates of diagnostic accuracy for CT scan combined with a clinical decision rule and D-dimer testing as compared with V/Q scan.

Ultrasonography

Ultrasonography of the lower extremity is commonly used as a diagnostic adjunct when PE is suspected. Although it can be a useful part of a diagnostic strategy for PE[105] when used in combination with other studies, it may miss up to 71% of patients with PE when it is the sole diagnostic modality used.[106]

Formal or bedside echocardiography may also be a useful adjunctive study in the setting of suspected PE. Echocardiographic signs of acute PE include right ventricular dilatation and hypokinesia, paradoxic systolic septal motion, pulmonary artery dilatation, and peak tricuspid regurgitation velocity greater than 2.7 m/s.[107] Echocardiography has been shown to have a sensitivity ranging from 51% to 93% and a specificity from 82% to 90% for acute PE.[108-110] Perrier and colleagues[109] found that by combining right-ventricular dilatation and tricuspid regurgitation velocity greater than 2.7 m/s, they achieved a sensitivity of 67% and specificity of 94%.

V/Q Scan

As compared with the gold standard of pulmonary angiography, the V/Q scan has been found to have an overall diagnostic accuracy of anywhere from 15% to 86% when combined with a clinical scoring system.[111] V/Q scans are read as normal, low probability, intermediate probability, or high probability of PE, and the study is most useful at the extremes. Scans read as normal essentially exclude the diagnosis of PE, whereas high-probability scans have an 85% to 90% positive predictive value.[104] Although normal and high-probability V/Q scans have powerful prognostic value, the poor overall performance stems from the large number of patients who have indeterminate results. For patients with scans interpreted as low or intermediate probability, significant diagnostic uncertainty remains.

Summary of Diagnostic Testing

The diagnosis of PE can be challenging and requires a high index of suspicion. The most common approach uses a combination of a clinical decision rule, D-dimer testing, and CT angiography, with or without lower extremity ultrasound studies. However, if the clinical suspicion is high and the diagnostic study of choice is not available, empiric anticoagulation may be indicated.

Missed PE is a major source of medical malpractice lawsuits.[112] Malpractice cases of DVT/PE generally fall into 1 of 4 categories: (1) failure to use appropriate prophylaxis for DVT; (2) failure to diagnose DVT/PE; (3) failure to treat DVT/PE correctly; and (4) unexpected side effects of medications used for treatment of DVT/PE.[113] Proper prophylaxis is rarely the responsibility of the EP, but the other 3 issues are often encountered in the ED. Given the varied manifestations of PE and the potential dire consequences of missed diagnosis, a high index of suspicion is warranted. All patients who complain of dyspnea should be screened for PE risk factors, and validated clinical scoring systems should be used to guide testing and imaging. If no obvious historical risk factor emerges, then workup for an underlying cause is indicated in all new diagnoses of PE.

SUMMARY

EPs evaluate patients with dyspnea many times each shift. Although many of the serious causes are easily recognized and quickly treated, it is crucial to consider related underlying disease. Chronic untreated disease is often the precipitant in acute episodes of asthma, COPD, PE, and congestive heart failure, and the underlying disease can complicate otherwise straightforward therapies, such as decompression for spontaneous pneumothorax. EPs must always balance the efficiency of rapid evaluation and treatment of the most likely cause of dyspnea with the flexibility to consider other diagnoses when the presentation or progression of illness is atypical.

REFERENCES

1. Ruger JP, Lewis LM, Richter CJ. Identifying high-risk patients for triage and resource allocation in the ED. Am J Emerg Med 2007;25(7):794–8.
2. Berner ES, Graber ML. Overconfidence as a cause of diagnostic error in medicine. Am J Med 2008;121(Suppl 5):S2–23.
3. Blaivas M. Incidence of pericardial effusion in patients presenting to the emergency department with unexplained dyspnea. Acad Emerg Med 2001;8(12):1143–6.

4. Starling EH. Some points in the pathology of heart disease. Lancet 1897;1: 652–5.
5. Roy CL, Minor MA, Brookhart MA, et al. Does this patient with a pericardial effusion have cardiac tamponade? JAMA 2007;297(16):1810–8.
6. Cornily J, Pennec P, Castellant P, et al. Cardiac tamponade in medical patients: a 10-year follow-up survey. Cardiology 2008;111(3):197–201.
7. Maisch B, Seferović PM, Ristić AD, et al. Guidelines on the diagnosis and management of pericardial diseases executive summary; the Task force on the diagnosis and management of pericardial diseases of the European society of cardiology. Eur Heart J 2004;25(7):587–610.
8. Curtiss EI, Reddy PS, Uretsky BF, et al. Pulsus paradoxus: definition and relation to the severity of cardiac tamponade. Am Heart J 1988;115(2):391–8.
9. Spodick DH. Acute cardiac tamponade. N Engl J Med 2003;349(7):684–90.
10. Ikematsu Y. Incidence and characteristics of dysphoria in patients with cardiac tamponade. Heart Lung 2007;36(6):440–9.
11. Krisanda TJ. Atrial fibrillation with cardiac tamponade as the initial manifestation of malignant pericarditis. Am J Emerg Med 1990;8(6):531–3.
12. Tintinalli JE, Peacock FW, Wright MA. Emergency medical evaluation of psychiatric patients. Ann Emerg Med 1994;23(4):859–62.
13. Kanich W, Brady WJ, Huff JS, et al. Altered mental status: evaluation and etiology in the ED. Am J Emerg Med 2002;20(7):613–7.
14. Mandavia DP, Hoffner RJ, Mahaney K, et al. Bedside echocardiography by emergency physicians. Ann Emerg Med 2001;38(4):377–82.
15. Tayal VS, Kline JA. Emergency echocardiography to detect pericardial effusion in patients in PEA and near-PEA states. Resuscitation 2003;59(3):315–8.
16. Beaulieu Y. Bedside echocardiography in the assessment of the critically ill. Crit Care Med 2007;35(Suppl 5):S235–49.
17. Wenzel SE, Busse WW. Severe asthma: lessons from the Severe Asthma Research Program. J Allergy Clin Immunol 2007;119(1):14–21 [quiz 22–3].
18. Moore WC, Peters SP. Severe asthma: an overview. J Allergy Clin Immunol 2006; 117(3):487–94 [quiz 495].
19. Magadle R, Berar-Yanay N, Weiner P. The risk of hospitalization and near-fatal and fatal asthma in relation to the perception of dyspnea. Chest 2002;121(2): 329–33.
20. Marquette CH, Saulnier F, Leroy O, et al. Long-term prognosis of near-fatal asthma. A 6-year follow-up study of 145 asthmatic patients who underwent mechanical ventilation for a near-fatal attack of asthma. Am Rev Respir Dis 1992;146(1):76–81.
21. Getahun D, Demissie K, Rhoads GG. Recent trends in asthma hospitalization and mortality in the United States. J Asthma 2005;42(5):373–8.
22. Miller MK, Lee JH, Miller DP, et al. Recent asthma exacerbations: a key predictor of future exacerbations. Respir Med 2007;101(3):481–9.
23. Lugogo NL, Kraft M. Epidemiology of asthma. Clin Chest Med 2006;27(1): 1–15, v.
24. Ford JG, Meyer IH, Sternfels P, et al. Patterns and predictors of asthma-related emergency department use in Harlem. Chest 2001;120(4):1129–35.
25. Barnes N. Most difficult asthma originates primarily in adult life. Paediatr Respir Rev 2006;7(2):141–4.
26. Prys-Picard C. Many asthma deaths may be preventable. Thorax 2006;61(3). Available at: http://thorax.bmj.com/cgi/content/extract/61/3/195. Accessed June 6, 2009.

27. Taylor DR, Bateman ED, Boulet L, et al. A new perspective on concepts of asthma severity and control. Eur Respir J 2008;32(3):545–54.
28. Rodrigo GJ, Rodrigo C. Rapid-onset asthma attack: a prospective cohort study about characteristics and response to emergency department treatment. Chest 2000;118(6):1547–52.
29. Woodruff PG, Emond SD, Singh AK, et al. Sudden-onset severe acute asthma: clinical features and response to therapy. Acad Emerg Med 1998; 5(7):695–701.
30. Arnold AG, Lane DJ, Zapata E. The speed of onset and severity of acute severe asthma. Br J Dis Chest 1982;76(2):157–63.
31. Ramnath VR, Clark S, Camargo CA. Multicenter study of clinical features of sudden-onset versus slower-onset asthma exacerbations requiring hospitalization. Respir Care 2007;52(8):1013–20.
32. Molfino NA, Nannini LJ, Martelli AN, et al. Respiratory arrest in near-fatal asthma. N Engl J Med 1991;324(5):285–8.
33. Sur S, Crotty TB, Kephart GM, et al. Sudden-onset fatal asthma. A distinct entity with few eosinophils and relatively more neutrophils in the airway submucosa? Am Rev Respir Dis 1993;148(3):713–9.
34. Restrepo RD, Peters J. Near-fatal asthma: recognition and management. Curr Opin Pulm Med 2008;14(1):13–23.
35. Bijl-Hofland ID, Cloosterman SG, Folgering HT, et al. Relation of the perception of airway obstruction to the severity of asthma. Thorax 1999;54(1):15–9.
36. Choi IS, Chung S, Han E, et al. Effects of anti-asthma therapy on dyspnea perception in acute asthma patients. Respir Med 2006;100(5):855–61.
37. Kleis S, Chanez P, Delvaux M, et al. Perception of dyspnea in mild smoking asthmatics. Respir Med 2007;101(7):1426–30.
38. Tatum AM, Greenberger PA, Mileusnic D, et al. Clinical, pathologic, and toxicologic findings in asthma deaths in Cook County, Illinois. Allergy Asthma Proc 2001;22(5):285–91.
39. von Leupoldt A, Kanniess F, Dahme B. The influence of corticosteroids on the perception of dyspnea in asthma. Respir Med 2007;101(6):1079–87.
40. Rodrigo GJ. Predicting response to therapy in acute asthma. Curr Opin Pulm Med 2009;15(1):35–8.
41. Emerman CL, Cydulka RK. Factors associated with relapse after emergency department treatment for acute asthma. Ann Emerg Med 1995;26(1):6–11.
42. Gaskell H, Derry S, Andrew Moore R, et al. Prevalence of anaemia in older persons: systematic review. BMC Geriatr 2008;8:1.
43. Guralnik JM, Eisenstaedt RS, Ferrucci L, et al. Prevalence of anemia in persons 65 years and older in the United States: evidence for a high rate of unexplained anemia. Blood 2004;104(8):2263–8.
44. Hoffman R. Hoffman: hematology: basic principles and practice. Philadelphia: Churchill Livingstone; 2008.
45. Weiskopf RB, Viele MK, Feiner J, et al. Human cardiovascular and metabolic response to acute, severe isovolemic anemia. JAMA 1998;279(3):217–21.
46. Goldman L, Ausiello D. Approach to the anemias. In. Philadelphia: Saunders/Elsevier; 2007.
47. Brannon ES, Merrill AJ, Warren JV, et al. The cardiac output in patients with chronic anemia as measured by the technique of right atrial catheterization. J Clin Invest 1945;24(3):332–6.
48. Sheth TN, Choudhry NK, Bowes M, et al. The relation of conjunctival pallor to the presence of anemia. J Gen Intern Med 1997;12(2):102–6.

49. Nardone DA, Roth KM, Mazur DJ, et al. Usefulness of physical examination in detecting the presence or absence of anemia. Arch Intern Med 1990;150(1):201–4.

50. Tefferi A. Anemia in adults: a contemporary approach to diagnosis. Mayo Clin Proc 2003;78(10):1274–80.

51. Crapo JD, Glassroth J, Karlinsky JB, et al. Baum's Textbook of Pulmonary Diseases. 7th edition. Philadelphia: Lippincott Williams & Wilkins; 2004. p. 1364–65.

52. Sahn SA, Heffner JE. Spontaneous pneumothorax. N Engl J Med 2000;342(12): 868–74.

53. Baumann MH, Strange C, Heffner JE, et al. Management of spontaneous pneumothorax: an American College of Chest Physicians Delphi consensus statement. Chest 2001;119(2):590–602.

54. Melton LJ, Hepper NG, Offord KP. Incidence of spontaneous pneumothorax in Olmsted County, Minnesota: 1950 to 1974. Am Rev Respir Dis 1979;120(6): 1379–82.

55. Bense L, Eklund G, Wiman LG. Smoking and the increased risk of contracting spontaneous pneumothorax. Chest 1987;92(6):1009–12.

56. Baumann MH. Management of spontaneous pneumothorax. Clin Chest Med 2006;27(2):369–81.

57. Henry M, Arnold T, Harvey J. BTS guidelines for the management of spontaneous pneumothorax. Thorax 2003;58(Suppl 2):ii39–52.

58. Mason RJ, Broaddus VC, Murray JF, et al. Murray and Nadel's textbook of respiratory medicine. 4th edition. Philadelphia: Elsevier Saunders; 2005. p. 2193–210.

59. Heffner JE, Huggins JT. Management of secondary spontaneous pneumothorax: there's confusion in the air. Chest 2004;125(4):1190–2.

60. Videm V, Pillgram-Larsen J, Ellingsen O, et al. Spontaneous pneumothorax in chronic obstructive pulmonary disease: complications, treatment and recurrences. Eur J Respir Dis 1987;71(5):365–71.

61. Dines DE, Clagett OT, Payne WS. Spontaneous pneumothorax in emphysema. Mayo Clin Proc 1970;45(7):481–7.

62. Vail WJ, Alway AE, England NJ. Spontaneous pneumothorax. Dis Chest 1960; 38:512–5.

63. O'Connor AR, Morgan WE. Radiological review of pneumothorax. BMJ 2005; 330(7506):1493–7.

64. Bradley M, Williams C, Walshaw MJ. The value of routine expiratory chest films in the diagnosis of pneumothorax. Arch Emerg Med 1991;8(2):115–6.

65. Blaivas M, Lyon M, Duggal S. A prospective comparison of supine chest radiography and bedside ultrasound for the diagnosis of traumatic pneumothorax. Acad Emerg Med 2005;12(9):844–9.

66. Lichtenstein DA, Mezière G, Lascols N, et al. Ultrasound diagnosis of occult pneumothorax. Crit Care Med 2005;33(6):1231–8.

67. Soldati G, Testa A, Sher S, et al. Occult traumatic pneumothorax: diagnostic accuracy of lung ultrasonography in the emergency department. Chest 2008; 133(1):204–11.

68. Qureshi NR, Gleeson FV. Imaging of pleural disease. Clin Chest Med 2006; 27(2):193–213.

69. Simon BC, Paolinetti L. Two cases where bedside ultrasound was able to distinguish pulmonary bleb from pneumothorax. J Emerg Med 2005;29(2):201–5.

70. Kelly A, Kerr D, Clooney M. Outcomes of emergency department patients treated for primary spontaneous pneumothorax. Chest 2008;134(5):1033–6.

71. Ayed AK, Chandrasekaran C, Sukumar M. Aspiration versus tube drainage in primary spontaneous pneumothorax: a randomised study. Eur Respir J 2006; 27(3):477–82.

72. Zehtabchi S, Rios CL. Management of emergency department patients with primary spontaneous pneumothorax: needle aspiration or tube thoracostomy? Ann Emerg Med 2008;51(1):91–100, 100.e1.

73. Wakai A, O'Sullivan RG, McCabe G. Simple aspiration versus intercostal tube drainage for primary spontaneous pneumothorax in adults. Cochrane Database Syst Rev 2007;(1):CD004479.

74. Chan SS. The role of simple aspiration in the management of primary spontaneous pneumothorax. J Emerg Med 2008;34(2):131–8.

75. Soulsby T. British Thoracic Society guidelines for the management of spontaneous pneumothorax: do we comply with them and do they work? J Accid Emerg Med 1998;15(5):317–21.

76. Apostolakis E, Koniari I. Re-expansion pulmonary oedema: is its prevention possible? Interact Cardiovasc Thorac Surg 2008;7(3):489–90.

77. Mahfood S, Hix WR, Aaron BL, et al. Reexpansion pulmonary edema. Ann Thorac Surg 1988;45(3):340–5.

78. Mahajan VK, Simon M, Huber GL. Reexpansion pulmonary edema. Chest 1979; 75(2):192–4.

79. Sohara Y. Reexpansion pulmonary edema. Ann Thorac Cardiovasc Surg 2008; 14(4):205–9.

80. Matsuura Y, Nomimura T, Murakami H, et al. Clinical analysis of reexpansion pulmonary edema. Chest 1991;100(6):1562–6.

81. Beng ST, Mahadevan M. An uncommon life-threatening complication after chest tube drainage of pneumothorax in the ED. Am J Emerg Med 2004; 22(7):615–9.

82. Rizkallah J, Man SFP, Sin DD. Prevalence of pulmonary embolism in acute exacerbations of COPD: a systematic review and metaanalysis. Chest 2009;135(3): 786–93.

83. Horlander KT, Mannino DM, Leeper KV. Pulmonary embolism mortality in the United States, 1979-1998: an analysis using multiple-cause mortality data. Arch Intern Med 2003;163(14):1711–7.

84. Carson JL, Kelley MA, Duff A, et al. The clinical course of pulmonary embolism. N Engl J Med 1992;326(19):1240–5.

85. Goldhaber SZ, Grodstein F, Stampfer MJ, et al. A prospective study of risk factors for pulmonary embolism in women. JAMA 1997;277(8):642–5.

86. Stein PD, Beemath A, Matta F, et al. Clinical characteristics of patients with acute pulmonary embolism: data from PIOPED II. Am J Med 2007;120(10):871–9.

87. Tamariz LJ, Eng J, Segal JB, et al. Usefulness of clinical prediction rules for the diagnosis of venous thromboembolism: a systematic review. Am J Med 2004; 117(9):676–84.

88. Chunilal SD, Eikelboom JW, Attia J, et al. Does this patient have pulmonary embolism? JAMA 2003;290(21):2849–58.

89. Wells PS, Ginsberg JS, Anderson DR, et al. Use of a clinical model for safe management of patients with suspected pulmonary embolism. Ann Intern Med 1998;129(12):997–1005.

90. Wells PS, Anderson DR, Rodger M, et al. Excluding pulmonary embolism at the bedside without diagnostic imaging: management of patients with suspected pulmonary embolism presenting to the emergency department by using a simple clinical model and d-dimer. Ann Intern Med 2001;135(2):98–107.

91. Wolf SJ, McCubbin TR, Nordenholz KE, et al. Assessment of the pulmonary embolism rule-out criteria rule for evaluation of suspected pulmonary embolism in the emergency department. Am J Emerg Med 2008;26(2):181–5.
92. Kline JA, Courtney DM, Kabrhel C, et al. Prospective multicenter evaluation of the pulmonary embolism rule-out criteria. J Thromb Haemost 2008;6(5):772–80.
93. Stein PD, Terrin ML, Hales CA, et al. Clinical, laboratory, roentgenographic, and electrocardiographic findings in patients with acute pulmonary embolism and no pre-existing cardiac or pulmonary disease. Chest 1991;100(3):598–603.
94. McGinn S, White PD. Acute cor pulmonale resulting from pulmonary embolism: its clinical recognition. JAMA 1935;104(17):1473–80.
95. Pollack ML. ECG manifestations of selected extracardiac diseases. Emerg Med Clin North Am 2006;24(1):133–43, vii.
96. Sinha N, Yalamanchili K, Sukhija R, et al. Role of the 12-lead electrocardiogram in diagnosing pulmonary embolism. Cardiol Rev 2005;13(1):46–9.
97. Ferrari E, Imbert A, Chevalier T, et al. The ECG in pulmonary embolism. Predictive value of negative T waves in precordial leads–80 case reports. Chest 1997; 111(3):537–43.
98. Richman PB, Loutfi H, Lester SJ, et al. Electrocardiographic findings in Emergency Department patients with pulmonary embolism. J Emerg Med 2004; 27(2):121–6.
99. Frost SD, Brotman DJ, Michota FA. Rational use of D-dimer measurement to exclude acute venous thromboembolic disease. Mayo Clin Proc 2003;78(11): 1385–91.
100. Stein PD, Hull RD, Patel KC, et al. D-dimer for the exclusion of acute venous thrombosis and pulmonary embolism: a systematic review. Ann Intern Med 2004;140(8):589–602.
101. Drucker EA, Rivitz SM, Shepard JA, et al. Acute pulmonary embolism: assessment of helical CT for diagnosis. Radiology 1998;209(1):235–41.
102. Perrier A, Howarth N, Didier D, et al. Performance of helical computed tomography in unselected outpatients with suspected pulmonary embolism. Ann Intern Med 2001;135(2):88–97.
103. Stein PD, Fowler SE, Goodman LR, et al. Multidetector computed tomography for acute pulmonary embolism. N Engl J Med 2006;354(22):2317–27.
104. Anderson DR, Kahn SR, Rodger MA, et al. Computed tomographic pulmonary angiography vs ventilation-perfusion lung scanning in patients with suspected pulmonary embolism: a randomized controlled trial. JAMA 2007;298(23): 2743–53.
105. Roy P, Colombet I, Durieux P, et al. Systematic review and meta-analysis of strategies for the diagnosis of suspected pulmonary embolism. BMJ 2005; 331(7511):259.
106. Turkstra F, Kuijer PM, van Beek EJ, et al. Diagnostic utility of ultrasonography of leg veins in patients suspected of having pulmonary embolism. Ann Intern Med 1997;126(10):775–81.
107. Madan A, Schwartz C. Echocardiographic visualization of acute pulmonary embolus and thrombolysis in the ED. Am J Emerg Med 2004;22(4):294–300.
108. Nazeyrollas P, Metz D, Jolly D, et al. Use of transthoracic Doppler echocardiography combined with clinical and electrocardiographic data to predict acute pulmonary embolism. Eur Heart J 1996;17(5):779–86.
109. Perrier A, Tamm C, Unger PF, et al. Diagnostic accuracy of Doppler-echocardiography in unselected patients with suspected pulmonary embolism. Int J Cardiol 1998;65(1):101–9.

110. Grifoni S, Olivotto I, Cecchini P, et al. Utility of an integrated clinical, echocardio-graphic, and venous ultrasonographic approach for triage of patients with suspected pulmonary embolism. Am J Cardiol 1998;82(10):1230–5.
111. Value of the ventilation/perfusion scan in acute pulmonary embolism. Results of the prospective investigation of pulmonary embolism diagnosis (PIOPED). The PIOPED Investigators. JAMA 1990;263(20):2753–9.
112. Laack TA, Goyal DG. Pulmonary embolism: an unsuspected killer. Emerg Med Clin North Am 2004;22(4):961–83.
113. Fink S, Chaudhuri TK, Davis HH. Pulmonary embolism and malpractice claims. South Med J 1998;91(12):1149–52.

Pitfalls in Evaluating the Low-Risk Chest Pain Patient

Ian D. Jones, MD[a,b,c,*], Corey M. Slovis, MD[a,d,e]

KEYWORDS

- Acute coronary syndrome • Atypical chest pain
- Chest pain in the elderly • Electrocardiogram
- Low-risk chest pain • Risk stratification

One of the most common causes of patients visiting an emergency department (ED) is a chief complaint of chest pain. Nationwide, more than 6 million ED visits a year involve patients presenting with chest pain, which is more than 5% of all ED visits. Only abdominal pain is seen more commonly.[1]

Chest pain has multiple causes ranging from benign to immediately life-threatening (**Box 1**). Immediately life-threatening causes of chest pain include acute coronary syndrome (ACS, defined as a spectrum of disease ranging from unstable angina to acute myocardial infarction [AMI]), pulmonary embolus, aortic dissection, tension pneumothorax, pericarditis with pericardial tamponade, and esophageal rupture. Less immediately life-threatening are pneumonia, anxiety, and musculoskeletal and gastrointestinal (GI, esophageal spasm, biliary colic, peptic ulcer disease) causes of chest pain. In a large percentage of patients, the cause of their chest pain is never found. The challenge for the physician evaluating a patient with acute chest pain is to rule out potential life-threatening causes and to formulate a diagnostic and management strategy that will allow for rapid and safe disposition of the patient.

In the case of most life-threatening causes of chest pain, rapidly available diagnostic tests clearly and reliably make or disprove the diagnosis. For example, when the physician considers a diagnosis of tension pneumothorax, pericardial tamponade,

[a] Department of Emergency Medicine, Vanderbilt University Medical Center, 1313 21st Avenue, South 703 Oxford House, Nashville, TN 37232-4700, USA
[b] Department of Biomedical Informatics, Vanderbilt University Medical Center, 1313 21st Avenue, South 703 Oxford House, Nashville, TN 37232-4700, USA
[c] Adult Emergency Department, Vanderbilt University Medical Center, 1313 21st Avenue, South 703 Oxford House, Nashville, TN 37232-4700, USA
[d] Metro Nashville Fire Department, Nashville, USA
[e] Nashville International Airport, Nashville, USA
* Corresponding author. Department of Emergency Medicine, Vanderbilt University Medical Center, 1313 21st Avenue, South 703 Oxford House, Nashville, TN 37232-4700
E-mail address: ian.jones@vanderbilt.edu (I.D. Jones).

Emerg Med Clin N Am 28 (2010) 183–201
doi:10.1016/j.emc.2009.10.002
0733-8627/09/$ – see front matter © 2010 Elsevier Inc. All rights reserved.

Box 1
Immediately life threatening causes of chest pain

Acute Coronary Syndrome (including unstable angina and acute myocardial infarction)

Pulmonary Embolism

Pericarditis with Tamponade

Tension Pneumothorax

Aortic Dissection

Esophageal Rupture

---

or aortic dissection, tests such as a chest radiograph, chest computed tomography (CT), or bedside ultrasonography can be used to make a rapid and definitive diagnosis. Although historically a diagnostic challenge, the diagnosis of pulmonary embolism has also become more straightforward with the development of diagnostic strategies using a combination of clinical probability, D-dimer testing, lower extremity venous compression ultrasonography, or high-resolution multidetector pulmonary CT angiography (CTA). Recent studies have shown that this strategy can be used reliably and safely to exclude the diagnosis of pulmonary embolism.[2,3]

Although the diagnosis of chest pain is becoming more straightforward with many of these causes, the diagnosis remains problematic when chest pain arises from ACS. This is especially true in patients thought by the clinician to be at low risk of cardiac ischemia.

There is considerable literature that has attempted to define the patient population with low-risk chest pain and a newer body of literature that has begun to define a subset of patients at very low risk of cardiac ischemia. The focus of this article will be on defining these patient populations and identifying potential pitfalls in the recognition and management of the patient with low-risk chest pain.

SCOPE OF THE PROBLEM

Heart disease is the leading cause of death for men and women. In 2005, cardiac ischemia was responsible for 20% of all deaths in the United States.[4] The number of new and recurrent myocardial infarctions (MIs) presenting to hospitals is estimated to be 935,000 per year. The direct and indirect cost of coronary artery disease (CAD) in the United States is estimated to be more than 165 billion dollars in 2009.[4] Because of the high prevalence of ischemic heart disease and the overwhelming morbidity, mortality, and cost associated with its management, there is no other disease process seen in the ED that has been more extensively investigated.

Numerous studies have demonstrated a fairly high rate of patients with missed cardiac ischemia who were discharged from the ED. This rate has been reported to vary from 2% to 4%, with significantly higher rates at individual centers.[5–7] Furthermore, patients discharged from an ED with undiagnosed cardiac ischemia have a high likelihood of death with mortality ranging between 10% and 25%.[7]

The significant morbidity and mortality associated with missing MI results in the highest overall cost to insurers of any missed diagnosis in emergency medicine.[8,9] Compounding this problem are the variable practice patterns amongst individual physicians in the management of patients with low-risk chest pain due to their fear of litigation. The literature has shown that emergency physicians' fear of being sued for missed ACS leads to considerable increased testing and inappropriate admission for patients in the population with low-risk chest pain.[10]

It is critically important that the emergency physician understand that a large percentage of patients defined as "low risk" in the literature are not at low enough risk to discharge home without further testing. The difficulty for the emergency physician is balancing clinical judgment, appropriate testing strategies, and evidence-based principles to manage this group of patients in a safe and cost-effective manner.

CHARACTERIZING PATIENTS DISCHARGED FROM THE ED WITH MISSED CARDIAC ISCHEMIA

In an attempt to define the type of patient who is inadvertently discharged with a missed diagnosis of cardiac ischemia, many important studies have identified the same or similar factors that lead to misdiagnosis. Lee and colleagues[6] found that patients sent home with missed MI were younger, had atypical symptoms, and were less likely to have a history of prior angina or known CAD. Additionally, roughly half of these patients had missed signs of ischemia on initial electrocardiogram (ECG). McCarthy and colleagues[7] had similar findings albeit with a lower incidence of misinterpreted ECGs. Several of these patients were diagnosed with ischemia but were thought to have stable rather than unstable angina. In a large multicenter study, Pope and colleagues[5] had similar findings and also found a continuing trend showing decreasing rates of misinterpreted signs of ischemia on ECG. They identified several, additional, significant factors in patients with missed cardiac ischemia, including women younger than 55 years and a 2-fold increase in inappropriate discharge of patients of nonwhite race.

In a recent multicenter study of missed MI in Canada, Schull and colleagues[11] found a high disparity in the number of missed MIs that inversely correlated to overall ED volume. The overall rate of missed MI in this study was 2-fold higher in low-volume facilities and ranged from 0% in EDs with the highest volume of patients to a staggering 29% at one low-volume facility. The conclusion was that higher-volume facilities with improved expertise and access to testing and consultants have the greatest ability to detect patients with cardiac ischemia.

In addition to facility volume, data in the literature demonstrate that physicians with greater experience are less likely to miss ACS. One study of litigation against emergency physicians for missed MI showed that the average number of years of ED experience was 2.6 years for those missing the diagnosis versus 5.1 years of ED experience for controls. Furthermore, physicians sued for a missed diagnosis were less likely to document cardiac risk factors or chest pain descriptors or, in some cases, even obtain an ECG.[9]

In summary, patients discharged from EDs with missed ischemia are generally younger or have atypical symptoms. Women and individuals of nonwhite race make up a larger percentage of these patients. Although a trend is seen in decreasing misinterpretation of the initial ECG, it continues to be a problem. Facilities with lower volumes of patients and physicians with less experience of working in an ED also have higher incidence of inadvertent discharge of these patients (**Box 2**).

DEFINING THE PATIENT WITH LOW-RISK AND VERY LOW-RISK CHEST PAIN

There is no single prospectively validated study or, for that matter, body of literature that defines comprehensively the patient with low-risk chest pain or specifies what an acceptable miss rate might be. In the eyes of the individual physician, the patient, and the patient's family, the miss rate should be low; ideally approaching zero. Clearly, this is a very difficult, if not impossible, task to accomplish, arising from several issues. Foremost is the complete lack of standardized reporting guidelines for studies

---

Box 2
Characteristics associated with increased inadvertent discharge of a patient with missed cardiac ischemia

Younger patient age

Atypical symptoms

Women

Nonwhite race

Physician inexperience

Lower-volume EDs

Failure to detect ischemia on initial ECG

Failure to obtain an ECG

Data from Refs.[5–9,11]

---

evaluating risk stratification in patients with potential ACS, which makes comparisons between studies difficult, and hence, no single risk stratification tool has gained widespread use in day-to-day clinical practice.[12]

There are several studies in the literature that have proposed various risk stratification schemes to identify patients with low-risk chest pain. All these studies have sought to identify a group of patients who are unlikely to have cardiac ischemia and/or AMI and therefore do not need intensive management or hospital admission. Several more recent studies have gone a step further in identifying a very low-risk subset of patients (<1% likelihood of ACS) who may be safe for discharge from the ED without additional testing beyond an ECG, thorough history and physical examination, assessment of cardiac risk factors, and if indicated, cardiac biomarkers.[13–15]

RISK STRATIFICATION

In the 1960s, the focus of a chest-pain evaluation centered on the diagnosis of AMI as evidenced by history, physical examination, and ECG findings. In 1963, coronary care units (CCUs) were developed in the United States primarily to treat lethal arrhythmias associated with AMI with pharmacologic management and early defibrillation. Before this time, one-third of patients admitted to hospitals with AMI died there. Because of the high mortality associated with AMI at the time, a concept of precoronary care was evolving. In 1967, Bernard Lown and colleagues[16] published an article advocating early monitoring in emergency wards and "immediate hospitalization on mere suspicion of myocardial infarction." At the same time, the use of cardiac biomarkers, first identified in the mid 1950s, and stress testing were still in their infancy and had not gained widespread clinical use. It was not until 1979 that the World Health Organization (WHO) officially recognized the application of an increase and decrease of cardiac biomarkers in the diagnosis of AMI.[17] Because of the difficulty in making a clear-cut diagnosis of AMI at the time and of working with less reliable data elements, very large numbers of patients with chest pain were admitted to the nations CCUs, most of whom did not have AMI.

Toward the end of this era, the first decision-making tools were developed to assist with risk stratification in patients presenting with chest pain. In 1982, Goldman and colleagues[18] published a computer-based algorithm to assist in identifying ED patients having an AMI. This tool was intended to aid the clinician in making the diagnosis of AMI and to decrease admission to CCUs in patients identified as low risk. However, it did not address the issues of unstable angina or of patients who were safe to discharge home from the ED.

As it became clear that there was a need to exclude the entire spectrum of ACS and in the face of the extreme cost of admitting large numbers of patients with chest pain to CCUs, the focus shifted to the development of chest-pain units where patients could be evaluated with a combination of ECG, biomarkers, and exercise stress testing. During this time, the focus of risk stratification models changed to include the diagnosis of cardiac ischemia in addition to AMI. In 1998, Selker and colleagues[19] published the Acute Cardiac Ischemia Time-Insensitive Predictive Instrument (ACI-TIPI) using the combination of age, sex, presence of chest pain, and ST-segment abnormalities to predict the likelihood of ACS. Although the tool was proven to be useful in triaging patients with higher-risk chest pain needing admission, it also lacked an adequate degree of sensitivity to be used by itself in the decision to discharge a patient with chest pain home without additional testing. A subsequent review of the sensitivity of the Goldman and the ACI-TIPI chest-pain stratification models has shown that the sensitivity of Goldman's risk score for detecting AMI is 90% and the ACI-TIPI for detecting cardiac ischemia is 86% to 95%.[20] Clearly, neither of these models provides the sensitivity to identify a group of patients that can be safely discharged home without additional evaluation.

An additional risk stratification tool, the thrombolysis in MI (TIMI) risk score, was published in 2000 and was originally validated on a high-risk patient population with known unstable angina or non–ST-elevation MI.[21] The tool, based on a 7-point scale, incorporates various elements, including age, risk factors, chest pain, prior CAD, use of aspirin in the previous week, positive biomarkers and ECG changes, and it was used to predict major ischemic complications at 14 days. Use of the TIMI risk score has been studied retrospectively and prospectively to assist in risk stratification in the ED of patients with low-risk chest pain.[22,23] Although the tool is excellent for identifying the highest-risk patients, those with a TIMI risk score of zero had an unacceptably high 30-day major ischemic complication rate of 1.7% to 2.1%, making its use problematic in identifying patients needing no further evaluation.[22,23] Recent efforts to improve the sensitivity of the TIMI risk score by combining a low score with a clear-cut alternative noncardiac diagnosis have also been evaluated. The results of this study demonstrated that the addition of a clear-cut noncardiac diagnosis in patients with lower TIMI risk scores did not significantly reduce major ischemic complications at 30 days.[24] Thus, the TIMI risk score does not have the sensitivity to identify patients who can be sent home from the ED without further diagnostic testing.

Later, Sanchis and colleagues[13] proposed a risk score with a primary end point of death or AMI within 1 year. This risk score improves on the original TIMI risk score and includes the cardiac biomarker troponin and a chest-pain score based on previously validated elements of the chest-pain history. A small subset of this population (17%) with a risk score of zero was deemed to be at very low risk and had no reported adverse outcomes at 1 year. However, individuals characterized as low risk by this model with a score of one had a 1-year adverse outcome rate of 3.1%.

An analysis of a subset of patients enrolled in the Rule Out Myocardial Infarction Using Coronary Artery Tomography (ROMICAT) Study has compared the sensitivity of the Goldman, TIMI, and Sanchis models in detecting ACS in ED patients with chest pain deemed to be candidates for CTA.[25] In this subset of patients, none of these models was sufficiently sensitive in detecting ACS, with all three having sensitivities falling to less than 90%.

The holy grail in the management of the patient with low-risk chest pain is identifying a subset of patients (deemed to be very low risk) who need no additional evaluation beyond a thorough history, ECG, and if indicated, cardiac biomarkers. The Vancouver Chest Pain Rule[14] has recently proposed a risk stratification model that includes age less than 40 years, no history of CAD, and a normal initial ECG result to define a very low-risk group. In addition, a very low-risk subset of individuals older than 40 years was also identified. In patients older than 40 years, further criteria were applied along with the characteristics described earlier. These included a combination of low-risk chest-pain characteristics (nonradiating pain and pain reproduced by palpation or pain described as pleuritic) combined with an initial creatine kinase MB (CK-MB) value less than 3.0 μg/L or if the CK-MB was higher than this threshold, lack of ischemic changes on repeat ECG or upward trending CK-MB or troponin value at 2 hours. Patients fitting into these criteria were deemed to be at very low risk of ACS. In this study, the sensitivity for detecting this very low-risk population was reported to be 98.8%. Furthermore, one-third of patients with chest pain evaluated in this particular study fit these criteria.

Hess and colleagues[26] reviewed 8 ED, chest-pain, decision prediction rules, including the Vancouver and Sanchis rules. After reviewing the methodology of the studies and evaluating the sensitivity and specificity of each for detecting ACS, the authors of this study have concluded that none of these models can be recommended for use in clinical practice.

It is important for the physician to understand that many early risk-stratification models were derived using high-risk patients. It is equally important that the emergency physician not equate low-risk chest pain to "no risk."

As of early 2009, no single study in the literature has been prospectively validated for adequate sensitivity to identify a subset of patients at low enough risk for discharge from the ED without further testing that may include exercise treadmill testing, nuclear scintigraphy, or coronary CTA.

CLINICAL HISTORY

The patient's history is one of the most important pieces of information available to the clinician evaluating acute chest pain in the ED. The quality, location, duration, and modifying factors associated with a patient's chest pain are critically important in establishing the correct diagnosis. Although certain aspects of the clinical history are important in identifying patients at high risk of ACS, the clinician must be aware of the pitfalls associated with placing too much reliance on symptoms thought to be less typical of the disease. This is especially true in higher-risk patients, including the elderly, patients with known CAD, diabetics, and women. Studies have repeatedly shown an increased incidence of missed ACS in patients because the physician viewed the patient's symptoms as atypical.

TYPICAL CHEST PAIN

Although some historians pointed to the possibility of earlier descriptions of angina in the medical literature, most agree that angina pectoris was first clearly described in 1768 by William Heberden.[27] Although Heberden had no knowledge of the pathophysiology of the condition, his classic description of angina pectoris included left-sided substernal pain, described as a strangling sensation worsened by exertion and relieved by rest, that radiated to the left arm. The condition was commonly seen in men older than 50 years, and as it progressed over time, the patients would invariably expire. Textbook descriptions of typical angina are variable. There is excellent information in the literature regarding elements of the chest-pain history increasing the likelihood that the pain is from cardiac ischemia. For example, pain radiating to the one or both arms significantly increases the likelihood of ACS.[28,29] Pain radiating to the right arm or both arms is far more predictive of ACS than pain radiating to the left arm. Furthermore, pain described as pressure only minimally increases the likelihood ratio that the pain is cardiac in nature.[29] Since Heberden's time, there has been a continual refinement in the accepted description of ischemic chest pain. Current guidelines published by The National Heart Attack Alert Program Coordinating Committee on recognition of symptoms potentially associated with cardiac ischemia describe the presentation as follows: Pain, if present, is described as pressure, tightness, or heaviness. It may radiate to the neck, jaw, shoulders, back, or one or both arms. The pain may also be described as indigestion or heartburn with associated nausea and/or vomiting. Additional symptoms in the absence of pain may include shortness of breath, weakness, dizziness, lightheadedness, or loss of consciousness.[30] This description serves as a useful tool and illustrates the wide constellation of symptoms associated with this disease process, many of which may be considered atypical by the inexperienced clinician.

ATYPICAL CHEST PAIN

Many clinicians use the presence of typical features in helping establish the diagnosis of ACS and atypical features to help disprove it. Unfortunately, the literature has proven that things are not quite so black-and-white. Webster's dictionary defines atypical to mean unusual or not ordinarily encountered. Symptoms referred to as atypical chest pain include those signs and symptoms that do not fit the classically described complaints typically associated with myocardial ischemia. There is currently no consensus opinion on what exactly defines "atypical" chest pain.[29] Lee and colleagues[31] reviewed the clinical history of nearly 600 patients presenting with chest pain and found that a combination 3 variables defined a low-risk group with no identified cases of ACS: (1) sharp or stabbing pain; (2) no history of angina; and (3) pain reproduced by palpation or position. Without this combination of variables, 5% of patients whose pain was described as sharp, stabbing, or pleuritic, or could be reproduced by palpation were diagnosed with AMI.[31] A separate study of patients meeting the diagnostic criteria for costochondritis found that 6% of patients actually had enzyme-proven MI.[32] Furthermore, atypical symptoms, such as burning pain and indigestion, long considered to be more suggestive of a GI cause by many physicians, has been shown to be equivalent to pressure in patients with documented myocardial ischemia.[28,29,31]

One of the major problems with an individual's chest-pain symptoms is that they are subjective and will always be so. Cultural and ethnic differences and language barriers in different patient populations further complicate the issue. Underlying diseases, such as psychiatric illness, further cloud the picture. In one illustrative study, an actress portrayed the same chest-pain history in a businesslike and then in a histrionic fashion. Physicians were nearly 5 times less likely to believe a cardiac cause of the patient's pain in the histrionic patient.[33] It is critically important that the clinician evaluating acute chest pain understand that many of the symptoms classically regarded as atypical may in fact be representative of ischemia or could even be typical myocardial ischemia. Multiple reviewers have all come to the same conclusion regarding a patient's history. Specifically, there is no single historical element that can be used to safely discharge a patient with potential ACS without additional testing. In patient with high-risk features, using the presence of atypical symptoms to exclude the diagnosis of ACS is fraught with danger.

ACS IN THE ABSENCE OF CHEST PAIN

Complicating an already difficult problem is the issue of silent ischemia. Fully 25% of patients in the Framingham study, arguably the most studied group of patients in history, have been found to have a Q-wave MI on routine annual ECGs that was so atypical in presentation that it escaped medical detection.[34] More than half of these patients had no recollection of the event, signifying a truly silent MI. More sobering is the finding of a recent study using delayed enhancement cardiovascular magnetic resonance imaging in high-risk patients that has indicated an incidence of unrecognized non–Q-wave infarction that is 3-fold higher than unrecognized Q-wave infarction.[35] Extrapolated to the entire population, this represents a staggering number of unrecognized MIs.

Studying the presenting symptoms of patients with recognized infarction, Canto and colleagues[36] reviewed the clinical presentation of more than 434,877 patients reported in the National Registry of Myocardial Infarction 2 database (NRMI-2) between 1994 and 1998 with a diagnosis of AMI. Thirty three percent of these patients did not have chest discomfort or arm, neck, or jaw pain on initial presentation to the hospital. AMI patients presenting without chest pain were, on average, 7 years older and had a higher population of women and diabetics than these patients presenting with chest pain. Brieger and colleagues[37] reviewed more than 20,000 cases of ACS in the Global Registry of Coronary Events (GRACE) database. In this population, 8.4% did not have chest pain at presentation and almost a quarter of these were not recognized to have ACS on their initial presentation. The most common symptom in the absence of chest pain was dyspnea followed by diaphoresis, nausea, and syncope. Similar to Canto's findings, this group of patients was also far more likely to be elderly, female, hypertensive, diabetic, or have a history of congestive heart failure.

To summarize, the greatest pitfall for the emergency physician in evaluating a patient with ACS in the absence of chest pain is failing to consider the diagnosis of cardiac ischemia entirely. Specific symptoms by themselves in the absence of chest pain may in fact be anginal equivalents in certain patient populations. If the patient fits the criteria described earlier, such as an elderly diabetic with syncope or an 80-year-old man with unexplained dyspnea, the physician must have a high degree of suspicion and include ACS high on their differential diagnosis and must manage the patient aggressively.

PRECIPITATING FACTORS

There are several activities that may precipitate acute ischemia. Culic[38] performed a meta analysis reviewing 17 different studies covering more than 10,000 patients with AMI and identified several important triggers. In this review, nearly 35% of patients with AMI were performing some kind of physical activity. Patients were found to be eating in 8.2% of cases and 6.8% of patients reported emotional stress before the event. The study also found that 20% of patients were awakened from sleep.

The important factor demonstrated here is that the physician should not discount emotional stress or eating as precipitating factors and assign an alternate cause for the patient's symptoms, such as anxiety or GI cause.

RELIEVING FACTORS

Many individuals incorrectly assume that because a patient's chest pain is relieved with nitroglycerine, the pain is more likely to be cardiac in nature. In examining this question, Henrikson and colleagues[39] found a higher incidence of relief of chest pain in patients without ACS than those with active ischemia. Steele and colleagues[40] also found that nitroglycerine relieved chest pain in 66% of patients who were ultimately diagnosed with noncardiac chest pain. This data shows that chest-pain relief by nitroglycerine had no value in predicting or disproving ACS. Similarly, physicians have used the GI cocktail (a mixture of antacids and viscous lidocaine) to prove the likelihood of a GI cause and disprove the presence of ACS. There is no recent literature supporting the use of the GI cocktail for differentiating these types of pain, but the practice persists. Many physicians believe that burning substernal pain relieved by antacids is clearly caused by esophagitis or gastritis. Subsequent studies have actually shown that "burning" chest pain or pain described as "indigestion" may be as strong a descriptor of ischemia as chest pressure.[28,31] In a small descriptive study, Wrenn and colleagues[41] found indiscriminate use of the GI cocktail for various ED complaints. In this subset, a significant portion of patients who were subsequently admitted with possible myocardial ischemia reported total or partial relief after administration of a GI cocktail.

In summary, chest-pain relief with either nitroglycerine or GI cocktail does nothing to improve the diagnostic accuracy for ACS and should not be used to influence decision making.

CARDIAC RISK FACTORS

There are a large number of conditions and behaviors that have traditionally been associated with the development of CAD. These classic risk factors are advanced age, male sex, diabetes mellitus, smoking, hypertension, hypercholesterolemia, and the presence of premature coronary disease in a first-degree relative. In addition to these well-recognized risk factors, a host of other conditions are known to be associated with the development of CAD, whereas others are now known to be involved in AMI in patients with normal coronary arteries (**Box 3**). It would seem intuitive that assessing risk factors or risk-factor burden can guide a physician's disposition of an individual patient and many physicians use the presence or absence of cardiac risk factors to guide management. Jayes and colleagues[42] examined whether the presence of classic cardiac risk factors had significant predictive value in diagnosis of acute ischemia in the ED. The findings of this study showed that except for diabetes and a positive family history in male patients, classical risk factors were of little additional value in predicting ischemia. Although these 2 risk factors were found to be important, they conferred only a 2-fold increase in risk for acute ischemia. This was far less than the relative risk of a compelling history or ECG abnormalities.[42] Nearly 20% of patients with known ischemic heart disease do not have conventional risk factors of CAD, which illustrates the potential pitfalls of over-reliance on risk factors in the acute setting.[43] The clinician must be aware that risk factors predict the development of CAD over a lifetime and do not correlate at all well with the risk of ischemia in a patient with acute chest pain.

One possible exception to this rule is the absence of cardiac risk factors in patients younger than 40 years. Several studies have shown that patients younger than 40 years without identifiable risk factors are at low risk of ACS.[14,15,44]

In looking at overall risk-factor burden, Han and colleagues[44] found increasing likelihood of ACS as the total number of risk factors increased. This was especially

---

Box 3
Risk factors of CAD

Classic or traditional risk factors

    Advanced age

    Male sex

    Hypertension

    Diabetes mellitus

    Hypercholesterolemia

    Premature CAD in a first-degree relative

    Cigarette smoking

Nontraditional risk factors

    HIV

    Systemic lupus erythematosus

    End-stage renal disease

    Cocaine

    Type A personality

    Genetic and acquired thrombophilias

---

important in patients younger than 40 years. However, in patients older than 40 years, absence of risk factors was insufficient in itself to rule out ACS.

In patients older than 40 years, cardiac factors are of very little use in the acute setting in the diagnosis of ACS. Hence, they should not be used to alter physicians' judgment in this patient population.

GENDER DIFFERENCES

In general, men develop coronary disease 7 to 10 years earlier than women. Clear differences do exist in the presentation of ACS between men and women. In a study of 1450 patients with documented MI, Goldberg and colleagues[45] defined differences in symptom presentation based on gender. Findings from the study showed that men were less likely to complain of neck, back, or jaw pain and were less likely to present with nausea. Canto and colleagues[46] confirmed these findings and found a higher proportion of women with ACS reporting indigestion, fatigue, palpitations, and weakness. Women with ACS also have a higher total number of associated symptoms and risk factors than men and generally present at a more advanced age.[46,47] Amongst individuals with advanced disease, women were less likely to be treated aggressively and had a higher mortality.[47]

CHEST PAIN AND ACS IN YOUNG ADULTS

CAD is uncommon in individuals younger than 40 years, and in the United States, CAD in this age group has a prevalence of 0.8% in men and women.[4] It is important to be aware that MIs do occur with some frequency in younger patients and approximately 6% to 10% occur in patients younger than 45 years.[48] Most of these patients (80%) are men and have single-vessel coronary disease. Up to 20% of these patients do not have coronary atherosclerosis.[48] Berenson and colleagues[49] studied the presence of coronary atherosclerosis in young adults at autopsy to identify risk factors for the development of CAD. In this population, elevated body mass index, hyperlipidemia, hypertension, and smoking were all strongly correlated with the development of premature CAD. Prior studies have also strongly linked poorly controlled diabetes to premature coronary atherosclerosis.[49]

In a study of clinical characteristics and outcomes of ED patients younger than 40 years with chest pain, Walker and colleagues[50] found a 4.7% incidence of ACS. Within this group, however, a population at very low risk of ACS was identified. Amongst this group of patients with chest pain and no history of cocaine use, individuals without a known history of CAD, a normal ECG result, no classic cardiac risk factors, and normal cardiac biomarker levels were found to have had less than 0.5% risk of ACS. Marsan and colleagues[15] prospectively validated Walker's original study. In this group, an adverse 30-day outcome was defined by the need for bypass surgery, angioplasty, or by AMI or death. Once again, the overall incidence of ACS in this cohort was not insignificant, with 5.4% of patients in the study being diagnosed with ACS, and the very low-risk patient group (normal ECG results, normal enzyme levels, and no cardiac risk factors) was found to have a very low rate (0.14%) of adverse events at 30 days.

In summary, the physician should be acutely aware of the potential for ACS in younger patients and that age, by itself, cannot and should not be used to assign a patient to a very low-risk group. Roughly 5% of patients younger than 40 years presenting with chest pain have cardiac ischemia. Although young patients are less likely to present with ACS, those with a compelling history and cardiac risk factors, either traditional or nontraditional, should prompt a careful evaluation.

CARDIAC ISCHEMIA IN THE ELDERLY

The elderly patient population stands to gain the most from rapid recognition of and intervention in ACS, yet studies continue to indicate lower use of invasive treatments and cardiovascular medications amongst this patient population.[51] AMI carries a significantly higher risk of death in the elderly patient; 82% of patients who die from CAD are aged 65 years or older and one-third of deaths in this population are a result of ischemic heart disease.[4]

Difficulties arise in the evaluation of elderly patients with ACS primarily due to an increasing number of vague and atypical symptoms and the wide constellation of complaints that are associated with ACS in this patient group. ACS may also accompany another acute incident in the elderly, such as a fall or a cerebrovascular accident, and may therefore be missed. Age-related neurologic diseases, such as dementia, further cloud this picture. In a study of a large population of Medicare beneficiaries with unstable angina, Canto and colleagues[52] found that more than half had presentations that were categorized as atypical. These complaints included dyspnea, nausea, diaphoresis, syncope, or pain primarily localized to the arm, neck, jaw, or abdomen. Data from the NRMI has shown that only 60% of patients 85 years or older had no chest pain on initial presentation.[51] Amongst patients presenting with ACS in the absence of chest pain, up to 25% are missed on initial presentation.[37] Despite the importance of obtaining a rapid ECG, recent literature has demonstrated that the elderly are less likely to have an ECG performed in a timely fashion or to receive appropriate initial care.[53]

Most physicians recognize the elderly to be at high risk of ACS. The major pitfall in this group of patients is the wide variety of atypical presentations that may be seen and the physician's failure to recognize that these symptoms may be arising from cardiac ischemia.

THE PHYSICAL EXAMINATION

As medicine has advanced, many think that the physical examination has taken on a less important role than sophisticated imaging and laboratory testing in a patient's evaluation. Although the physical examination is extremely important for many disease processes, it is of little benefit in establishing a diagnosis of ACS in the patient with low-risk chest pain, and results are often normal. Physical signs associated with ACS, such as heart failure, are rare in most patients with ACS. The most common finding in acute ischemia is the presence of a fourth heart sound.[54] However, the noisy ED environment is often a difficult place to hear subtle and often fleeting heart sounds. Furthermore, more recent information from a study using digitally recorded heart sounds on patients with chest pain showed no statistical association between abnormal heart sounds and ACS.[55] The physical examination is of limited use in establishing a diagnosis of ACS; its value however lies in assisting with finding or excluding an alternate diagnosis.

PHYSICIANS INITIAL IMPRESSION AND JUDGMENT

To perform initial risk stratification of patients presenting with acute chest pain, physicians must rely on various immediately available data elements, including the patient's chest pain history, risk factor profile, physical examination, and initial ECG. Miller and colleagues[56] studied whether the physician's initial impression of noncardiac chest pain based on these data elements was sufficient information to send the patient home without further testing. The results of this study looked at physicians' impressions for 17,737 patients with chest pain older than 18 years enrolled in the multicenter chest-pain registry, Internet Tracking Registry of Acute Coronary Syndromes (i*trACS). In this study, patients were assigned to several categories, including definite unstable angina or AMI and high-risk, low-risk, or noncardiac chest pain. After the initial evaluation, physicians assigned 20.8% of patients to this noncardiac group. These patients had further evaluations, including biomarkers and stress testing, at the discretion of the treating physician. Adverse outcomes, including AMI, revascularization at 30 days, or cardiac death, were measured. Findings within this noncardiac chest-pain group showed that 2.8% had a definite cardiac event at 30 days. Further analysis of these patients showed that those who had adverse outcomes were older and more likely to have traditional risk factors of CAD or known CAD.

In another study, Hollander and colleagues[57] examined the relationship between the physician impression of a clear-cut alternative diagnosis and 30-day adverse outcomes for chest pain. After initial ED evaluation, including biomarkers if requested, physicians were asked if the patient had a clear-cut alternative diagnosis, such as gastroesophageal reflux, musculoskeletal pain, or other noncardiac cause. In this study 30% of patients were thought to have a clear-cut alternative chest-pain diagnosis, yet at 30 days, 4% had an adverse cardiac outcome.

Although physician judgment is critically important and can be used to improve risk stratification, it must be tempered with the evidence that in patients with advancing age, known CAD or risk-factor burden, an impression in itself, is not enough information to safely send a patient home without further testing.

THE INITIAL ECG

Electrical activity in the heart was first recognized in the mid 1800s. In 1920, ST elevation was first described in association with a patient having an AMI.[58] Today, the 12-lead ECG continues to be the single most important and most rapidly available diagnostic test used in the management of the patient with chest pain.

Any ECG changes should be considered important. Studies of patients discharged from the ED with a missed diagnosis of myocardial ischemia have shown that a major reason is misinterpretation of the ECG.[5–7] Virtually all risk stratification schemes assign higher risk to patients with abnormal ECG results.

Objective findings such as ST depression on presentation carry significant mortality. In one study of more than 250,000 patients in the NRMI database, patients with ST depression had an in-hospital mortality of 15.5%, which was equivalent to that of patients with an ST-segment elevation myocardial infarction (STEMI).[59] Furthermore, any T-wave abnormalities, including T-wave inversion and flattening, carry higher risks of cardiovascular events at 30 days.[60]

Several studies in the not-so-distant past have suggested that a normal or nonspecific ECG result portends low morbidity and mortality, and deferred outpatient testing in this patient population was recommended. Approximately 50% of patients with unstable angina and non–Q-wave MI do not have significant abnormalities on ECG. Welch and colleagues[61] reviewed initial ECG findings from the NRMI database in 391,208 patients with documented AMI. Within this patient population, 7.8% had a normal ECG result and 35.2% had nonspecific ECG findings on initial presentation. Based on this data, it is clear that a normal or nonspecific ECG finding cannot, by itself, be used to rule out ischemia.

Testing the hypothesis that the sensitivity of the ECG would be greater on symptomatic patients, Chase and colleagues[62] examined the prognostic value of a normal or nonspecific ECG obtained while the patient was experiencing chest pain. The results of this study indicated that patients with normal or nonspecific ECG findings obtained during pain had similar 30-day adverse outcome rates to those whose ECG had been obtained after their pain had subsided.

A normal or nondiagnostic ECG has been shown to be one of the most likely reasons that a patient was discharged with missed cardiac ischemia. The physician managing a patient with acute chest pain should recognize that an ECG represents a single snapshot in the patient's presentation and may be normal or nondiagnostic even in the face of active ischemia. Furthermore, ECG findings are often dynamic in patients with ACS. Strategies, such as continuous ST-segment trend monitoring and aggressive use of serial ECGs, may be of help but are less useful if a patient's pain has resolved. Physicians should not rely on a normal ECG alone in disposition of patients without further evaluation.

CARDIAC BIOMARKERS

Cardiac biomarkers are an essential component in the initial workup of patients with possible ischemic chest pain. The first cardiac biomarkers were identified in 1954 but did not gain widespread clinical use for more than 20 years.[17] Through the 1970s, assays were plagued with issues with sensitivity and it was not until the age of immunoassays in the 1980s that the use of cardiac biomarkers realized their full potential.

Today, the gold standard biomarker for diagnosing AMI is troponin[63] and immunoassays for cardiac troponin. Troponin T and I can be used to detect myocardial necrosis with a high degree of sensitivity.

An early investigation[64] looked at the prognostic value of a negative troponin T or troponin I value at presentation in ED patients with acute chest pain. In this study, the investigators concluded that patients with negative troponin values were at low risk and could safely be discharged from the ED with no additional testing. Several studies performed since then have shown that this is clearly not the case. Subsequent evaluations of the prognostic value by 2 larger studies have found that a normal initial troponin value had low sensitivity for predicting cardiac events.[65,66] Hence, although both studies found a normal troponin value to be beneficial in risk stratification, it does not assure a favorable prognosis and cannot be used by itself to guide management in the low-risk patient population.

The literature has shown that the use of serial biomarkers can assist in detection of ACS. Fesmire and colleagues[67] have devised a protocol using a combination of ECG findings, comparison of 2-hour serial cardiac biomarkers, and physician judgment with a sensitivity that approaches 85% for detecting ACS in high- and low-risk patients. An upward trend in biomarkers has been shown to have significant power for detecting ACS. Some physicians have incorporated the increased discriminatory power of serial markers in decision making to discharge low-risk patients without further workup. The authors caution against this practice without further testing in all but patients determined to be at very low risk.

Many physicians continue to obtain troponin and CK-MB. Storrow and colleagues[68] looked at the odds ratio (OR) for ACS with discordant values of CK-MB and troponin. Both groups of patients, one found to have elevated troponin and normal CK-MB level and the other, normal troponin and elevated CK-MB level, were at higher risk of ACS (OR 4.8 and 2.2, respectively). Additionally, the finding of elevated CK-MB level with a normal total CK value was also associated with a higher incidence of ACS.

In summary, a single normal cardiac biomarker level cannot be used to rule out ACS. Although serial biomarkers can improve the detection of ACS, the physician should use careful judgment of the patient population on which they can be used without further testing. Finally, the finding of discordant biomarkers identifies higher-risk groups that should undergo further testing.

PRIOR NEGATIVE CARDIAC WORKUP

A frequent issue facing the emergency physician is a patient who presents to the ED with chest pain who has undergone a prior stress test or cardiac catheterization. Although cardiac catheterization remains the gold standard in diagnosing CAD and there is excellent literature on the favorable short-term prognosis of discharged patients who have undergone stress testing of all types, there is little information in the literature on the management of patients who return to the ED after a negative result in chest-pain workup.

In cases where the stress test result is abnormal or catheterization shows disease, the management is more straightforward. Patients who have known disease should never be considered low risk. In patients where a prior workup had negative results, the issue becomes more complex.

The 3-year event rate for patients with prior negative stress testing results has been reported as being between 5% and 15% in several small studies.[69,70] A negative stress test result by itself does not rule out coronary disease. A stress test can be considered valid during the time it is performed to rule out ischemia as the cause of a patient's chest pain during that visit. As a result, many physicians have a low threshold for repeating stress testing on subsequent chest-pain evaluations. In the only study examining the impact of a prior negative stress test result on physician management patterns for patients returning to the ED with chest pain, it was found that patients were admitted with a prior negative stress test result at the same rate as those who had never had a stress test.[71]

Many physicians take comfort in a prior normal cardiac catheterization and a belief that this portends very low risk for the patient re-presenting with chest pain. A small study of 17 patients with angiographically normal coronaries found that only 2 (11.7%) had developed coronary disease at the time of repeat angiogram (averaging 9 years between procedures).[72] A later study covering 1-year events rates in 7656 patients with mild CAD (<50% stenosis) or normal coronary arteries pooled from 3 large randomized trials found a serious event rate (defined as death or AMI) of 3.3% and 1.2% in these 2 groups, respectively.[73] These data are at odds with many physicians' belief that a normal angiogram equates to no short-term risk of ACS. It has been known for many years that by their very nature, angiograms may miss clinically important lesions,[74] and hence, the clinician should not be overly reliant on the results of a prior normal angiogram if clinical concern is sufficient.

In summary, although a prior negative angiogram may be helpful in risk stratification, in a patient with a compelling history or in a high-risk clinical situation, it cannot be used alone to discharge a patient without further testing.

SUMMARY

Risk stratification and management of the patient with low-risk chest pain continues to be challenging despite considerable effort on the part of numerous investigators. At least, there is now evidence that a specific subset of young patients can be defined as a very low-risk group in whom further testing may not be necessary. For all other patients, the physician must have a high index of suspicion for ACS and understand the myriad of often subtle and atypical presentations of ischemic heart disease, especially in certain patient populations such as the elderly.

Although the initial history, ECG, and biomarkers are critically important, obtaining serial ECGs and biomarkers improves sensitivity in detecting ACS. However, physicians must always keep in mind that for many patients with atypical symptoms, relying on normal or unchanged ECG findings, negative cardiac biomarker levels, or the absence of cardiac risk factors, is not enough to safely discharge a patient without further workup. Hence, some type of objective testing such as exercise treadmill testing, nuclear scintigraphy, stress echocardiography, or coronary CTA, should be strongly considered before, or soon after, discharge in all patients who do not have a clearly explained reason for their chest pain.

REFERENCES

1. Pitts SR, Niska RW, Xu J, et al. National hospital ambulatory medical care survey: 2006 emergency department summary. Natl Health Stat Report 2008;(7):1–38.
2. Anderson DR, Kahn SR, Rodger MA, et al. Computed tomographic pulmonary angiography vs ventilation-perfusion lung scanning in patients with suspected pulmonary embolism: a randomized controlled trial. JAMA 2007;298(23): 2743–53.
3. Anderson DR, Kovacs MJ, Dennie C, et al. Use of spiral computed tomography contrast angiography and ultrasonography to exclude the diagnosis of pulmonary embolism in the emergency department. J Emerg Med 2005;29(4):399–404.
4. Lloyd-Jones D, Adams R, Carnethon M, et al. Heart disease and stroke statistics–2009 update: a report from the American Heart Association Statistics Committee and Stroke Statistics Subcommittee. Circulation 2009;119(3):480–6.
5. Pope JH, Aufderheide TP, Ruthazer R, et al. Missed diagnoses of acute cardiac ischemia in the emergency department. N Engl J Med 2000;342(16):1163–70.

6. Lee TH, Rouan GW, Weisberg MC, et al. Clinical characteristics and natural history of patients with acute myocardial infarction sent home from the emergency room. Am J Cardiol 1987;60(4):219–24.
7. McCarthy BD, Beshansky JR, D'Agostino RB, et al. Missed diagnoses of acute myocardial infarction in the emergency department: results from a multicenter study. Ann Emerg Med 1993;22(3):579–82.
8. Freas GC. Medicolegal aspects of acute myocardial infarction. Emerg Med Clin North Am 2001;19(2):511–21.
9. Rusnak RA, Stair TO, Hansen K, et al. Litigation against the emergency physician: common features in cases of missed myocardial infarction. Ann Emerg Med 1989;18(10):1029–34.
10. Katz DA, Williams GC, Brown RL, et al. Emergency physicians' fear of malpractice in evaluating patients with possible acute cardiac ischemia. Ann Emerg Med 2005;46(6):525–33.
11. Schull MJ, Vermeulen MJ, Stukel TA. The risk of missed diagnosis of acute myocardial infarction associated with emergency department volume. Ann Emerg Med 2006;48(6):647–55.
12. Hollander JE. Risk stratification of emergency department patients with chest pain: the need for standardized reporting guidelines. Ann Emerg Med 2004; 43(1):68–70.
13. Sanchis J, Bodi V, Nunez J, et al. New risk score for patients with acute chest pain, non-ST-segment deviation, and normal troponin concentrations: a comparison with the TIMI risk score. J Am Coll Cardiol 2005;46(3):443–9.
14. Christenson J, Innes G, McKnight D, et al. A clinical prediction rule for early discharge of patients with chest pain. Ann Emerg Med 2006;47(1):1–10.
15. Marsan RJ Jr, Shaver KJ, Sease KL, et al. Evaluation of a clinical decision rule for young adult patients with chest pain. Acad Emerg Med 2005;12(1):26–31.
16. Lown B, Vasaux C, Hood WB Jr, et al. Unresolved problems in coronary care. Am J Cardiol 1967;20(4):494–508.
17. Dolci A, Panteghini M. The exciting story of cardiac biomarkers: from retrospective detection to gold diagnostic standard for acute myocardial infarction and more. Clin Chim Acta 2006;369(2):179–87.
18. Goldman L, Weinberg M, Weisberg M, et al. A computer-derived protocol to aid in the diagnosis of emergency room patients with acute chest pain. N Engl J Med 1982;307(10):588–96.
19. Selker HP, Beshansky JR, Griffith JL, et al. Use of the acute cardiac ischemia time-insensitive predictive instrument (ACI-TIPI) to assist with triage of patients with chest pain or other symptoms suggestive of acute cardiac ischemia. A multicenter, controlled clinical trial. Ann Intern Med 1998;129(11):845–55.
20. Lau J, Ioannidis JP, Balk EM, et al. Diagnosing acute cardiac ischemia in the emergency department: a systematic review of the accuracy and clinical effect of current technologies. Ann Emerg Med 2001;37(5):453–60.
21. Antman EM, Cohen M, Bernink PJ, et al. The TIMI risk score for unstable angina/ non-ST elevation MI: a method for prognostication and therapeutic decision making. JAMA 2000;284(7):835–42.
22. Pollack CV Jr, Sites FD, Shofer FS, et al. Application of the TIMI risk score for unstable angina and non-ST elevation acute coronary syndrome to an unselected emergency department chest pain population. Acad Emerg Med 2006;13(1):13–8.
23. Chase M, Robey JL, Zogby KE, et al. Prospective validation of the thrombolysis in myocardial infarction risk score in the emergency department chest pain population. Ann Emerg Med 2006;48(3):252–9.

24. Campbell CF, Chang AM, Sease KL, et al. Combining thrombolysis in myocardial infarction risk score and clear-cut alternative diagnosis for chest pain risk stratification. Am J Emerg Med 2009;27(1):37–42.
25. Manini AF, Dannemann N, Brown DF, et al. Limitations of risk score models in patients with acute chest pain. Am J Emerg Med 2009;27(1):43–8.
26. Hess EP, Thiruganasambandamoorthy V, Wells GA, et al. Diagnostic accuracy of clinical prediction rules to exclude acute coronary syndrome in the emergency department setting: a systematic review. CJEM 2008;10(4):373–82.
27. Heberden W. Some account of a disorder of the breast. Med Trans Roy Coll of Phys 1772;2:59–67.
28. Goodacre SW, Angelini K, Arnold J, et al. Clinical predictors of acute coronary syndromes in patients with undifferentiated chest pain. QJM 2003;96(12):893–8.
29. Swap CJ, Nagurney JT. Value and limitations of chest pain history in the evaluation of patients with suspected acute coronary syndromes. JAMA 2005;294(20): 2623–9.
30. Emergency department: rapid identification and treatment of patients with acute myocardial infarction. National Heart Attack Alert Program Coordinating Committee, 60 Minutes to Treatment Working Group. Ann Emerg Med 1994; 23(2):311–29.
31. Lee TH, Cook EF, Weisberg M, et al. Acute chest pain in the emergency room. Identification and examination of low-risk patients. Arch Intern Med 1985; 145(1):65–9.
32. Disla E, Rhim HR, Reddy A, et al. Costochondritis. A prospective analysis in an emergency department setting. Arch Intern Med 1994;154(21):2466–9.
33. Birdwell BG, Herbers JE, Kroenke K. Evaluating chest pain. The patient's presentation style alters the physician's diagnostic approach. Arch Intern Med 1993; 153(17):1991–5.
34. Kannel WB, Abbott RD. Incidence and prognosis of unrecognized myocardial infarction. An update on the Framingham study. N Engl J Med 1984;311(18): 1144–7.
35. Kim HW, Klem I, Shah DJ, et al. Unrecognized non-Q-wave myocardial infarction: prevalence and prognostic significance in patients with suspected coronary disease. PLoS Med 2009;6(4):e1000057.
36. Canto JG, Shlipak MG, Rogers WJ, et al. Prevalence, clinical characteristics, and mortality among patients with myocardial infarction presenting without chest pain. JAMA 2000;283(24):3223–9.
37. Brieger D, Eagle KA, Goodman SG, et al. Acute coronary syndromes without chest pain, an underdiagnosed and undertreated high-risk group: insights from the global registry of acute coronary events. Chest 2004;126(2):461–9.
38. Culic V. Acute risk factors for myocardial infarction. Int J Cardiol 2007;117(2): 260–9.
39. Henrikson CA, Howell EE, Bush DE, et al. Chest pain relief by nitroglycerin does not predict active coronary artery disease. Ann Intern Med 2003;139(12):979–86.
40. Steele R, McNaughton T, McConahy M, et al. Chest pain in emergency department patients: if the pain is relieved by nitroglycerin, is it more likely to be cardiac chest pain? CJEM 2006;8(3):164–9.
41. Wrenn K, Slovis CM, Gongaware J. Using the "GI cocktail": a descriptive study. Ann Emerg Med 1995;26(6):687–90.
42. Jayes RL Jr, Beshansky JR, D'Agostino RB, et al. Do patients' coronary risk factor reports predict acute cardiac ischemia in the emergency department? A multicenter study. J Clin Epidemiol 1992;45(6):621–6.

43. Khot UN, Khot MB, Bajzer CT, et al. Prevalence of conventional risk factors in patients with coronary heart disease. JAMA 2003;290(7):898–904.
44. Han JH, Lindsell CJ, Storrow AB, et al. The role of cardiac risk factor burden in diagnosing acute coronary syndromes in the emergency department setting. Ann Emerg Med 2007;49(2):145–52, 152 e141.
45. Goldberg RJ, O'Donnell C, Yarzebski J, et al. Sex differences in symptom presentation associated with acute myocardial infarction: a population-based perspective. Am Heart J 1998;136(2):189–95.
46. Canto JG, Goldberg RJ, Hand MM, et al. Symptom presentation of women with acute coronary syndromes: myth vs reality. Arch Intern Med 2007;167(22): 2405–13.
47. Dey S, Flather MD, Devlin G, et al. Sex-related differences in the presentation, treatment and outcomes among patients with acute coronary syndromes: the Global Registry of Acute Coronary Events. Heart 2009;95(1):20–6.
48. Choudhury L, Marsh JD. Myocardial infarction in young patients. Am J Med 1999; 107(3):254–61.
49. Berenson GS, Srinivasan SR, Bao W, et al. Association between multiple cardiovascular risk factors and atherosclerosis in children and young adults. The Bogalusa Heart Study. N Engl J Med 1998;338(23):1650–6.
50. Walker NJ, Sites FD, Shofer FS, et al. Characteristics and outcomes of young adults who present to the emergency department with chest pain. Acad Emerg Med 2001;8(7):703–8.
51. Alexander KP, Newby LK, Cannon CP, et al. Acute coronary care in the elderly, part I: Non-ST-segment-elevation acute coronary syndromes: a scientific statement for healthcare professionals from the American Heart Association Council on Clinical Cardiology: in collaboration with the Society of Geriatric Cardiology. Circulation 2007;115(19):2549–69.
52. Canto JG, Fincher C, Kiefe CI, et al. Atypical presentations among Medicare beneficiaries with unstable angina pectoris. Am J Cardiol 2002;90(3): 248–53.
53. Alexander KP, Roe MT, Chen AY, et al. Evolution in cardiovascular care for elderly patients with non-ST-segment elevation acute coronary syndromes: results from the CRUSADE National Quality Improvement Initiative. J Am Coll Cardiol 2005; 46(8):1479–87.
54. Craddock LD. The physical examination in acute cardiac ischemic syndromes. J Emerg Med 1991;9(1–2):55–60.
55. Miller C, Warner RA, Hoekstra JW. The utility of electronically recorded S3 and S4 gallops to predict cardiac events in emergency department patients with chest pain [abstract]. Ann Emerg Med 2006;48(4):46.
56. Miller CD, Lindsell CJ, Khandelwal S, et al. Is the initial diagnostic impression of "noncardiac chest pain" adequate to exclude cardiac disease? Ann Emerg Med 2004;44(6):565–74.
57. Hollander JE, Robey JL, Chase MR, et al. Relationship between a clear-cut alternative noncardiac diagnosis and 30-day outcome in emergency department patients with chest pain. Acad Emerg Med 2007;14(3):210–5.
58. Pardee H. An electrocardiographic sign of coronary artery obstruction. Arch Intern Med 1920;26:244–57.
59. Pitta SR, Grzybowski M, Welch RD, et al. ST-segment depression on the initial electrocardiogram in acute myocardial infarction-prognostic significance and its effect on short-term mortality: A report from the National Registry of Myocardial Infarction (NRMI-2, 3, 4). Am J Cardiol 2005;95(7):843–8.

60. Lin KB, Shofer FS, McCusker C, et al. Predictive value of T-wave abnormalities at the time of emergency department presentation in patients with potential acute coronary syndromes. Acad Emerg Med 2008;15(6):537–43.
61. Welch RD, Zalenski RJ, Frederick PD, et al. Prognostic value of a normal or nonspecific initial electrocardiogram in acute myocardial infarction. JAMA 2001;286(16):1977–84.
62. Chase M, Brown AM, Robey JL, et al. Prognostic value of symptoms during a normal or nonspecific electrocardiogram in emergency department patients with potential acute coronary syndrome. Acad Emerg Med 2006;13(10):1034–9.
63. Alpert JS, Thygesen K, Antman E, et al. Myocardial infarction redefined–a consensus document of The Joint European Society of Cardiology/American College of Cardiology Committee for the redefinition of myocardial infarction. J Am Coll Cardiol 2000;36(3):959–69.
64. Hamm CW, Goldmann BU, Heeschen C, et al. Emergency room triage of patients with acute chest pain by means of rapid testing for cardiac troponin T or troponin I. N Engl J Med 1997;337(23):1648–53.
65. Kontos MC, Anderson FP, Alimard R, et al. Ability of troponin I to predict cardiac events in patients admitted from the emergency department. J Am Coll Cardiol 2000;36(6):1818–23.
66. Sanchis J, Bodi V, Llacer A, et al. Risk stratification of patients with acute chest pain and normal troponin concentrations. Heart 2005;91(8):1013–8.
67. Fesmire FM, Hughes AD, Fody EP, et al. The Erlanger chest pain evaluation protocol: a one-year experience with serial 12-lead ECG monitoring, two-hour delta serum marker measurements, and selective nuclear stress testing to identify and exclude acute coronary syndromes. Ann Emerg Med 2002;40(6):584–94.
68. Storrow AB, Lindsell CJ, Han JH, et al. Discordant cardiac biomarkers: frequency and outcomes in emergency department patients with chest pain. Ann Emerg Med 2006;48(6):660–5.
69. Smith SW, Jackson EA, Bart BA, et al. Incidence of myocardial infarction in emergency department chest pain patients with a recent negative stress imaging test [abstract]. Acad Emerg Med 2005;12:51.
70. Walker JG, Galuska M, Vega D, et al. Significant coronary artery disease in emergency chest pain patients with recent negative cardiac stress testing [abstract]. Ann Emerg Med 2008;52(4):s90.
71. Nerenberg RH, Shofer FS, Robey JL, et al. Impact of a negative prior stress test on emergency physician disposition decision in ED patients with chest pain syndromes. Am J Emerg Med 2007;25(1):39–44.
72. Pitts WR, Lange RA, Cigarroa JE, et al. Repeat coronary angiography in patients with chest pain and previously normal coronary angiogram. Am J Cardiol 1997; 80(8):1086–7.
73. Bugiardini R, Manfrini O, De Ferrari GM. Unanswered questions for management of acute coronary syndrome: risk stratification of patients with minimal disease or normal findings on coronary angiography. Arch Intern Med 2006;166(13):1391–5.
74. Topol EJ, Nissen SE. Our preoccupation with coronary luminology. The dissociation between clinical and angiographic findings in ischemic heart disease. Circulation 1995;92(8):2333–42.

The High-Risk Airway

Robert J. Vissers, MD[a,b,*], Michael A. Gibbs, MD, FACEP[c,d]

KEYWORDS

• Emergency • Airway • Difficult • Failed • Intubation

There are few conditions in emergency medicine as potentially challenging and high-risk as the difficult or failed airway. Time is often limited, the patient's condition may be critical, and a failed airway has the potential for significant morbidity or death. The emergency physician must be able to rapidly identify the potential for a difficult or failed airway and plan accordingly. Underlying cardio-respiratory compromise or the acute condition itself may predispose the patient to physiologic insults during airway management. Anticipation and management of these risks can prevent worsening of the existing medical condition. Fortunately, there are methods to quickly identify the potentially difficult or failed airway. Preparation and pretreatment strategies may mitigate the potential risks of airway management in some conditions. Finally, there are a myriad of airway devices, many of which are new to emergency medicine, that can assist with the identification, management, and rescue of the high-risk airway. Once a difficult airway is anticipated, the clinician can choose a strategy and technique based on the reason for the airway being potentially difficult and on whether oxygenation can be maintained.

IDENTIFICATION OF THE HIGH-RISK AIRWAY

The first step in the management of the high-risk airway is recognizing its potential presence. Although all emergency airway management could arguably be considered high risk, the vast majority of emergent airways are managed successfully, with good outcomes, particularly when using established principles and techniques, such as rapid sequence induction (RSI). Airways that could be described as being at higher risk of failure or complication generally fall into 3 categories: the difficult airway, the failed airway, and the physiologically compromised patient's airway.

The 3 conditions can be defined as follows: (1) The difficult airway is defined by anatomical characteristics that predict, through pre-intubation assessment, the

[a] Emergency Department, Legacy Emanuel Hospital, 2801 North Gantenbein Avenue, Portland, OR 97227, USA
[b] Department of Emergency Medicine, Oregon Health Sciences University, Portland, OR 97227, USA
[c] Department of Emergency Medicine, Maine Medical Center, 22 Bramhall Street, Portland, ME 04102-3175, USA
[d] Department of Emergency Medicine, Tufts University School of Medicine, Boston, MA 02110, USA
* Corresponding author.
E-mail address: rvissers@comcast.net (R.J. Vissers).

Emerg Med Clin N Am 28 (2010) 203–217
doi:10.1016/j.emc.2009.10.004
0733-8627/09/$ – see front matter © 2010 Elsevier Inc. All rights reserved.

potential for difficulty with bag-mask ventilation, difficult laryngoscopy and intubation, or difficulty with placement of a rescue airway; (2) The failed airway is defined by difficulties encountered after airway management has been attempted. In emergency airway management, the failed airway has been defined as failure to maintain acceptable oxygen saturations following laryngoscopic attempts or 3 failed attempts by an experienced provider, even when saturations can be maintained; (3) The physiologically compromised patient is one whose underlying medical condition potentially increases the risk of morbidity from airway management.[1]

It is critical that providers assess the potential for a high-risk airway before initiating any emergency airway management. By definition, these airways can be associated with significant urgency; however, this assessment and identification can be performed rapidly in almost all situations, the rare exception being the arrested or near-arrest patient. Once a high-risk airway is identified, an understanding of why it is high risk can help define the optimal management, mitigate potential morbidity, and identify appropriate rescue strategies.

The Difficult Airway

The difficult airway has been defined by the American Society of Anesthesiologists (ASA) as difficulty with mask ventilation, difficulty with tracheal intubation, or both.[2] This has been further defined as follows: (1) more than 2 attempts at intubation with the same laryngoscopic blade have been made; (2) a change in blade or use of intubation stylet is required; or (3) an alternative intubation technique or rescue is required. Although these criteria are helpful at quantifying the presence of the difficult airway in anesthesia practice, the actual incidence of difficult airways in emergency practice is less clear. Difficulty visualizing the vocal cords during laryngoscopy (Cormack grade 3 or 4 view) has been estimated to occur in 14% to 25% of trauma patients intubated in the emergency department (ED).[3,4] First-attempt failure during RSI in the ED occurs about 10% to 23% of the time, however the need for more than 2 attempts is about 3%.[5–7] The failure rate for RSI in the ED is approximately 1%.[7–9]

More important to the clinician is the ability to predict a potentially difficult airway before the initiation of a paralytic agent. Although the presence of a potentially difficult airway is not an absolute contraindication to RSI, early identification allows for appropriate planning and a rescue strategy. In some cases, anticipated difficulty may present too great a risk for paralytics and require an "awake look" or fiberoptic intubation to avoid the rare but dangerous "cannot intubate, cannot ventilate" scenario in a paralyzed patient. Before any attempt at airway management, an assessment of potential difficulties with bag-valve-mask (BVM) ventilation, laryngoscopy and intubation, and possible rescue must be performed. It is important that the clinician consider the difficulty with direct laryngoscopy and the potential for successful bag-mask ventilation and airway rescue.[10] Once the potential for difficulty is identified, optimal management can be determined based on airway difficulty and anatomy, operator experience, and availability of alternative devices.

The ability to successfully perform BVM ventilation should be considered before proceeding with RSI. The presence of two of the following 5 factors is predictive of difficult BVM: facial hair, obesity, edentulous patient, advanced age, and snoring.[11,12] In most circumstances, bag-mask ventilation is the primary rescue following a failed attempt. It is critical for the emergency physician to master this important skill and have facility with techniques to overcome difficulties.

Multiple external features are also associated with difficult laryngoscopy and intubation. These features include facial hair, obesity, a short neck, small or large chin, buckteeth, high arched palate, and any airway deformity due to trauma, tumor, or inflammation. In some cases, particularly when there is anatomic disruption from injury, the difficulty is obvious. However, a focused clinical examination of the airway anatomy is needed to identify the more common, subtle predictors of intubation difficulty. In the emergency setting, a practical, systematic, and rapid evaluation of the airway is needed to predict a potentially poor laryngoscopic view before the initiation of neuromuscular blockade, and from this evaluation, a management plan is established.

The "LEMON" mnemonic represents one such assessment that is simple, quick, and can be performed on any emergency patient.[1] This approach, based on known independent predictors, was first introduced by Murphy and Walls[13] as a tool for the identification of difficult laryngoscopy and intubation. Subsequent studies have demonstrated that this approach can be performed successfully in the emergent setting and has proven to have predictive value.[14] The "LEMON" mnemonic has also been recommended as a method of evaluating airway difficulty in the most recent Advanced Trauma Life Support (ATLS) guidelines.[15] The LEMON mnemonic represents the following 5 elements requiring assessment.

Look externally
The initial impression of potential airway difficulty is based on obvious anatomic distortion or external features associated with difficulty.

Evaluate airway geometry (the 3-3-2 rule)
Measuring the geometry of the airway can predict the clinician's ability to align the oral, pharyngeal, and tracheal axes. The mandibular opening in an adult should be at least 4 cm, or 2 to 3 fingerbreadths. The ability of the mandible to accommodate the tongue can be estimated by the distance between the mentum and the hyoid bone, which should be 3 to 4 fingerbreadths. A smaller mandible is less likely to accommodate the tongue, which can impair visualization during laryngoscopy. An unusually large mandible can elongate the oral axis. A high, anterior larynx may be present if the space between the mandible and top of the thyroid cartilage is narrower than 2 fingerbreadths.

Mallampati score
The degree to which the tongue obstructs the visualization of the posterior pharynx on mouth opening has some correlation with the visualization of the glottis.[16] Simply put, the less posterior pharynx seen, the less likely it is that the cords may be fully visualized.

Obstruction or obesity
Obstruction is often readily apparent and may be the indication for emergent airway management. It is important to appreciate where the obstruction is occurring, because this will dictate the airway management options. The speed of progression is another important consideration in determining a management strategy.

Neck mobility
Neck immobility also interferes with the ability to align the visual axes by preventing the desired "sniffing position." Neck immobility may be imposed by the presence of a cervical collar. If there is no suspicion of cervical injury, atlanto-occipital extension should be assessed, even in the uncooperative patient.

If difficulty with bag-mask ventilation or laryngoscopy suggests the potential for a failed airway, the clinician must then consider the likely success of rescue techniques, such as supraglottic blind insertion devices or a subglottic surgical airway.

Airway devices that may serve as alternatives to RSI or as rescue devices in the failed airway, are discussed later, as are strategies in management and device selection.

The Failed Airway

The failed airway in emergency management has been defined as (1) inability to maintain adequate oxygenation following a failed intubation attempt; or (2) three failed attempts at intubation by an experienced provider, even if oxygenation can be maintained.[1] The rate of failed airways in the emergent setting is approximately 1%, and may be higher in trauma patients.[7,8] Ideally, the failed airway is prevented through assessment of airway difficulty and appropriate patient selection for RSI. However, despite optimal evaluation and preparation, failed airways are likely to occur, particularly in the emergent setting. Therefore any clinician providing emergent airway management must have facility with rescue devices and surgical airways.

The Physiologically Challenging Airway

There are patients in whom airway management poses a high risk because of their underlying chronic or acute medical condition, regardless of their airway anatomy. Although the technical aspect of intubation is predicted to be successful and a failed airway is unlikely, the procedure itself poses an increased risk of hypoxia, hypotension, or exacerbation of an underlying condition. Patients who have respiratory or hemodynamic compromise before the procedure are at particular risk. There are also certain conditions that may be exacerbated by the drugs used to facilitate rapid sequence intubation and by the physiologic effects secondary to the procedure itself. Many of these undesirable effects may be prevented or mitigated through recognition of the risk, adequate preoxygenation, and attention to drug selection.

Patients with raised intracranial pressure, reactive airways disease, and cardiac ischemia may suffer exacerbation of the condition from the direct physiologic effects of laryngoscopy. Although there remains some controversy over the true impact on outcome, the clinician should consider the use of pretreatment agents that may potentially mitigate the undesirable effects of intubation when the underlying condition calls for it.[17] A discussion of the individual pretreatment agents and their specific indications is beyond the scope of this article. Of greater importance is adequate preoxygenation, which should begin as soon as intubation becomes a consideration. Preoxygenation is recommended in all patients being intubated, including those with no apparent hypoxia. The displacement of nitrogen with oxygen in the alveolar space creates a potential reservoir of oxygen, which may prevent hypoxia for several minutes of apnea. This varies with the physiologic state of the patient, and hypoxia develops quicker in children, pregnant women, obese patients, and associated hyperdynamic states.[18] Optimal preoxygenation is particularly critical in patients with high-risk airways, because of underlying respiratory compromise or need for more "apnea time" when the potential for failed intubation exists.

TOOLS TO MANAGE AND RESCUE THE HIGH-RISK AIRWAY

The number of airway tools available to the emergency physician has exploded in the past decade. In some cases, this represents an adoption of devices that have had a long history of use and success within the specialty of anesthesia. This explosion may follow some modification that enhanced the effectiveness in the emergency setting, such as lower cost, increased durability, or ability to protect the airway. The disposable intubating laryngeal mask airway (I-LMA; Laryngeal Mask Company, Henley on Thames, UK) is a good example of this. The proliferation of lower-cost, durable, and easy-to-use fiberoptic devices is another recent phenomenon that is changing the approach to high-risk airway management in the ED. Finally, the development of educational courses focused on teaching these skills to emergency providers have probably played an important role.

Although several devices are listed in this section, it is not possible for emergency physicians to have facility with all techniques, nor is it likely that all these devices would be available because of the associated cost. The first "rescue" from failed intubation or bag-mask ventilation should usually be better laryngoscopic and bag-mask ventilation technique. Following that, the emergency physician should be comfortable using an intubating stylet, and have at least 1 supraglottic rescue device and 1 surgical airway technique in their armamentarium. Facility with a fiberoptic or video laryngoscopic device is becoming increasingly desirable.

Airway Management Tools
1. Bag-mask ventilation
2. Direct laryngoscopy
   a. Endotracheal tube introducers
3. Supraglottic rescue devices
   a. Blind insertion devices
      i. Double-balloon esophageal airways
      ii. LMAs
   b. Direct visualization
      i. Video laryngoscopy
      ii. Flexible fiberoptics
      iii. Fiberoptic stylets
4. Subglottic rescue devices
   a. Retrograde intubation
   b. Transtracheal jet ventilation
   c. Percutaneous cricothyrotomy
   d. Open surgical cricothyrotomy

Bag-Mask Ventilation

Bag-mask ventilation is a critical skill for the emergency provider and remains the first-line rescue in a failed intubation attempt. Maintaining oxygenation should take priority over repeated attempts at laryngoscopy.[19,20] An inability to adequately ventilate with a BVM is usually solved by better positioning, and if possible, exaggerating the head tilt, chin lift, and jaw thrust into the mask. A tighter seal with 2-person bagging and the use of oral and nasal airways to improve patency are often all that is required to achieve ventilation. A poor seal due to a beard may be improved with a lubricant, and keeping dentures in place can facilitate BVM ventilation. Cricoid pressure (Sellick maneuver) has been shown to impair bag-mask ventilation in some patients and may need to be eased or released when bagging is difficult.[21]

Direct Laryngoscopy

The most common reasons for intubation failure in direct laryngoscopy are inadequate equipment preparation and poor patient positioning. Optimizing patient position and laryngoscopic technique should be the first step following a failed attempt. Direct cricoid pressure in the unconscious or paralyzed patient has been recommended to prevent passive regurgitation of gastric contents and reduce gastric insufflation during active bag-mask ventilation. However, its effectiveness in RSI is in question, and cricoid pressure has been shown to impair laryngoscopic view and insertion of the tube over an endotracheal introducer. Therefore, in the case of difficult laryngoscopy, cricoid pressure should be released.

A maneuver to enhance visualization of the anterior glottis involves the application of backward-upward-rightward pressure on the thyroid cartilage (not the cricoid ring).[22,23] In a technique called bimanual laryngoscopy, the intubator manipulates the larynx with the right hand until ideal visualization is achieved, and then an assistant maintains this position. Attempts at blind passage are usually met with failure and anoxia and should be discouraged. When the emergency provider experiences a failed intubation attempt, measures should be taken to improve the chance of success on repeat attempts, and simultaneously, preparation for a possible rescue airway must be considered. Just as important is the ability to recognize when further attempts at laryngoscopy are unlikely to succeed or should be abandoned in favor of an alternative management strategy. Persistence in laryngoscopy beyond 3 attempts has been associated with low success and increased morbidity and mortality and should be discouraged.[20,24]

ENDOTRACHEAL TUBE INTRODUCER

An important and underused aid to intubation with direct vision is an endotracheal tube introducer or intubating stylet. Also called the "gum elastic bougie," the endotracheal tube introducer, is a semirigid or malleable, blunt-tipped stylet, which can assist with tube placement in the emergent intubation. These introducers are typically 70 cm long and made of plastic, and they use a deflection of the distal tip to facilitate insertion when the glottis cannot be fully visualized, specifically in Cormack grade 2 (arytenoids) and grade 3 (epiglottis only) views.[25] The introducer is inserted into the trachea with the right hand while maintaining visualization with the laryngoscope. Insertion in the trachea can also be appreciated through the tactile sensation of the tip moving over the tracheal rings. Using a Seldinger technique, the endotracheal tube (6.0 mm inner diameter or greater) is then threaded over the introducer into the trachea, and the introducer is removed. Difficulty in passing the tube through the glottis, usually reflects a failure to maintain the best possible laryngoscopic view throughout the procedure. Gentle 90° clockwise and counterclockwise rotation of the endotracheal tube may overcome resistance to passing the tube through a more favorable alignment of the beveled tip.

Supraglottic

Blind
There are several extraglottic devices that can be used as rescue airways in the failed intubation or as an alternative to emergency endotracheal intubation for less experienced providers, such as prehospital providers. These devices share a steep learning curve, are inserted blindly, and, because of their extraglottic placement, do not provide a definitive protected airway.

The laryngeal mask airway (LMA), and some similar devices are truly supraglottic in their placement, which is distinct from the double-balloon devices that are sometimes considered retroglottic, because they enter the upper esophagus. Initially introduced in 1981, the LMA has enjoyed widespread use in anesthetic practice because of its ease of use, and it is considered less invasive than an endotracheal tube. The primary drawback to the traditional LMA in the emergent setting is that it does not provide a definitive, protected airway in the nonfasted emergency patient. However, the advent of the disposable LMA Fastrach (Laryngeal Mask Company, Henley on

Thames, UK) or I-LMA represents a device that is easy to insert, is very successful at achieving ventilation, and can be converted to a protected airway by the placement of an endotracheal tube through the I-LMA.[26,27] The intubation success rate is about 95%; however, the highest success rates are achieved when the endotracheal tubes provided with the device are used in conjunction with fiberoptics.[27–29] Because of its high success and the ability to convert to an endotracheal intubation, the I-LMA is the preferred extraglottic rescue device in the ED.

Double-balloon airways represent the other type of blindly inserted, extraglottic airway device. The Combitube (Kendall-Sheridan Catheter Corp, Argyle, NY, USA) and the King LT(King Systems Corporation, Noblesville, IN, USA) are the most common types used in the emergency setting; however, other similar devices include the Rüsch Easytube (Teleflex Medical, Kernen, Germany), the Laryngeal Tube (VBM Medizintechnik, Sulz, Germany), the Airway Management Device (AMD; Nagor Ltd, Douglas, Isle of Man; Biosil Ltd, Cumbernauld, UK), and the Cobra Perilaryngeal Airway (Cobra PLA; Engineered Medical Systems, Indianapolis, IN, USA). Designed to be placed into the esophagus, one balloon seals it and the other balloon is inflated in the oropharynx. Ventilation takes place through an outlet positioned between the 2 balloon cuffs, which have effectively sealed off the larynx. Most of the experience with these devices is in the prehospital setting, because they are relatively inexpensive and disposable and have a high success rate and a quickly learned technique.[30,31] These devices are not considered a definitive airway and do not provide optimal protection from aspiration, which, however, seems to be a rare event.[32] The King LT differs from the Combitube in that it uses a single pilot balloon to inflate both cuffs, and the newer designs allow gastric aspiration through an open distal tip. There is a more extensive literature on the Combitube, but the King LT seems promising and has been rapidly adopted in many prehospital settings.[33,34]

Direct vision

Video laryngoscopy represents the most promising recent addition to the airway tools available in the management of the high-risk airway.[35] The operator, using a blade and handle similar to the traditional laryngoscope, performs the intubation watching a video screen, rather than looking into the oropharynx. Through the placement of a micro video camera in the tip of the blade, the distal image is transmitted to an external monitor. This magnified view enhances visualization and, in some cases, provides views that cannot be obtained through direct laryngoscopy. Video laryngoscopy can be performed in a neutral neck position and in patients with reduced oral opening. This is a particular advantage in patients with potentially difficult airways or restricted cervical spine mobility.[36,37] There are educational advantages in shared visualization and in the ability to record the video-assisted intubation for future viewing. Video laryngoscopy is a technique for the high-risk airway and for low-risk emergent intubations, thus allowing the operators to gain experience and skill. Other video laryngoscopes incorporate a smaller video monitor onto the handle of the device similar to conventional laryngoscopes, and they may represent a more intuitive design.

Several studies have demonstrated high success rates and improved Cormack-Lehane views with video laryngoscopy compared with direct laryngoscopy.[38,39] Despite the relative paucity of studies, the popularity and rapid adoption of video laryngoscopy suggests that these devices will play an increasingly important role in emergent airway management. Devices that incorporate an antifog mechanism are desirable for improved visualization. Some video laryngoscopes offer a single-use disposable blade, which reduces the downtime needed for sterilization and may be preferred in the emergent setting. Several devices now have blade sizes available for all ages. There are limited data comparing different products, however one study demonstrated a first-attempt success difference between devices when no stylet was used.[39] When a stylet was used, the difference was not significant and success of all the devices went up. There was significant improvement in the Cormack-Lehane view and in the success of all devices when compared with direct laryngoscopy.

The technique for video laryngoscopy differs from traditional laryngoscopy, in that a midline insertion is preferred and a tongue sweep is not needed. The ideal view is usually obtained by insertion into the vallecula, much like a Macintosh blade, and gentle tilting of the handle.

Flexible fiberoptics are a useful option for the assessment of airway difficulty and for facilitating intubation when there are anatomic limitations that may prevent visualization of the vocal cords using traditional laryngoscopy. Although the fiberoptic scope requires some facility and practice, it is an increasingly important skill for the emergency physician that can be mastered through instruction and simulation.[40,41] The most common role for flexible fiberoptics in the ED should be in the evaluation of airway difficulty, which also creates opportunity for operator experience. Intubation over the scope in a difficult airway crisis can be life-saving but requires a higher degree of technical skill. Timely assistance from consultants with fiberoptic skills may also be needed in the absence of equipment or a skilled provider in the ED.

Clinical indications for flexible fiberoptics include conditions that prevent opening or movement of the mandible, massive tongue swelling from angioedema, upper airway infections, congenital anatomic abnormalities, and cervical spine immobility. The most common relative contraindications to fiberoptic intubation are insufficient time and impaired visualization from blood or secretions. The procedure requires preparation and usually a compliant, spontaneously breathing patient. Patients in need of an immediate airway, patients with near-complete obstructions, and those who cannot be ventilated to maintain saturations are poor candidates for this procedure.

Topical anesthesia, an antisialogogue, sedation, and if the nasal route is used, a topical vasoconstrictor are all essential pharmacologic adjuncts to a successful fiberscopic procedure. The nasal route is usually preferred, because the scope is easier to keep in the midline and it enters the glottis at a less acute angle. Because oral obstruction is a common indication for fiberoptic intubation, the nasal route may be required. However, if the oral route is used, a breakaway bite block, such as a Berman intubating airway, is recommended to prevent damage to the scope and keep it midline.

Flexible fiberoptics can be useful in converting a rescue airway, such as an I-LMA, to an endotracheal intubation. In the case of the I-LMA, the success rate approaches 99%.[29] Recent advances, such as enhanced visualization with complementary metal-oxide semiconductor video technology, improved antifogging, and better durability, have made this technology more accessible to the emergency environment. Ease of use, the absence of available consulting expertise, and growing indications all contribute to an increasingly important role for flexible fiberoptics in emergency airway management.

Fiberoptic stylets are devices that incorporate fiberoptics into a hand-held rigid or malleable stylet. The endotracheal tube is mounted on the stylet and indirect visualization of the glottis is achieved through an eyepiece on the handle. The operator sees from the perspective of the tip of the stylet or tube. Although their diagnostic capabilities do not replace those of a flexible fiberoptic scope, these devices can be useful when direct visualization of the larynx is impossible due to neck immobility, reduced oral opening, or an anterior larynx, and they are usually much less expensive than traditional fiberoptics.[42–44] Blood and excessive secretions can impair visualization.

Subglottic

Although the need to perform a surgical airway in an emergent setting is rare (about 1% of emergency airways), there are clinical circumstances, specifically the "cannot oxygenate, cannot intubate" scenario, where a surgical airway may be the only option and the final end-point in all difficult airway algorithms. Therefore all emergency airway managers need to have immediate access to and familiarity with a surgical airway technique. Regardless of the technique used, all emergent surgical airways access the subglottic airway through the cricothyroid membrane.[45,46]

Cricothyrotomy, using either an open surgical technique or an over-the-wire Seldinger technique, is the recommended surgical airway in the emergent setting. Individual experience is limited; however, case series, cadaveric studies, and simulation models all suggest that this is a technique that can be successfully learned and translated into clinical practice. Both techniques can be performed in less than a minute and have similar learning curves and success rates.[47,48] The open technique may be more successful in obese patients. There are commercially available kits that have the necessary equipment to perform an open or Seldinger cricothyrotomy.[45]

Needle cricothyrotomy with percutaneous transtracheal jet ventilation can be performed emergently as a temporizing surgical airway. This technique can be effective at providing oxygenation, is easy to perform and does not have an age restriction, and therefore is the surgical airway of choice in young children. There are several disadvantages compared with the cricothyrotomy techniques described earlier. Ventilation may not be possible unless supraglottic patency can be maintained. Airway protection is not present and suctioning is not possible. Barotrauma is common and displacement or obstruction of the catheter is more likely. Retrograde tracheal intubation is another option that has been used when conventional airway approaches fail. This procedure is time-consuming and is not an alternative to cricothyrotomy in the patient who cannot be intubated or ventilated. Because of this limitation and the recent advent of alternative airway devices, retrograde tracheal intubation is rarely used in the emergent setting.

APPROACH TO THE MANAGEMENT OF THE HIGH-RISK AIRWAY

The number of airway rescue devices available continues to grow at a staggering pace. It is important for clinicians to stay abreast of these technological advances and invest when investment is needed. Even more vital is the notion that the emergency physician must develop and use a well thought-out plan for managing the difficult airway and failed airway. A thoughtful strategy based on patient characteristics that incorporates appropriate preparation and uses the optimal technique is always more important than the tools themselves.

Because ED failed airways are low-frequency events that almost always unfold rapidly and without the luxury of time to plan, it makes sense to use decision-making tools to help frame one's thinking. Several algorithms have been proposed to address this vexing problem. The ASA's difficult airway algorithm works well in the controlled, operating room setting but is difficult to apply in the ED.[2] Another approach geared to the emergency setting uses vertically oriented algorithms that provide a logical framework for dealing with the difficult and the failed airway.[49]

There are elements common to most recommended algorithms that are critical to successful airway management. Despite the urgency often associated with emergent airway management, appropriate preparation and attention to optimal oxygenation are important. This includes an assessment of airway difficulty, a preconceived strategy, and the identification of an appropriate rescue device if a failed airway

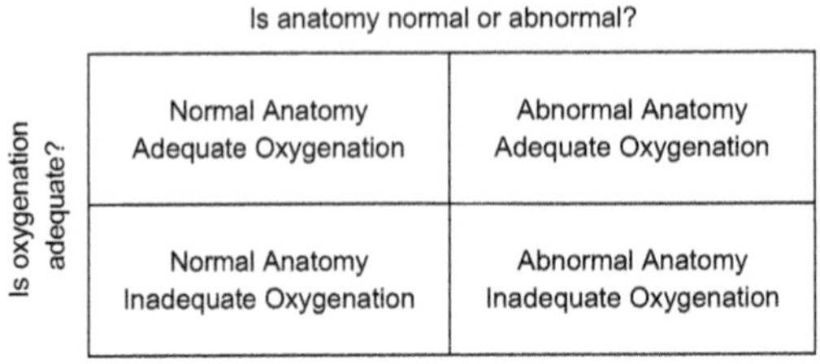

Is anatomy normal or abnormal?

	Normal Anatomy Adequate Oxygenation	Abnormal Anatomy Adequate Oxygenation
	Normal Anatomy Inadequate Oxygenation	Abnormal Anatomy Inadequate Oxygenation

(left vertical axis label: Is oxygenation adequate?)

Fig. 1. Difficult airway grid.

occurs. The use of an awake look, commonly used in anesthesia, is an increasingly important technique in emergent difficult airway assessment, and it is becoming easier to perform with the increased availability of fiberoptic airway devices. Recognizing the need for help from other consultants or colleagues, if available, can be the key to success in some circumstances. Finally, the ability to anticipate and perform a subglottic, surgical airway is an important skill that all airway managers must possess.

It can be challenging to determine the most appropriate airway device for the particular airway scenario. To some degree, the selection of the tool to use will be determined or at least limited by what is available and the skill set of the clinician. Despite the large number of airway devices beyond traditional laryngoscopy that are available to the airway manager, they tend to fall into a few categories. There are supraglottic devices, which can be further divided into blind insertion devices, such as the I-LMA, and direct visualization, fiberoptic devices; and there are subglottic techniques, which are invasive airways, usually obtained through the cricothyroid membrane. One of the authors, M.A. Gibbs, has developed an approach using a 4-box grid (**Fig. 1**) and a series of principles and solutions that apply to each patient category. Using this approach can help develop an appropriate plan and potential rescue device. Patients with difficult or failed airways can be categorized by the answers to 2 basic questions:

1. Is airway anatomy normal or abnormal?
2. Is oxygenation adequate (ie, O2 saturations>90%)?

In the context of this grid, an abnormal anatomy implies disrupted or altered anatomy, not just an anticipated difficulty in visualizing the glottis. Causes of a difficult airway with abnormal anatomy include trauma, burns, hematoma, cancer, abscess, foreign body, and angioedema. Causes of a difficult airway with normal anatomy include obesity, a small mouth, and a high anterior larynx.

Principles and solutions for each box on the grid are listed below followed by illustrative case examples. It is important to recognize that although these principles are generalizable, the solutions will vary based on skill level and equipment availability.

Table 1
Normal anatomy + adequate oxygenation

Principles	Solutions
You have time	Hand-held fiberoptics are available:
No need for a surgical airway	Any of these should work
Blind-insertion devices appropriate	Hand-held fiberoptics are not available:
Hand-held fiberoptics ideal	First choice, I-LMA[25–29]; second choice, intubating
Cuffed tube the goal	stylet

Table 2 Normal anatomy + inadequate oxygenation	
Principles	**Solutions**
No time	Hand-held fiberoptics are available:
Multiple attempts with blind-insertion devices inappropriate	Limited attempts with these, then surgical
	Hand-held fiberoptics are not available:
Use what is known best	Limited attempts with I-LMA, then surgical
Surgical airway if first rescue plan fails	

Case Example 1

Consider a morbidly obese patient who presents to the ED after an overdose. He has stable vital signs but is obtunded and not protecting his airway. Airway dimensions and anatomy are normal. Oxygen saturations are greater than 95% on supplemental oxygen. Following sedation and paralysis, the glottis cannot be visualized despite 3 attempts with repositioning. Oxygenation can be maintained with BVM ventilation.

This case illustrates 2 key features (**Table 1**): First, because oxygenation can be maintained, one has some time. Second, there is nothing anatomically wrong with the airway; it just cannot be seen. Blind insertion devices are therefore safe and would be a reasonable choice. Hand-held fiberoptic devices that provide a direct view of the glottis are an even better choice.

Case Example 2

Now consider the same overdose patient who has been paralyzed and sedated. Aspiration is evident after the first attempt at laryngoscopy, and it is difficult oxygenating the patient even with adequate positioning and an oral airway.

The key difference between this scenario and Case 1 is that one no longer has time (**Table 2**). One's "device menu" is essentially the same, but multiple attempts with any of these rescue devices are neither possible nor appropriate. In this situation, limited attempts (1–2 at most) using the rescue device with which one has the most experience and therefore the highest likelihood of success, should be one's first move. If this is unsuccessful, a surgical airway is the next step.

Case Example 3

Consider a patient with Ludwig angina in the setting of a severe dental infection. The patient has stable vital signs and an oxygen saturation of 98%. On physical examination, there is significant trismus and a large submandibular abscess. Because of progressive swelling, a decision is taken to intubate the patient before transfer to a tertiary center.

Table 3 Abnormal anatomy + adequate oxygenation	
Principles	**Solutions**
Blind insertion device risky	Hand-held fiberoptics are available:
Direct airway visualization preferred	Limited attempts with fiberoptic
Fiberoptic okay if not obscured by blood	Surgical airway if unsuccessful
Surgical airway backup	Hand-held fiberoptics are not available:
	Surgical airway

Table 4
Abnormal airway + inadequate oxygenation

Principles	Solutions
No time	Hand-held fiberoptics are available:
Blind insertion devices contraindicated	One attempt with fiberoptic
Fiberoptic okay if not obscured by blood	Surgical airway if unsuccessful
Surgical often the best first choice	Hand-held fiberoptics are not available:
	Surgical airway

This case illustrates several important concepts (**Table 3**): First, one has some but not much time. Second, blind insertion devices are not recommended in the setting of significantly altered airway anatomy, because these are unlikely to be successful and may cause additional injury during insertion attempts. Third, a direct view of the glottis using a fiberoptic device is preferred. Fourth, if fiberoptic devices are to work, the airway must be reasonably clear of blood and secretions.

Case Example 4

Consider a patient with a gunshot wound to the mouth. The mandible is blown apart and blood is pouring into the airway. Oxygen saturations are dropping and the patient is impossible to bag.

The key message here is not to outsmart oneself. Because the likelihood of failure with most techniques is so high, it can be easily argued that an immediate surgical airway is the only answer in this case (**Table 4**).

SUMMARY

The high-risk airway can be anatomically difficult, at risk of intubation failure, and physiologically challenging. By anticipating these challenges and planning accordingly, the emergency physician can increase the likelihood of a successful outcome. Facility with some of the alternative airway devices is an integral part of high-risk airway management. However, thoughtful preparation, knowing when to avoid RSI, using fiberoptics and video laryngoscopy when appropriate, and finally, choosing the correct rescue strategy in the failed airway, remain the key elements in managing the high-risk airway.

REFERENCES

1. Murphy MF, Walls RM. Identification of the difficult and failed airway. In: Walls RM, Murphy MF, editors. Manual of emergency airway management. 3rd edition. Philadelphia: Lippincott Williams & Wilkins; 2008. p. 81–93.
2. Caplan RA, Benumof JL, Berry FA, et al. Practice guidelines for management of the difficult airway: an updated report by the American Society Anesthesiologists Task Force on Management of the Difficult Airway. Anesthesiology 2003;98: 1269–77.
3. Graham CA, Beard D, Henry JM, et al. Rapid sequence intubation of trauma patients in Scotland. J Trauma 2004;56:1105–11.
4. Heath KJ. The effect of laryngoscopy of different cervical spine immobilization techniques. Anaesthesia 1994;49:843–5.
5. Sagarin MJ, Barton ED, Chang YM, et al. Airway management by U.S. and Canadian emergency medicine residents: a multicenter analysis of more than 6,000 endotracheal intubation attempts. Ann Emerg Med 2005;46:328–36.

6. Levitan RM, Rosenblatt B, Meiner EM, et al. Alternating day emergency medicine and anesthesia resident responsibility for management of the trauma airway: a study of laryngoscopy performance and intubation success. Ann Emerg Med 2004;43:48–53.

7. Sackles JC, Laurin EG, Rantapaa AA, et al. Airway management in the emergency department: a one-year study of 610 tracheal intubations. Ann Emerg Med 1998;31:325–32.

8. Bair AE, Filbin MR, Kulkami R, et al. Failed intubation in the emergency department: analysis of prevalence, rescue techniques, and personnel. J Emerg Med 2002;23:131–40.

9. Tayal VS, Riggs RW, Marx JA, et al. Rapid-sequence intubation at an emergency medicine residency: success rate and adverse events during a two-year period. Acad Emerg Med 1999;6:31–7.

10. Murphy M, Hung O, Launcelott G, et al. Predicting the difficult laryngoscopic intubation: are we on the right track? Can J Anaesth 2005;52:231–5.

11. Langeron O, Masso E, Huraux C, et al. Prediction of difficult mask ventilation. Anesthesiology 2000;92:1229.

12. Kheterpal S, Han R, Tremper KK, et al. Incidence and predictors of difficult and impossible mask ventilation. Anesthesiology 2006;105:885.

13. Murphy MF, Walls RM. The difficult and failed airway. In: Walls RM, Murphy MF, Luten RC, et al, editors. Manual of emergency airway management. 1st edition. Philadelphia: Lippincott, Williams and Wilkins; 2000. p. 31–9.

14. Reed MJ, Dunn MJ, McKeown DW, et al. Can an airway assessment score predict difficulty at intubation in the emergency department? Emerg Med J 2005;22:99–102.

15. Kortbeck JB. ATLS. J Trauma 2008;64:1638.

16. Lee A, Fan LTY, Gin T, et al. A systematic review (meta-analysis) of the accuracy of the Mallampati tests to predict the difficult airway. Anesth Analg 2006;102:1867.

17. Caro DA, Bush S. Pretreatment agents. In: Walls RM, Murphy MF, editors. Manual of emergency airway management. 3rd edition. Philadelphia: Lippincott Williams & Wilkins; 2008. p. 222–33.

18. Benumof JL, Dagg R, Benumof R. Critical hemoglobin desaturation will occur before return to an unparalyzed state following 1mg/kg of intravenous succinylcholine. Anesthesiology 1997;87:979–82.

19. Dorges V, Wenzel V, Knacke P, et al. Comparison of different airway management strategies to ventilate apneic, nonpreoxygenated patients. Crit Care Med 2003;313:800–4.

20. Peterson GN. Management of the difficult airway. A closed claims analysis. Anesthesiology 2005;103:33.

21. Hartsilver EL, Vanner RG. Airway obstruction with cricoid pressure. Anaesthesia 2000;55:208–11.

22. Levitan RM, Kinkle WC, Levin WJ, et al. Laryngeal view during laryngoscopy: a randomized trial comparing cricoid pressure, backward-upward-rightward pressure, and bimanual laryngoscopy. Ann Emerg Med 2006;47:548.

23. Knill RL. Difficult laryngoscopy made easy with a "BURP". Can J Anaesth 1993;84:419–21.

24. Mort TC. Emergency tracheal intubation: complications associated with repeated laryngoscopic attempts. Anesth Analg 2004;99:607–13.

25. Dogra S, Falconer R, Latto IP. Successful difficult intubation. Tracheal tube placement over a gum elastic bougie. Anaesthesia 1990;45:774–6.

26. Parmet JL, Colonna-Romano P, Horrow JC, et al. The laryngeal mask airway reliably provides rescue ventilation in cases of unanticipated difficult tracheal intubation along with difficult mask ventilation. Anesth Analg 1998;87:661–5.

27. Rosenblatt WH, Murphy M. The intubating laryngeal mask: use of a new venti-lating-intubating device in the emergency department. Ann Emerg Med 1999; 33:234–8.
28. Fukutome T, Amaha K, Nakazawa K, et al. Tracheal intubation through the intubat-ing laryngeal mask airway (LMA-Fastrach) in patients with difficult airways. Anaesth Intensive Care 1998;26:387–91.
29. Ferson DZ, Rosenblatt WH, Johansen MJ, et al. Use of the LMA-Fastrach in 254 patients with difficult-to-manage airways. Anesthesiology 2001;95:1175–81.
30. Ochs M, Vilke GM, Chan TC, et al. Successful prehospital airway management by EMT-Ds using the combitube. Prehosp Emerg Care 2000;4:333–7.
31. Rumball CJ, MacDonald D. The PTL, combitube, laryngeal mask and oral airway: a randomized prehospital comparative study of ventilatory device effectiveness and cost-effectiveness in 470 cases of cardiopulmonary arrest. Prehosp Emerg Care 1997;1:1–10.
32. Mercer MH. An assessment of protection of the airway from aspiration of oropha-ryngeal contents using the Combitube airway. Resuscitation 2001;51:135–8.
33. Dorges V, Ocker H, Wenzel V, et al. The laryngeal tube: a new simple airway device. Anesth Analg 2000;90:1220–2.
34. Winterhalter M, Kirchhoff K, Groschel W, et al. The laryngeal tube for difficult airway management: a prospective investigation in patients with pharyngeal and laryngeal tumors. Eur J Anaesthesiol 2005;22:678–82.
35. Sakles JC, Brown CA. Video laryngoscopy. In: Walls M, Murphy MF, Luten RC, editors. Manual of emergency airway management. 3rd edition. Philadelphia: Lippincott, Williams & Wilkins; 2008. p. 167–84.
36. Robitaille A, Williams SR, Tremblay MH, et al. Cervical spine motion during tracheal intubation with manual in-line stabilization: direct laryngoscopy versus GlideScope videolaryngoscopy. Anesth Analg 2008;106:935.
37. Cooper RM. Use of a new videolaryngoscope (GlideScope) in the management of a difficult airway. Can J Anaesth 2003;50:611.
38. Cooper RM, Pacey JA, Bishop MJ, et al. Early clinical experience with a new vid-eolaryngoscope (GlideScope) in 728 patients. Can J Anaesth 2005;52:191.
39. van Zundert A, Maassen R, Lee R, et al. A Macintosh laryngoscope blade for vid-eolaryngoscopy reduces stylet use in patients with normal airways. Anesth Analg 2009;109:825.
40. Wheeler M, Roth AG, Dsida RM, et al. Teaching residents pediatric fiberoptic intu-bation of the trachea: traditional fiberscope with an eyepiece versus a video-as-sisted technique using a fiberscope with an integrated camera. Anesthesiology 2004;101:842.
41. Naik VN, Matsumoto E, Houston P, et al. Fiberoptic orotracheal intubation on anesthetized patients: Do manipulation skills learned on a simple model transfer into the operating room? Anesthesiology 2001;95:343.
42. Turkstra TP, Craen R, Gelb A, et al. Cervical spine motion: a fluoroscopic comparison of Shikani Optical Stylet vs Macintosh laryngoscope. Can J Anaesth 2007;54:441.
43. Kovacs G, Law JA, Petrie D. Awake fiberoptic intubation using an optical stylet in an anticipated difficult airway. Ann Emerg Med 2007;49:81–3.
44. Greenland KB, Liu G, Tan H, et al. Comparison of the Levitan FPS Scope and the single-use bougie for simulated difficult intubation in anaesthetised patients. Anaesthesia 2007;62:509.
45. Vissers RJ, Bair AE. Surgical airway techniques. In: Walls M, Murphy MF, editors. Manual of emergency airway management. 3rd edition. Philadelphia: Lippincott, Williams & Wilkins; 2008. p. 193–220.

46. Bair AE, Panacek EA, Wisner DH, et al. Cricothyrotomy: a 5-year experience at one institution. J Emerg Med 2003;24:151–6.
47. Eisenberger P, Laczika K, List M, et al. Comparison of conventional surgical versus seldinger technique emergency cricothyrotomy performed by inexperienced clinicians. Anesthesiology 2000;92:687–90.
48. Chan TC, Vilke GM, Bramwell KJ, et al. Comparison of wire-guided cricothyrotomy versus standard surgical cricothyrotomy technique. J Emerg Med 1999;17:957–62.
49. Walls RM. The emergency airway algorithms. In: Walls RM, Murphy MF, editors. Manual of emergency airway management. 3rd edition. Philadelphia: Lippincott Williams & Wilkins; 2008. p. 9–22.

Pitfalls in First-Trimester Bleeding

Susan B. Promes, MD, FACEP[a],*, Flavia Nobay, MD[b]

KEYWORDS

• First trimester • Pregnancy • Emergency department
• Vaginal bleeding

Vaginal bleeding during pregnancy is a significant event in a woman's life. It warrants a thoughtful emergency department (ED) evaluation with careful attention to avoid pitfalls that may pose unexpected consequences. There are many reasons for vaginal bleeding during pregnancy. The differential of vaginal bleeding in gravid women varies immensely depending primarily on the stage of the pregnancy. Some diagnoses are serious and pose significant health risks; others are less of an issue from a medical perspective. Regardless of the cause, any gravid patient with vaginal bleeding can be emotionally upset.

The focus of this article is first-trimester bleeding. Vaginal bleeding during the first 3 months of pregnancy is a common event. It is important that emergency physicians recognize patients with vaginal bleeding who may have an adverse outcome if misdiagnosed or not treated appropriately in the ED. Causes of first-trimester vaginal bleeding include implantation bleeding, spontaneous abortions (SABs), ectopic pregnancy, and lesions involving the female reproductive system and perineal area infections.

Patients may not always recognize that they are pregnant, so it is critical to order a pregnancy test on any woman of childbearing age presenting to an ED with vaginal bleeding, spotting, or lower abdominal pain. Also, childbearing age in the modern area of fertility treatment has changed dramatically and should be taken to mean all women who still menstruate. The various pregnancy tests have limitations. There are two general classes of pregnancy tests: quantitative and qualitative. Serum β-hCG tests are generally quantitative and provide clinicians with a numeric β-hCG value that can be followed over time. Early in a normal pregnancy, this value is expected to double approximately every 2 to 3 days. Qualitative tests, alternatively, are generally used for screening purposes. Urine pregnancy tests are qualitative tests and give a provider a "yes" or "no" answer to the question, "Is this patient pregnant?" The

[a] Department of Emergency Medicine, University of California San Francisco, 505 Parnassus Avenue, Room M-24, Box 0203, San Francisco, CA 94143-0203, USA
[b] Department of Emergency Medicine, University of Rochester, 601 Elmwood Avenue, Box 655, Rochester, NY 14642, USA
* Corresponding author.
E-mail address: susan.promes@ucsf.edu (S.B. Promes).

Emerg Med Clin N Am 28 (2010) 219–234
doi:10.1016/j.emc.2009.10.005
0733-8627/09/$ – see front matter © 2010 Elsevier Inc. All rights reserved.

newer generation of urine pregnancy tests detect low levels of β-hCG, approximately in the range of 25 to 50 IU/L, so are excellent pregnancy screening tools.[1] Some authors have suggested that dilute urine with a specific gravity of less than 1.015 may produce a false-negative result; however, urine immunoassays currently used are extremely sensitive and produce a positive result even when testing dilute urine.[2] Instructions should be followed explicitly, however, with regard to length of time to read a test result after the urine is added in order to avoid a false-negative result. Another potential pitfall with respect to pregnancy tests is a false-negative result as a result of the high-dose hook effect. When patients have a high β-hCG, as with patients with a hydatidiform mole (or molar pregnancy), the test can be overwhelmed by the high concentration of β-hCG and result in false-negative urine and serum β-hCG test results. If a diagnosis of molar pregnancy is entertained for a patient, dilution of the serum or urine sample is key because high levels of the substrate can overwhelm the assays.[3] A final comment about pitfalls with respect to serum pregnancy tests and ectopic pregnancies is that quantitative β-hCG levels are not helpful alone in differentiating a failing intrauterine pregnancy (IUP) from an ectopic pregnancy.[4]

One common cause of first-trimester vaginal bleeding is implantation bleeding. It reportedly occurs in up to one-third of pregnant women early in their pregnancy. Implantation bleeding occurs approximately 4 weeks after a woman's last menstrual period. The bleeding is a result of a fertilized egg implanting and invading the wall of the endometrial cavity. Implantation bleeding is generally not copious and often described as simply a small amount of pinkish or brownish blood on a woman's undergarments although frank blood can be expelled from the vagina. It is not heavy, and the duration of this type of vaginal bleeding is less than expected from a woman's normal menses. Cramping and backaches do not usually accompany implantation bleeding. Implantation bleeding is a benign process. The pitfall lies in attributing vaginal bleeding in the first trimester to the implantation process when it is actually something more serious.

Ectopic pregnancy, in contrast to implantation bleeding, is a life- and fertility-threatening condition. This is a diagnosis clinicians should not miss. Unfortunately, missed and delayed diagnoses of ectopic pregnancy are not infrequent. In one study published in 1980, it was reported that ectopic pregnancies were missed 50% of the time on their first medical consultation.[5] With the advent of ED-focused bedside ultrasound and increasingly sensitive urine pregnancy tests, this statistic hopefully has improved but there are no recent studies evaluating this. Unfortunately, ectopic pregnancies are increasing. In the United States, the incidence of ectopic pregnancy increased from 4.5 per 1000 reported pregnancies in 1970 to 19.7 per 1000 pregnancies in 1992, equating to 2% of reported pregnancies and 9% of pregnancy-related deaths.[6] Heterotopic pregnancies are also on the rise. A heterotopic pregnancy is the coexistence of an IUP and an ectopic pregnancy. The occurrence is rare (1 in 2600 pregnancies) but the incidence increases dramatically with fertility treatments.[7] With the advent of bedside ultrasound and β-hCG tests, the incidence of ruptured ectopic pregnancies and fatality rates have declined from 35.5 deaths per 10,000 ectopic pregnancies in 1970 to 3.8 deaths per 10,000 in 1989.[8]

Implantation of a fertilized egg normally occurs in the superior and posterior walls of the uterine cavity. Simply defined, an ectopic pregnancy is any pregnancy that occurs outside the uterus generally in the female reproductive track and less commonly in the abdominal cavity. Symptoms of an ectopic pregnancy develop as the pregnancy grows and distorts surrounding tissue or ruptures causing hypotension or peritoneal irritation. Patients at greatest risk for ectopic pregnancy are women who have anatomic abnormalities, such as scarring or functional abnormalities with their fallopian tubes. Pelvic inflammatory disease secondary to sexually transmitted infections is the most common risk factor for ectopic pregnancy (**Box 1**). The most common location for an ectopic pregnancy is the fallopian tube, hence the term, *tubal pregnancy*. Nontubal sites of ectopic pregnancies (abdomen, ovary, and cervix) are rare and account for less than 2% of ectopic pregnancies (**Fig. 1**).[9] An ectopic pregnancy, if not recognized and treated, can cause tubal rupture or intra-abdominal bleeding depending on the location of the ectopic pregnancy.

The most common presenting symptoms for ectopic pregnancy are abdominal pain and vaginal bleeding. Because they are not always present, however, it is imperative that clinicians have a high index of suspicion for this diagnosis in patients with risk factors or patients who present with hypotension with no obvious cause. The classic triad of abdominal pain, delayed menses, and vaginal bleeding is, unfortunately, not sensitive for ectopic pregnancy. Pain is the most common symptom, followed by vaginal bleeding, in patients with ectopic pregnancy.[10] A physical examination in ectopic pregnancies is unreliable. A woman may or may not have a mass or tenderness on examination and vaginal bleeding may be minimal, yet a patient can be critically ill. Vital signs of patients with ruptured ectopic pregnancies also may be normal, and paradoxic bradycardia is common. Hemodynamic variables do not correlate well with blood loss in patients with ruptured ectopic pregnancies. Therefore, it is important not to be falsely reassured by normal vital signs.[11]

With the use of ultrasound in an ED diagnostic algorithm, the goal of emergency practitioners is to exclude ectopic pregnancy by documenting IUP. Any patients in whom IUP cannot be established must be assumed to have ectopic pregnancy until proved otherwise. Rh status should be determined and a quantitative β-hCG concentration measured in all pregnant women who receive evaluation for possible ectopic pregnancy. Serum β-hCG should not be used, however, to decide if an ultrasound is needed—this is a potential pitfall in the evaluation of pregnant women with first-trimester pain or bleeding. In a normal pregnancy, an IUP should be reliably seen on transabdominal ultrasound with β-hCG levels greater than or equal to 2500 mIU/mL and on transvaginal ultrasound with β-hCG levels greater than or equal to 1500 mIU/mL. These β-hCG values are termed the discriminatory zone. These levels were derived for predicting IUP, however, and are not of use to exclude ectopic pregnancy in the ED setting. Women who present to the ED with pain or vaginal bleeding

---

Box 1
Risk factors for ectopic pregnancy

Pelvic inflammatory disease

Previous ectopic pregnancy

Previous pelvic/abdominal surgery

Previous tubal surgery

Infertility and infertility treatments

Smoking

Intrauterine device use

In utero diethylstilbestrol (DES) exposure

Data from Ankum WM, Mol BW, Van der Veen F, Bossuyt PM. Risk factors for ectopic pregnancy: a meta-analysis. Fertil Steril 1996;65(6):1093–9.

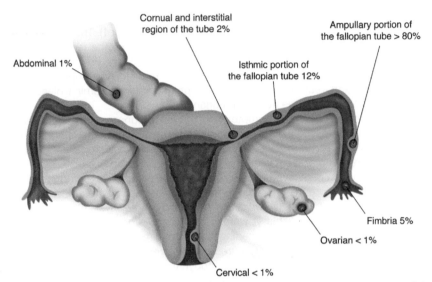

Fig. 1. Potential ectopic pregnancy sites. (*Adapted from* Breen JL. A 21 year survey of 654 ectopic pregnancies. Am J Obstet Gynecol 1970;106(7):1004–19; with permission.)

and serum β-hCG levels less than 1500 mIU/mL are at twice the risk of ectopic pregnancy compared with those who have levels above this value.[12]

The approach to ED ultrasound is a focused, bedside study to answer a specific question: Is there an IUP? If the answer is "yes" (definitive IUP is present), appropriate follow-up is arranged. If the answer is "no" (no definitive IUP), a formal ultrasound (by the radiology department) should be performed and an obstetric consultation obtained.[13]

The American College of Emergency Physicians in a policy statement lists pelvic ultrasound as a primary indication for ED practitioners to evaluate for the presence of IUP.[14] A complete ED study should include the following. The uterus should be examined in at least two planes, the short and long axis, to avoid missing findings. The most common indicator of an IUP used in emergency medicine is the visualization of a true gestational sac. The uterus should be scanned from the fundus to the cervix confirming that it is actually the uterus being scanned rather than a gestational reaction from a large ectopic pregnancy.[14] If an IUP is noted, there should be an all-encompassing ring of myometrium, also known as myometrial mantle, of at least 5 mm surrounding the IUP. If the appropriate myometrial mantle does not surround the pregnancy, the diagnosis of an interstitial pregnancy must be entertained. The cul-de-sac should also be examined for free fluid. A large amount of free fluid is abnormal and suspicious for an ectopic pregnancy in the right clinical setting (**Fig. 2**). Although a formal ultrasound includes an evaluation of the adnexa, it is beyond the scope of the focused bedside ultrasound done by most emergency physicians. If no IUP noted, an ectopic pregnancy exists until proved otherwise and a formal ultrasound is warranted (**Table 1**). Another pitfall in the diagnosis of ectopic pregnancy is not performing a quick focused assessment with sonography for trauma (FAST) examination in addition to a pelvic ultrasound. This is recommended to look for free fluid, which might suggest a ruptured ectopic pregnancy (**Figs. 3** and **4**). An emergent obstetrics-gynecology consultation is imperative for all patients with proved ectopic pregnancy. Those patients with a concerning history and physical examination and indeterminate

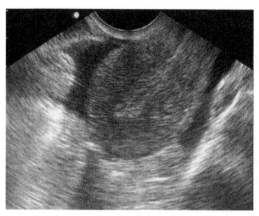

Fig. 2. Transvaginal ultrasound of an empty uterus and free fluid in the pelvis, which is concerning for an ectopic pregnancy in a patient with a positive pregnancy test.

or nondiagnostic ultrasound should be discussed with an obstetrician-gynecologist before final disposition. All patients with a positive pregnancy test and vaginal bleeding who are discharged home need close follow-up and repeat β-hCG in 48 to 72 hours.

There are two primary options for treating patients with a confirmed ectopic pregnancy: medical or surgical management. Methotrexate inhibits the formation of nucleotides necessary to synthesize DNA and RNA. It is recommended only for use in the patients with the following characteristics: hemodynamic stability, no active bleeding or signs of hemoperitoneum, unruptured ectopic pregnancy less than 3.5 cm in size, and a β-hCG level of less than 15,000 mIU/mL.[15] The dose recommended is 50 mg/m^2 intramuscularly once and can be repeated on follow-up if β-hCG levels are not declining as expected. The success of this treatment option is dependent on the size of the ectopic pregnancy and β-hCG level with smaller ectopic pregnancies and lower β-hCG levels having a higher success rate. A side effect of methotrexate

Table 1
Transvaginal ultrasound findings in ectopic pregnancy

Ultrasound Finding	Likelihood Ratio of Ectopic Pregnancy
Ectopic cardiac activity	>100
Ectopic gestational sac	23
Ectopic mass and free fluid	9.9
Free fluid	4.4
Ectopic mass	3.6
No IUP	2.2
Normal adnexal region	0.55
IUP	0.07

Data from Moi BW, Van der Veen F, Bossoyt PM. Implementation of probabilistic decision rules improves the predictive values of algorithms in the diagnostic management of ectopic pregnancy. Hum Reprod 1999;14:2855–62.

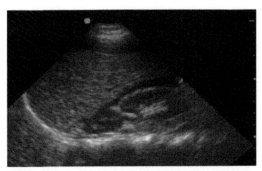

Fig. 3. FAST examination demonstrating free fluid in the splenorenal interface of a patient with an ectopic pregnancy. (*Courtesy of* Nathiel Tiesman, MD, Alameda County Medical Center, Highland General Hospital. Oakland (CA).)

is gastrointestinal discomfort, although before abdominal pain is attributed to methotrexate use, patients must be re-evaluated for a ruptured or persistent ectopic pregnancy.[16] Surgical management of ectopic pregnancy is generally used for patients who refuse or have contraindications to medical treatment, have failed medical treatment, or are clinically unstable.

The consequences of missing the diagnosis of ectopic pregnancy can be catastrophic. Emergency medicine physicians should be keenly aware of several pitfalls, such as failing to perform a pregnancy test in any woman with pain, bleeding, or other symptoms consistent with pregnancy or failing to perform an ultrasound because there is no palpable mass on examination. There may be rare occasions of patients with a highly concerning presentation when, in spite of a negative urine pregnancy test, a serum β-hCG proves elevated. Other pitfalls include failing to appreciate the amount of blood loss a patient has suffered or feeling reassured in the pregnant woman who has passed tissue when the ultrasound does not demonstrate an IUP—it can be difficult to differentiate an ectopic pregnancy from a SAB. Finally, no discussion of ectopic pregnancy is complete without mentioning heterotopic pregnancy—the coexistence of an IUP and an ectopic pregnancy. The occurrence is rare (1 in 2600 pregnancies) but the incidence increases dramatically with fertility treatments.[7]

The majority of miscarriages occur during the first trimester. In a study in which daily urinary β-hCG levels were determined, the total rate of pregnancy loss after implantation was 31%. Seventy percent of these losses occurred before the pregnancy was detected clinically.[17] In an ED, most patients with potential miscarriages are recognized with a complaint of vaginal bleeding and abdominal pain. SAB is the most common complication of early pregnancy and the prevalence is dependent on several factors (**Box 2**). SABs occur for a variety of reasons. One-third are blighted ovums in which no embryo or yolk sac is found in the gestational sac. In the remaining two-thirds, embryos are found and 50% of these have had a spontaneous chromosomal abnormality. The remainder of the SABs are attributed to trauma, host factors (unfavorable uterus), and unknown causes.[18]

Many studies have found a slightly increased risk of adverse outcomes, such as miscarriage, preterm birth, premature rupture of membranes, and fetal growth restrictions in patients with first-trimester bleeding. The increased risk is minimal when bleeding is light and confined to the first trimester, in particular the first 6 weeks. The risk of later complications is increased when the bleeding is heavy, subchorionic

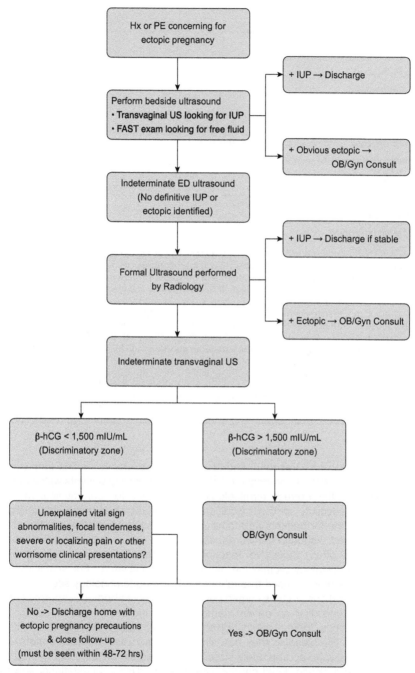

Fig. 4. Rule-out ectopic pregnancy algorithm. (*Adapted from* Reardon TF, Joing SA. First trimester pregnancy. In: Ma OJ, Mateer JR, Blaivas M, editors. Emergency ultrasound. 2nd edition. China: McGraw-Hill; 2008; with permission.)

Box 2
Risk factors associated with miscarriage

Maternal age

Early gestation

Increasing parity

First pregnancies

History of previous pregnancy loss

Toxins (tobacco, caffeine, alcohol, or cocaine abuse)

Nonsteroidal anti-inflammatory drugs

Low folate levels

Maternal body mass index <18 or >25 kg/m^2

Celiac disease

Maternal infections

Data from Nybo Andersen AM, Wohfahrt J, Christens P, et al. Maternal age and fetal loss: population based register linkage study. BMJ 2000;320:1708; Harger JH, Archer DF, Marchese, SG, et al. Etiology of recurrent pregnancy losses and outcomes of subsequent pregnancy. Obstet Gynecol 1983;62:574; Tata L, Card RT, Logan RFA, et al. Fertility and pregnancy events in women with celiac disease: a population-based cohort study. Gastroenterology 2005;128:849; ACOG practice bulletin. Management of recurrent pregnancy loss. Number 24, February 2001. American College of Obstetricians and Gynecologists. Int J Gynecol Obstet 2002;78:179; Chatenoud L, Parzzini F, di Cintio E. et al. Paternal and maternal smoking habits before conception and during the first trimester: in relation to spontaneous abortion. Ann Epidemiol 1998;8:520; Henricksen TB, Hjollund NH Jensen TK, et al. Alcohol consumption at the time of conception and spontaneous abortion. Am J Epidemiol 2004;160:661; Ness, RB, Grisso JA, Hirschinger, et al. Cocaine and tobacco use and the risk of spontaneous abortion. N Engl J Med 1999;340:333; George L, Mills JL, Johansson AL, et al. Plasma folate levels and risk of spontaneous abortion. JAMA 2002;288:1867.

---

hematoma is noted on ultrasound, and bleeding occurs later in the first trimester or into the second trimester of pregnancy.[19,20] When approaching patients with a potential miscarriage, the correct terminology is important for communication with colleagues and specialty services. Additionally, pregnancy loss is a highly charged and emotional time for patients and families regardless of whether or not the pregnancy was desired. Although the words, abortion and miscarriage, are interchangeable, there are often subjective reactions to them. Patients and geographic preference in terminology dictate the use of the nomenclature. For simplicity and medical clarity, abortion is used throughout the following terminology section.

Threatened abortions are thus named because the risk of abortion is approximately 35% to 50%, depending on patient demographics and severity of bleeding.[21] In threatened abortions, there is vaginal bleeding but the internal cervical os is closed on examination. The bleeding may be painless or associated with discomfort. The examination reveals an appropriately sized uterus given the gestational age and the cervix is long and closed. Fetal cardiac activity and advanced gestational age are positive predictors of progression to the second trimester.[22]

An inevitable abortion is manifest by an open cervical os and a cervix that is dilated. Frequently, products of conception are noted at the os or in the vaginal vault. Patients are often uncomfortable with abdominal cramps. Significant bleeding may occur in these patients as the uterus tries to expel the gestational products.

Incomplete abortions occur more rarely in the first 6 weeks of pregnancy compared with later in the first trimester. Products of conception are noted at the cervical os or in the vaginal vault. The amount of bleeding varies but can be severe enough to cause hypovolemic shock. Frequently, patients are in pain due to the nature of the uterine contractions. Ultrasound diagnosis is difficult because the endometrial stripe post pregnancy may be thickened and heterogeneous and there is no consensus as to what is considered acceptable thickness during miscarriage or immediately afterwards. This makes identifying retained gestational tissue challenging and is a potential pitfall.[23] Bleeding does not abate until the gestational products are removed or expelled. Without removal, these products can become a nidus for infection leading to a septic abortion.

When the entire gestational contents are expelled from the uterus, this is considered a completed abortion. More than one-third of all cases of first-trimester abortions are complete. If complete, the uterus is small and well contracted with a closed cervix, minimal vaginal bleeding, and mild cramping. Given the difficulty of ultrasonographically assessing the postaborted uterus, however, it is a potential pitfall to mistakenly call an incomplete abortion complete because of the problematic findings of the endometrial heterogeneity.

It is uncommon to diagnose missed abortions in the ED during the first trimester. Missed abortions occur when fetal demise occurs with retention of the gestational products for a prolonged period of time. Frequently, women with this condition have pregnancy-related symptoms that have resolved. Vaginal bleeding may occur and the cervical os is frequently closed. The uterus may or may not be appropriately sized depending on the length of time that the fetus has been nonviable. This terminology quickly is becoming obsolete as the way to date and view pregnancies has rapidly changed. Ultrasound and serial hormonal assays help date and time fetal demise much more quickly than in the past.

In the United States, septic abortions are not commonly seen in the first trimester. When they are diagnosed, however, they frequently are related to invasive procedures, such as chorionic villus sampling, amniocentesis, or self-administered abortions. They may also occur as a result of maternal bacteremia or incomplete SAB. Septic abortions occur when the gestational tissue or uterine support becomes infected. Patients frequently complain of abdominal pain, vaginal bleeding, fever, malaise, or purulent vaginal discharge. The physical examination may reveal tachycardia, hypotension, tachypnea, lower abdominal pain, and a tender, boggy uterus with a dilated cervix.[24] Septic abortions can be jointly classified as threatened, inevitable, or incomplete depending on the progression of the pregnancy. The infection frequently spreads from the endometrium through the myometrium to the to the peritoneum. The cause of the infection is usually polymicrobial, with *Escherichia coli* and other aerobic gram-negative rods frequently involved. Group B β-hemolytic streptococci, anaerobic streptococci, *Bacteroides* sp, and on occasion *Clostridium perfringens* are other organisms that can cause septic abortion. Because endotoxins can be released from the gram-negative bacilli, endotoxic shock may accompany septic abortion, particularly if it is caused by insertion of nonsterile agents into the uterine cavity. Rapid removal of the gestational products, supportive care, and intravenous broad-spectrum antibiotics to cover the organisms must be initiated immediately.

The clinical presentation of patients with SAB can be relatively benign or emergent when there is hemorrhage or sepsis. The presentation depends on maternal age, gestation, and circumstances of the abortion. Once pregnancy status is ascertained, pregnancy dates need to be obtained by evaluating for the last menstrual period. Constitutional symptoms, such as fevers, myalgias, rash, dizziness, or syncope, may help evaluate a septic abortion or hypovolemic shock in vaginal bleeding patients. The vaginal bleeding history may clue providers as to the timing of an abortion, the hemodynamic status, or potential future pregnancy related complications. Asking about the number and timing of changing sanitary pads and tampons can help clarify this issue. Patients should also be queried about the nature of the bleeding, focusing on clots, gestational tissue appearance, or fetal parts. Rhythmic contractions and cramping that start in the lower abdomen and move downward are indicative of uterine expulsion. Past medical history is also crucial in the prognosis of a current pregnancy. Pertinent information includes a history of sexually transmitted diseases and previous ectopic pregnancies or miscarriages.

The physical examination in pregnant patients with vaginal bleeding includes a careful abdominal examination to identify peritoneal signs and midline tenderness. A firm versus boggy uterus should be noted. Making a transabdominal approximation of uterine size may help date a pregnancy but historical information on a patient's last period and ultrasound are best for this. The pregnant uterus is a pelvic structure and difficult to assess until the early second trimester.

The pelvic examination begins with inspection of the external genitalia, looking for lesions, in particular lesions caused by the human papillomavirus and herpes simplex virus, that could bleed. A speculum examination should focus on the rate and content of the vaginal bleeding. All clots in the vaginal vault should be removed to identify the exact source of bleeding. Distinguishing clot from gestational tissue is often challenging and can be a pitfall. A quick way to make this distinction is to place the clot/tissue in a clear urine cup filled with water. Shining a light underneath shows the classic splay of tissue feathers of chorionic villi versus a dissolving clot. Noting products of conception can rule in a miscarriage and rule out other life-threatening conditions, such as ectopic pregnancy. All tissue specimens should be sent to pathology for confirmation of gestational products if there is any doubt about tissue identification.

A sterile bimanual examination should be performed next to assess the vaginal vault, cervical os, and uterine size and consistency. Probing the internal os with a sterile gloved finger should be done to access whether or not the cervical os is open. An open internal os is highly indicative of an inevitable abortion. Another pitfall is inadvertently only evaluating the external os, which is often open in multigravid women. The internal os is 1 to 2 cm deeper than the external os on examination.

Diagnosis of a threatened miscarriage is increasingly accurate with today's technology and medical knowledge. As discussed previously, transvaginal ultrasound and β-hCG are critical in assessing fetal viability in first-trimester patients with vaginal bleeding. Although direct visualization of an open cervical os or the presence of embryonic tissue may be sufficient to diagnose an inevitable, incomplete, or complete abortion clinically, ultrasound can provide additional information to emergency medicine physicians (eg, heterotopic pregnancy, multiple gestations, and retained gestational products). Definitive diagnosis of nonviable IUP can be made based on transvaginal ultrasound criteria (**Box 3**). In addition, there are certain findings on ultrasound examination that predict an increased chance of subsequent SAB (**Box 4**).

A normal fetal heart rate of 120 to 160 beats per minute is a reassuring indicator. In one study, 90% to 96% of pregnancies with fetal cardiac activity and vaginal bleeding at 7 and 11 weeks of gestation resulted in an ongoing pregnancy with higher success rates occurring at the later gestational ages (**Table 2**).[22] Despite ultrasound's strength in the diagnosis of first-trimester vaginal bleeding patients, nondiagnostic transvaginal ultrasound can frequently occur in the first 6 weeks of pregnancy. β-hCG levels may aid in the diagnosis of viability of the pregnancy. A β-hCG level rising by 66% within

---

Box 3
Endovaginal ultrasound criteria for nonviable pregnancies

Absence of a gestational sac at a β-hCG of 3000 IU/mL or 38 days since onset of last menses

Absence of embryo with gestational sac of 25-mm mean diameter

Absence of a yolk sac when the gestational sac's mean diameter is 13 mm

Absence of an embryonic pole when the mean gestational sac diameter >18 mm transvaginally

Absence of embryonic cardiac activity in an embryo of crown-rump length >5 mm or >9 weeks' gestational age

Adapted from Filly R. Ultrasound evaluation during the first trimester. In: Callen PW, editor. Ultrasonography in obstetrics and gynecology. 3rd edition. Philadelphia: W. B. Saunders; 1994; with permission.

---

48 hours is suggestive of normal pregnancy progression when accompanied by relevant ultrasound findings.[25–27] Preliminary studies have shown that progesterone levels of less than 5 ng/mL with β-hCG levels of greater than 3000 IU/mL had a high incidence of being an ectopic pregnancy or a nonviable intrauterine gestation in 97% of women.[28]

There are three possible courses of management for SABs and occasionally combinations of these approaches are employed. These include surgical treatment (dilation and curettage [D&C] or evacuation), medical treatment (*misoprostol*), or expectant/conservative management.

Hormonal confirmation of pregnancy should be confirmed by urinalysis or by serum β-hCG. When indicated, it is reasonable to check hemoglobin level to establish a baseline and follow progression in patients who continue to bleed. A white count may be obtained in patients suspect for a septic abortion. The Rh status of any pregnant patients with vaginal bleeding should be checked. Anti-D immunoglobulin (RhoGAM) should be administered if patients are Rh negative, unless the father is also known to be Rh negative. 50 μg of RhoGAM is an acceptable dose in the first trimester given the small volume of red cells in the fetoplacental circulation and is sufficient to treat ABO incompatibility between mother and fetus. The Kleihauer-Betke test is not necessary, unless requested by obstetrics during consultation.

Fluid resuscitation with normal saline may be required in select patients based on clinical history, initial vital signs, symptoms, and laboratory evaluation.

Ultrasonographic confirmation of an IUP should be obtained. If this is confirmed and there is a fetal heat beat noted within the uterus, the patient may safely be discharged

---

Box 4
Ultrasound findings worrisome for future spontaneous abortion

Abnormal yolk sac

Low fetal heart rate

Small gestational sac for gestational age

Subchorionic hematoma

Adapted from Filly R. Ultrasound evaluation during the first trimester. In: Callen PW, editor. Ultrasonography in obstetrics and gynecology. 3rd edition. Philadelphia: W. B. Saunders; 1994; with permission.

Table 2			
Transvaginal sonographic findings in normal pregnancy			
Gestational Age in Weeks	Ultrasound Finding	Crown-Rump Length	β-hCG (mIU/mL)
5	Gestation sac	Not applicable	1500
5.5	Yolk sac	Not applicable	5000
6	Fetal pole	2–3 mm	13,000–15,000
6	Cardiac activity	5 mm	13,000–15,000

Data from Nordenholz, K, Abbott J, Bailitz J. First trimester pregnancy. In: Cosby KS, Kendall JL, editors. Practical guide to emergency ultrasound. Philadelphia: Lippincott Williams and Wilkins; 2006. p. 123–60.

with a diagnosis of threatened miscarriage. If a provider's institution is using progesterone and other novel markers of pregnancy outcome, this is the appropriate time to order these tests.

Surgical procedures provide definitive options for the inevitable and incomplete abortion: procedural options in the ED include ring forceps removal of products of conception. This often slows vaginal bleeding considerably.[29] Dilation with suction curettage (D&C), however, is the definitive procedure to prevent hemorrhage and infection with retained products of conception. The risks of this procedure include those of procedural sedation, uterine adhesions and perforation, and cervical trauma and infection.[30] D&C, although a common procedure worldwide, is not currently a procedure done by emergency medicine physicians; however, the procedure can be performed in an ED by obstetricians and gynecologists with the proper sedation and equipment. Most of these risks of D&C are small and related to improper technique or sedation.

Medical management with misoprostol, a prostaglandin analog, is currently the most commonly used therapy for inducing abortion in those with inevitable and missed abortions during the first trimester. Its safety and effectiveness have been established by many randomized controlled trials.[31] Of those patients given misoprostol, 71% had uterine expulsion by day 3 and 84% had expulsion by day 8. Use of this therapy should be done in conjunction with obstetrics.[32] Expectant management of inevitable SABs is also common given that the majority of failed pregnancies complete their expulsion within 1 to 2 weeks after fetal demise. Approximately 50% of patients choose expectant management when given the choice of surgical, medical, or expectant management. Expectant management is only available to first-trimester patients. A Cochrane database showed that although there was a higher rate of return for surgical procedures and bleeding, expectant management was the favorite of most women, with 50% of women choosing it.[29]

Approximately 50% of all pregnant patients who come to the ED with vaginal bleeding eventually miscarry. As there are no therapies to prevent a miscarriage, expectant management is the accepted course for all threatened abortions. Many of the traditional recommendations for preventing SABs, such as bed rest, pelvic rest, and avoidance of exercise, have been debunked.[33] The overall risk of miscarriage in the future increases with each current miscarriage. It has been reported that there is a 43% miscarriage rate after two previous SABs.[34] Patients should be given clear and specific instructions about what to expect in the next few days and guarded pregnancy prognosis should be specifically stated. It is a pitfall in management of threatened abortion patients not to have frank discussion of the risks of a failed pregnancy.

Understanding the emotional and physical toll on patients is paramount in this highly charged situation. Addressing the guilt that a patient has done something "wrong" to cause the miscarriage to happen is an important role of the provider in this situation. If a patient is persistently bleeding, discuss infection prevention and caution against insertion of foreign bodies into the vagina. Simple pain medications, such as acetaminophen and narcotics, should be adequate to treat pain. There is no role for antibiotics in a simple threatened abortion. Follow-up ultrasound or hormonal tests should be scheduled in conjunction with the obstetrics service. In general, 24- to 48-hour follow-up for moderately bleeding pregnant patients is recommended and 48 to 72 hours for lightly bleeding patients. Adjustments should be made for changes in a patient's condition.[34] In patients with inevitable abortion, consultation with an obstetric service should be made for surgical, medical, or expectant options. These patients should all have obstetric follow-up. Bleeding may be brisk in these patients, because the uterus is unable to fully contract. An ED physician may be able to improve the bleeding if the tissue at the os is removed. An incomplete abortion needs to be completed. If the bleeding is mild but persistent, next-day follow-up may be reasonable as long as the social situation and emotional state of the patient are stable and there is minimal intrauterine tissue remaining as diagnosed by ultrasound.[35] Frequently, obstetrics surgically completes the abortion at the time of presentation. Patients should be instructed to return to the ED for any concerning signs of hypovolemia or infection. Up to 80% of patients complete their abortions without intervention in the first trimester. D&C can decrease the need for further visits and procedures, specifically if the fetal pole or gestational sac is visible on sonogram.[35] Overall, completed abortions are safe to discharge. Patients are generally advised to have pelvic rest for 2 weeks post expulsion or evacuation of uterine contents and to complete one to two full cycles of their menses before retrying to become pregnant. There are no data to support these recommendations. Patients with septic abortions should be admitted for D&C and intravenous antibiotics. Oral regimens may be tried based on patient presentation; however, this should be done with extreme caution and only in conjunction with obstetrics service involvement.

Vaginal bleeding that occurs in pregnant patients that is not related to an ectopic, miscarriage or implantation bleeding is usually related to vaginal or cervical pathology or trauma. Vaginal lesions related to sexually transmitted diseases that may bleed are associated with human papilloma virus and herpes simplex virus. These lesions are readily identified on external vaginal examination. A careful examination must be done to ensure proper identification of these lesions. It is more difficult to assess the cervix where human papilloma virus lesions may bleed; however, minor bleeds occur. If these are new lesions, a routine sexually transmitted disease examination should be initiated in addition to controlling the bleeding. Cervical extropion is also prone to light bleeding when touched during coitus or speculum examination and easily abates without therapy. Again, the important aspect of any pregnant patient with vaginal bleeding is to confirm maternal hemodynamic stability and fetal viability.

Vaginal lacerations are also seen in pregnant women. There are two types: coital and traumatic (straddle injuries and foreign bodies). Both of these are extremely difficult to distinguish from vaginal bleeding coming from the uterus due to the volume of blood that can potentially obscure visualization of the origin. Given the vascularity of the perineum during pregnancy, these lacerations can be profound and result in hypovolemic shock and death. Coitus causing vaginal wall lacerations is well reported but, unfortunately, a high percentage of these are related to sexual aggression. Any patients with a vaginal laceration should be carefully probed about the nature of the sexual encounter with appropriate referral as needed. Vaginal packing helps temporarily in bleeding; however, definitive laceration care is required and frequently done in conjunction with obstetrics.[36]

Trauma in pregnancy is beyond the scope of this article except to mention a few key issues. First, uterine injury, hence, traumatic bleeding from the uterus, is rare in the first trimester because the bony pelvis protects the small gravid uterus. Abruptio placentae (premature separation of the placenta from the uterine wall) occurs commonly with blunt trauma.[37] This condition presents with vaginal bleeding, pain, uterine contractions, and fetal distress. If this diagnosis is suspected in a woman in her first trimester of pregnancy, an obstetrics consultation is warranted. Unfortunately, there is not much that can be done for a placental abruption in the first trimester other than employing expectant management because the fetus is not viable outside the uterus until approximately 23 weeks' gestation.[38] Administering RhoGAM is a must if the mother is Rh negative and having vaginal bleeding from trauma. Another key issue is that intimate partner violence increases during pregnancy.[39] If a woman presents to the ED with trauma, emergency physicians must have a high index of suspicion for potential abuse. In cases where abuse is confirmed or suspected, traumatic injuries should be cared for and the physician should engage social workers or counselors to assist the pregnant woman with the psychosocial issues surrounding the abusive relationship. If a provider practices in a state where mandatory reporting is expected, it is key to report any suspected or confirmed case of abuse.

In conclusion, vaginal bleeding in first-trimester pregnant patients can have life-threatening implications. The most worrisome cause of vaginal bleeding in first-trimester pregnant patients is ectopic pregnancy. The most important question that an ED physician needs to answer in a timely manner is, "Is there an IUP?" Once that question has been answered with the help of ultrasound and a β-hCG, then appropriate management plans can be implemented. There are many pitfalls possible in the

---

Box 5
Pitfalls in the diagnosis and treatment of first-trimester vaginal bleeding

Failing to order a pregnancy test

Premature reading of a urine pregnancy test result

Inadvertently examining only the external os instead of the internal os

Believing a patient passed tissue when it was simply blood clots

Not ordering or incorrectly interpreting a pelvic ultrasound

Failing to order RhoGAM in Rh-negative women

Forgetting to entertain the diagnosis of heterotopic pregnancy, especially in women with fertility problems

Not inquiring about intimate partner violence or abuse

Attributing abdominal pain in a patient on methotrexate to the medication rather than problems with the ectopic pregnancy itself

Not arranging close follow-up

Discharge instructions not complete

Potential outcome not explained to patient

Not inquiring about sexual assault and intimate partner violence in trauma to the pregnant patient

evaluation of first-trimester bleeding patients; however, with careful consideration and a thoughtful approach, many of these can be avoided (**Box 5**).

REFERENCES

1. Alfthan H, BjÖrses UM, Tiitinen A, et al. Specificity and detection limit of ten pregnancy tests. Scand J Clin Lab Invest 1993;53(Suppl 216):105–13.
2. Neinstein L, Harvey F. Effect of low urine specific gravity on pregnancy testing. J Am Coll Health 1998;47(3):138–9.
3. Tabas JA, Strehlow M, Isaacs E. A false negative pregnancy test in a patient with a hydatidiform molar pregnancy. N Engl J Med 2003;349(22):2172–3.
4. Abbott J, Emmans LS, Lowenstein SR. Ectopic pregnancy: ten common pitfalls in diagnosis. Am J Emerg Med 1990;8:515–22.
5. Brenner PF, Roy S, Mishell DR. Ectopic pregnancy—a study of 300 consecutive surgically treated cases. JAMA 1980;243(7):673–6.
6. Centers for Diseases Control and Prevention. Current trends in ectopic pregnancy—United States, 1990–1992. MMWR Morb Mortal Wkly Rep 1995;44:46–8.
7. Bright DA, Gaupp FB. Heterotopic pregnancy: a reevaluationn. J Am Board Fam Pract 1990;3:125–8.
8. Goldner TE, Lawson HW, Xia Z, et al. Surveillance for ectopic pregnancy—United States, 1970–1989. MMWR CDC Surveill Summ 1993;42:73–85.
9. Breen JL. A 21 year survey of 654 ectopic pregnancies. Am J Obstet Gynecol 1970;106(7):1004–19.
10. Stovall TG, Kellerman AL, Ling FW, et al. Emergency department diagnosis of ectopic pregnancy. Ann Emerg Med 1990;19:1098–103.
11. Hick JL, Rodgerson JD, Heegaard WG, et al. Vital signs fail to correlate with hemoperitoneum from ruptured ectopic pregnancy. Am J Emerg Med 2001;19(6): 488–91.
12. Kohn MA, Kerr K, Malkevich D, et al. Beta-human chrorionic gonadotropin levels and the likelihood of ectopic pregnancy in emergency department patients with abdominal pain or vaginal bleeding. Acad Emerg Med 2003;10:119–26.
13. Murray H, Baakdah H, Bardell T, et al. Diagnosis and treatment of ectopic pregnancy. CMAJ 2005;173(8):905–12.
14. ACEP Policy Statement. Emergency ultrasound imaging criteria compendium. American College of Emergency Physicians 2006. Available at: http://www. acep.org/acepmembership.aspx?id=32298. Accessed June 16, 2009.
15. American College of Obstetrics and Gynecologists. Medical management of tubal pregnancy. ACOG Practice Bulletin 3. Washington, DC: ACOG; 1998.
16. American College of Emergency Physicians. Clinical policy: critical issues in the initial evaluation and management of patients presenting to the emergency department in early pregnancy. Ann Emerg Med 2003;41:123–33.
17. Wilcox SJ, Weinberg CR, O'Conner JF, et al. Incidence of early loss of pregnancy. N Engl J Med 1988;319:189.
18. Fantel AG, Shepard TH. Morphological analysis of spontaneous abortuses. In: Bennet MJ, Edmonds DK, editors. Spontaneous and recurrent abortion. Oxford (UK): Blackwell Scientific Publications; 1987. p. 8.
19. Harville EW, Wilcox AJ, Baird DD, et al. Vaginal bleeding in very early pregnancy. Hum Reprod 2003;18:1944.
20. Weiss JL, Malone FD, Vidaver J, et al. Threatened abortion: a risk factor for poor pregnancy outcome, a population –based screening study. Am J Obstet Gynecol 2004;190:745.

21. Chung TK, Sahota DS, Lau TK, et al. Threatened abortion: predictions of viability based on signs and symptoms. Aust N Z J Obstet Gynaecol 1999;39:443.
22. Deaton JK, Honore GM, Huffman CS, et al. Early transvaginal ultrasound following an accurately dated pregnancy: the importance of finding a yolk sac or fetal heart motion. Hum Reprod 1997;12:2820.
23. Sawyer E, Ofuasia E, Ofili-Yebovi D, et al. The value of measuring endometrial thickness and volume on transvaginal ultrasound scan for the diagnosis of incomplete miscarriage. Ultrasound Obstet Gynecol 2007;29(2):205–9.
24. Stubblefield PG, Grimes DA. Septic abortion. N Engl J Med 1994;331:310–4.
25. Kadar N, Caldwell BV, Romero R. A method of screening for ectopic pregnancy and its indications. Obstet Gynecol 1981;58:162.
26. Dart RG, Mitterando Julie, Dart Linda M. Rate of change of serial beta human chorionic gonadotropin values as predictor of ectopic pregnancy in patients with indeterminate transvaginal ultrasound findings. Ann Emerg Med 1999;34: 703–10.
27. Barnhart KT, Sammel MD, Rinaudo PF, et al. Symptomatic patients with an early viable intrauterine pregnancy: HCG curves redefined. Obstet Gynecol 2004; 104:50.
28. Stovall TG, Ling FW, Anderson RN, et al. Improved sensitivity and specificity of a single measurement of serum progesterone over serial quantitative beta-human chorionic gonadotrophin in screening for ectopic pregnancy. Hum Reprod 1992; 7:723.
29. Nanda K, Peloggia A, Grimes D, et al. Expectant care versus surgical treatment for miscarriage. Cochrane Database Syst Rev 2006;(2):CD003518.
30. Demetroulis C, Saridogan E, Kunde D, et al. A prospective randomized control trial comparing medical and surgical treatment for early pregnancy failure. Hum Reprod 2001;16:365.
31. Neilson J, Hickey M, Vazquez J. Medical treatment for early fetal death (less than 24 weeks). Cochrane Database Syst Rev 2006;(3):CD002253.
32. Zhang J, Gilles JM, Barnhart K, et al. A comparison of medical management with misoprostol and surgical management for early pregnancy failure. N Engl J Med 2005;353:761.
33. Aleman A, Althabe F, Belizan J, et al. Bed rest during pregnancy for preventing miscarriage. Cochrane Database Syst Rev 2005;(2):CD003576.
34. Regan L, Braude PR, Trembath PL. Influence of past reproductive performance on risk of spontaneous abortion. BMJ 1989;299:541.
35. Luise C, Jermy K, May C, et al. Outcomes of expectant management of spontaneous first trimester miscarriage. BMJ 2002;324:873.
36. Sloin MM, Karimian M, Ilbeigi P. Nonobstetric lacerations of the vagina. J Am Osteopath Assoc 2006;106(5):271–3.
37. Fleming AD. Abruptio placentae. Crit Care Clin 1991;7:865–75.
38. Doyle LW. Outcome at 5 years of age of children 23–27 weeks gestation: refining the prognosis. Pediatrics 2001;108:134–41.
39. Amaro H, Fried L, Cabral H, et al. Violence during pregnancy and substance abuse. Am J Public Health 1990;80:575–9.

The Violent or Agitated Patient

Jennifer Rossi, MD[a], Megan C. Swan, MD[a],
Eric D. Isaacs, MD, FACEP, FAAEM[b,c],*

KEYWORDS

- Violent • Agitated • Sedation • Restraints
- Psychiatric • Substance abuse

Every day emergency providers encounter violent or agitated patients, from the cocaine-intoxicated teenager to the belligerent chronic alcoholic, from the actively psychotic schizophrenic to the combative trauma victim to the encephalopathic liver patient. The emergency department (ED) is a unique health care setting in that federal law, by way of emergency medicine treatment and active labor act (EMTALA), mandates the medical evaluation of every patient who presents to the ED. In addition, violent and agitated patients are often escorted to the ED against their will. Behavioral emergencies account for about 1 in 20 ED visits, and violence or agitation, regardless of the etiology, constitutes most of these presentations.[1] Despite efforts to maintain order, emergencies are frequently emotional and sometimes chaotic. These stressful situations are compounded by long wait times, the noise of the ED, and sometimes by family and friends who may also be agitated or intoxicated. All these factors can trigger or exacerbate violent tendencies and agitation in patients.

Agitated or altered patients are high risk because they may pose a physical threat to the staff, may harm themselves, and may have dangerous comorbidities and illnesses causing their violent behavior. The emergency physician must quickly limit these behaviors and identify and treat their etiology, while simultaneously protecting patients' rights and reducing the risks of injury to other patients and medical staff. Appropriate disposition must also be determined. This article guides physicians through these essential aspects of caring for this high-risk patient population.

CLINICAL VIGNETTE ONE

A 47-year-old homeless man presents to the ED complaining of low back pain. He is disheveled and unbathed. After a long wait, he is brought back to the clinical area and

[a] Division of Emergency Medicine, Stanford University School of Medicine, 701 Welch Road, Building C, Palo Alto, CA 94304, USA
[b] Department of Medicine, University of California, San Francisco, CA, USA
[c] Emergency Department, San Francisco General Hospital, 1001 Potrero Avenue, Room 1E21, San Francisco, CA 94110, USA
* Corresponding author.
E-mail address: Eric.Isaacs@emergency.ucsf.edu (E.D. Isaacs).

Emerg Med Clin N Am 28 (2010) 235–256
doi:10.1016/j.emc.2009.10.006
0733-8627/09/$ – see front matter © 2010 Elsevier Inc. All rights reserved.

emed.theclinics.com

placed on a bed. None of the staff is in a rush to assess this patient and he remains clothed. After a period of time, he becomes quite angry and pulls a knife from his waistband.

Prevention of Violence in the ED

High-risk work environment: protect thyself

Violence toward staff members is all too common; the ED has the highest rate of employee assault in the hospital, with nurses the most common victims.[2,3] A frequently quoted survey of ED directors from 170 teaching hospitals reported approximately one quarter used restraints daily, one fifth had at least one verbal threat per day, and one sixth had at least one threat with a weapon each month.[4] Furthermore, 17 respondents reported a significant patient injury during restraint within the last 5 years, including one death, and 20 institutions reported involvement with litigation pertaining to restraint. Despite these statistics, only 51 institutions provided ED nurses with formal training in recognition and management of aggression and violence.[4] A survey of 171 randomly selected attending emergency physicians in Michigan found that 75% experienced at least one verbal threat in the previous year, 28% reported being physically assaulted, 12% were confronted outside the ED, and 3.5% were stalked.[5]

Formal security plans can decrease assaults against hospital employees. There are three levels of such management, as summarized in **Table 1**.[6] The California Hospital Safety and Security Act (Assembly Bill 508) mandates that hospitals in this state have a comprehensive security plan including environmental modifications of the physical layout, employee education and training, use of security and law enforcement, and surveillance of violent events. Besides California, only Washington State has passed a similar initiative. Available data indicate that such plans work: pre-enactment and postenactment employee assault rates in California EDs decreased 48% compared with rates in New Jersey, where state-based government workplace violence initiatives do not exist.[7]

High risk: concealed weapons and dangerous examination room environment

Prevention of violence starts outside the emergency facility's door and continues to the gurney. Departments should control access by protected entrances, metal detectors, and secured doors. This checkpoint can serve to prevent concealed weapons brought in by patients and visitors, and by persons with criminal intent, such as assailants searching to "finish off" a victim brought to the ED after a physical attack. Guards should enact standardized methods of removing concealed weapons from patients and visitors. Notably, however, although metal detectors and cameras decrease the number of weapons eventually confiscated in the clinical area, they have not been consistently shown to decrease the rate of assaults on physicians.[8] In addition, patients suffering major trauma usually arrive by ambulance and are usually not escorted through detector systems. In one large urban ED, over one quarter of these victims harbored a lethal weapon.[9]

Table 1 Steps to violence management	
Primary	Control Factors Leading to Violence
Secondary	Identify and respond to previolent and escalating behavior
Tertiary	Limit injury once violence is present

Data from Lavoie FW. Violence in emergency facilities. Acad Emerg Med 1994;1(2):166–8.

Other factors that may help reduce violent incidents include systems to alert staff when patients with a history of violence register at triage. When possible, rooming these patients quickly may limit frustration with long waiting times and can protect bystanders and decrease interaction with others in the waiting room that may incite aggression. Frequent updates on clinical course and anticipated length of stay and comfortable waiting rooms may help diffuse tension.

Fully clothed patients, such as the man in the first vignette, should not languish in the hallway. Once in the ED, patients should be instructed to change into a hospital gown. This action is crucial: (1) it allows for further search and removal of weapons; (2) patients are less likely to leave before evaluation is complete; and (3) it allows for a complete physical examination that uncovers sites of infections, trauma, and other clues to behavior. As personal belongings are tucked away, providing physical comforts, such as warm clothes, a blanket, and food, are simple acts that convey caring and help build patient-physician trust.

The setup of the examination room itself may facilitate safety. The perception of entrapment can fuel agitation. When possible, patients who are at high risk of violence should be placed in rooms with two exits so that both staff and the patient have unobstructed routes of exit. If there is only one exit, then the provider should position themselves so that neither their own nor the patient's exit is obstructed. Although a secluded area ensures sufficient privacy to conduct an interview and may also decrease stimuli and resulting tension, these needs must be balanced with the need for observation of patients who may pose a threat to themselves or others.

Provider personal safety is paramount. Any secluded space should not isolate the examiner from assistance. Providers should always remain in earshot of help and know the location of alarms or panic buttons when present in the clinical area. When the risk of patient violence outweighs the principle of patient privacy, station the assistance of others or security outside the door or at the bedside. Avoid arguing, turning one's back on the patient, crossing arms, or standing too close to patients at risk of violent behavior in the ED. Remove personal effects that may be used as a weapon. All dangling earrings, neckties, badge holders, and necklaces should be removed, and trauma shears, scalpels, and needles emptied from pockets before approaching the potentially violent individual.

Causes and Evaluation of Violence

High risk: not identifying organic and treatable causes of violence and agitation
The etiology of acute undifferentiated agitation is frequently unclear on presentation and complicates management. A thorough evaluation of each patient, every time they present to the ED, is essential to avoid missing a reversible organic cause of delirium manifesting as violence and agitation. Such diagnostic errors are all too common; almost 80% of patients found to have medical disease causing their agitated behavior were "medically cleared" by an emergency physician before discharge to a psychiatric facility.[10] The causes of violence and aggression can be roughly divided into organic (deriving from medical disorders, including substance abuse and other toxidromes); psychotic (schizophrenic, manic, delusional); and nonorganic nonpsychotic (personality disorders, impulse control disorders).

As with all critical patients, the first steps are to assess and secure hemodynamic and respiratory function and obtain vital signs (including temperature and blood glucose finger stick), monitoring equipment and an initial examination focused on airway, breathing, circulation, and neurologic status and level of consciousness. When intubation is necessary, a neurologic examination, with special attention to focal deficits and language function, should be attempted before paralysis and sedation.

When feasible, this may be done by one practitioner while a second prepares for intubation. Even in an uncooperative patient, testing of gross motor function, reflexes (including Babinski), and withdrawal to pain can be performed. To prevent catastrophic disability, if a head injury is in question, a cervical collar should be placed until a spinal injury is ruled out.

Once the stability of the patient is ensured, a comprehensive evaluation for etiology begins. It is a grave error to assume that all violent behavior is caused by intoxication or psychiatric disease, even in intoxicated patients and those with a history of a psychiatric diagnosis. Acute violent or agitated behavior may result from myriad causes including withdrawal, toxidromes, endocrinopathies, metabolic derangements, substance abuse, infections, and neurologic illnesses. Many of these causes are reversible. A number of reversible or potentially treatable conditions may present as delirium and can be remembered by the mnemonic "GOT IVS" (**Box 1**). Rare organic causes include brain tumors, brain infections, Wilson disease, Huntington disease, sleep disorders, thyroid disorders, hyperparathyroidism, vitamin deficiencies, and toxins. Less common substances implicated in violent tendencies include organophosphate poisoning and manganese poisoning. Brain tumors of the limbic system and hypothalamic areas of the brain can trigger personality changes and aggression or frank psychosis. The rapidity of onset of these symptoms is linked to the speed the tumor is growing. Associated symptoms included early morning headaches, seizures, visual disturbances, and nausea and vomiting. A variety of infections, most notably herpes simplex encephalitis, meningitis, and AIDS dementia, can cause bizarre or agitated behavior.

The crux of evaluation is the patient (or collateral) history. There are several clues that suggest that violent behavior is organic in origin: rapid in onset; no prior history of psychiatric disease (especially if older than 40 years old); visual-olfactory-tactile hallucinations; abnormal vital signs (ie, fever); cognitive deficits; slurred speech; confusion; substance abuse; disorientation; history of trauma; and physical evidence of trauma. Other key questions to consider include: What is the context of this violent or agitated behavior? Is their agitation only present in medical settings, the streets, at home, or all places? Is the violence directed outward at others or primarily in defense? Are there specific targets or random victims?

Whenever possible the provider should obtain corroborating information, because some patients may be unwilling or unable fully to answer. Even this information should be scrutinized, however, because sometimes family and friends may also have incentive not to reveal the truth. Authorities and prehospital care providers are additional

---

Box 1
GOT IVS diagnoses to be considered on presentation

G Glucose: hypoglycemia

O Oxygen: hypoxia

T Trauma: head injury, or bleeding

   Temperature: hyperthermia, hypothermia

I Infection: meningitis or sepsis

V Vascular: stroke or subarachnoid hemorrhage

S Seizure: postictal or status epilepticus

valuable sources and should be questioned thoroughly when they bring in an altered patient.

Physical examination may reveal the cause of agitation. A gross assessment of the mental status is performed concurrently with history-taking because patients may display signs of confusion, disorientation, memory problems, and racing or paranoid thoughts during basic questioning. Finer parts of the mental status examination can then be obtained as possible. In addition to assessing vital signs and neurologic status as discussed previously, providers should look for meningeal signs, marks of trauma, foci of infection, and evidence of seizure or a postictal state. Laboratory testing needed varies with each scenario, but all patients should have a blood glucose level documented. If encephalopathy is high on the differential, an ammonia level may be ordered. Other electrolytes that can alter mentation include sodium, blood-urea-nitrogen, and magnesium. An elevated white blood count may suggest an underlying infection or stress response. Chest radiographs should be obtained for patients suspected of pneumonia. Head CT can reveal tumors, intracranial hemorrhage, and subdural hematomas, all of which may cause agitation and violent behavior.

CLINICAL VIGNETTE TWO

A 21-year-old unrestrained passenger in a front-impact motor vehicle collision presents with mild headache, neck, and knee pain. Films are negative and the patient vomits 90 minutes after receiving morphine. Zofran is given but the patient pulls out the IV and demands to leave. A CT scan is ordered. How can this be accomplished safely?

The Violent Head-injured Patient

Agitation in the form of emotional lability and angry outbursts is well described in the recovery phase of traumatic brain injury (TBI), but agitation is also one of the earliest signs of increased intracranial pressure in the acute setting. As TBI and the possibility of increased intracranial pressure are recognized, the role of the emergency physician shifts to prevention of secondary injury. The presence of hypoxia or decreased perfusion causes significant additional insult to the injured brain in the hours or days after the primary event. Maintaining adequate oxygenation is important in treating all brain injuries, but the focus on maximizing the cerebral perfusion pressure by maintaining mean arterial pressure is particularly important in the treatment of TBI patients. Decisions about whether and how to sedate (and possibly paralyze and intubate) a potentially head-injured patient to safely obtain a diagnostic CT scan must incorporate the risks of respiratory depression and effect of hemodynamic status on an injured brain. The use of benzodiazapines, such as midazolam, and opioids, such as fentanyl (with caution for hypotension and decreased cerebral perfusion), is well-established, as is the use of etomidate for sedation in the setting of intubation. There are limited data on the use of atypical antipsychotics to control agitation in head-injured patients, although these medications are increasingly used to control acute agitation in patients with a history of psychotic spectrum disorders (see later). Finally, there has been some recent attention to the use of subdissociative doses of ketamine, given previous concern over potential increases in intracranial pressure in head-injured patients. A review of the literature shows that ketamine's deleterious effect on intracranial pressure was in dissociative doses in patients with obstruction of cerebrospinal fluid outflow. In patients with normal cerebrospinal fluid flow, there was minimal effect on intracranial pressure, and an increase in cerebral blood flow with resulting decreased ischemia may occur.[11–15]

Most head-injured patients do not require deep chemical restraint, but rather anxiolysis or a discrete period of procedural sedation for the purpose of diagnostic imaging and treatment. Mild sedation or anxiolysis is a drug-induced state that preserves basic cognitive functions and does not affect respiratory functions. Deeper or moderate sedation limits the patient's level of consciousness. These individuals may still have the ability to follow simple commands; however, their cardiopulmonary functions are concurrently limited and must be closely monitored throughout the medication's duration of effect. An end-tidal capnography monitor enables detection of subclinical respiratory depression and airway complications before the development of frank hypoventilation sooner than pulse oximetry alone and should be used in all circumstances possible.[16,17] Sometimes, chemical sedation is not necessary, as illustrated by the next vignette.

CLINICAL VIGNETTE THREE

The nurses come to ask for sedation orders for a 38-year-old helmeted mountain biker with neck pain who is in cervical spine precautions awaiting imaging studies. It is a busy day and the nurses note that his behavior has been escalating for the last 5 to 10 minutes.

Interview and De-escalation Techniques

This patient is at risk of a cervical spine injury and his agitation places him at risk of further injury. In addition, because his behavior may itself be the result of traumatic injury, providers must ensure that he is protected until further evaluation can be completed. Whereas chemical sedation is a possible treatment, these medications may mask the signs or symptoms of other developing injuries in the trauma patient. Instead, the provider should begin by reassessing the patient and addressing his concerns. Such de-escalation techniques can often calm rising agitation in patients, limit harm they cause themselves or others, and avert the need for physical or chemical restraints.

Providers should start the interview with a pleasant but firm introduction that includes name and position. Throughout, they should convey empathy to the patient through careful listening skills and positive language that indicates a sense of respect and positive regard. This may include consolatory tones. In contrast, hostile language, direct arguing, threatening, or ignoring the patient almost always exacerbate violent tendencies in patients. Disruptive behaviors should not be accepted by ED staff, but respect for the patient should be maintained. Small gestures, such as offering food or drink (if allowed), or acknowledging and responding to their discomfort develops the patient-provider relationship.

Concurrently, the provider must convey a sense of control and authority. Clear, consistent behavioral expectations and boundaries should be discussed as soon as a potential problem is identified. **Box 2** includes some warning signs of violence.

One overlooked "treatment" for escalating patients is pain control. Alleviating pain is crucial in all patients, but even more so in those who are agitated. Pain is the most common reason people come to the ED and is a factor in over half of all visits.[18] Physicians overall, however, notoriously undertreat pain.[19] This is a deficiency in treatment for any patient, and a big pitfall in patients already agitated or predisposed to violence. As pain persists, it induces a negative effect in the sufferer. This in turn can incite patients to become agitated, upset, and lash out at caregivers. Eliminating pain can help establish a therapeutic bond, decrease patient discomfort, and help diffuse escalating situations. For example, a trauma patient waiting for imaging is more apt to be cooperative if not in physical pain. Patients with florid psychosis, mania, delirium, or severe intoxication, however, are less likely to improve with pain control.

CLINICAL VIGNETTE FOUR

A 26-year-old man is brought in by police after he is found smashing car windows while running in the street. Four police officers were required to subdue the patient. His heart rate is 150 beats per minute, blood pressure is 184/96, and he is diaphoretic and agitated. He is yelling, "They are trying to kill me."

Substance abuse can directly cause and exacerbate violence in patients. **Box 2** summarizes the clues and risk factors for substance-related violence. Alcohol, cocaine, and amphetamines are common intoxications seen in the ED that are linked to violent behaviors.

Amphetamines are neuroexcitatory, primarily through increased neuronal dopaminergic activity. They inhibit dopamine reuptake and displace dopamine from storage vesicles in the terminal neuron resulting in increased dopamine in the synaptic cleft. This upregulation of dopamine in the brain can lead to agitation, aggression, violence, and psychoses. This is greatest in chronic abusers because of the long-term elevated dopamine levels. Amphetamines are linked to aggression because of three factors: (1) the disinhibition in the frontal cortex and impairment of executive functions, such as self-control; (2) neurotoxic effects triggering destruction of the dopaminergic and serotonergic pathways in the brain; and (3) the positive symptoms of psychosis, which increases fear and hostility toward others in their environment.[20] Of importance, chronic users are predisposed to violence regardless of whether they are currently intoxicated because of the long-term elevated dopamine levels. Methamphetamine users have a nine times greater risk of committing homicide than the rest of the population, even after controlling for concomitant substance abuse.[21]

Cocaine use also predisposes users to committing violent acts. Cocaine is a sympathomimetic agent that inhibits the reuptake of epinephrine and norepinephrine in the peripheral nervous system and augments the presynaptic release of norepinephrine.

Box 2
Risk factors for substance-related violence

Younger age

Male gender

Lower income

History of violence

Past juvenile detention

History of physical abuse by parent

Substance dependence only

Comorbid mental health and substance disorders

Victimization in past year

Unemployed and looking for work in the past

Data from Elbogen EB, Johnson SC. The intricate link between violence and mental disorder: results from the national epidemiologic survey on alcohol and related conditions. Arch Gen Psychiatry 2009;66:152–61.

The symptoms of acute cocaine intoxication include tachycardia, hypertension, and agitation.

Restraints: A High-risk Procedure for Both Patients and Staff

Indications and legal issues

Patients, such as the one in the vignette four, are unlikely to respond to verbal de-escalation techniques and require restraints. Physical and chemical restraints should be applied in situations when there is imminent risk that patients may harm others or may put themselves at risk of physical injury or delayed diagnosis and treatment. It is inappropriate and illegal to use restraints for punishment, retribution, coercion, or convenience.[22] The emergency physician must approach the decision to use restraints in a manner similar to that used with other therapeutics and carefully weigh the risks and benefits.

The 1982 Supreme Court case of *Youngberg v Romero* set the precedent that a physician may legally place a patient in restraints, imposing on their civil liberties, if that patient poses a risk to themselves or others. The Joint Commission published clear guidelines regarding the monitoring, documentation, and application of restraint.[23] The protection of the patient's rights, dignity, and well-being is of utmost importance. Practitioners must know their individual institution's policies.

High risk: Lack of Documentation Regarding the Initial and Continued Need for Patient Restraint and Continuous Patient Assessment

Although physicians may legally restrain patients if the appropriate indications arise, there are specific documentation and care requirements associated with restraint use. Both nurses and physicians must document the use of restraints, similar to the way they document other invasive procedures. A time-limited order for restraints must be on the chart before or shortly after restraints are applied. Chart documentation should be specific about the patient's presentation and reason for restraint, including the potential danger to the patient or others, the plan of care, and an assessment of the patient's decision-making capacity. Competent patients have the right to refuse restraints, as they may any medical treatment; the application of restraints is limited to those who lack judgment.[24] Standing orders or "as needed" PRN orders must never be issued. The Joint Commission outlines these time limitations for restraint orders: 4 hours for adults age 18 and over, 2 hours for adolescents ages 9 to 17, and 1 hour for children under age 9. They can be renewed, however, up to 24 hours.[23]

Nursing notes should indicate any injuries associated with the application of restraint; frequent reassessment of the patient's condition including vital signs, medical, and behavioral status; and the readiness for discontinuation of the restraint.

Physical Restraints

Systematic, consistent, protocol-driven, and practiced techniques best achieve safe application of physical restraints. Whenever possible, the physician should not participate in restraint placement to preserve the physician-patient relationship. The restraint team should ideally consist of at least five trained members, with an experienced leader. After the team is assembled, they should enter the room in unison as a show of force and tell the patient why restraints are to be placed. The leader should move to the head of the bed, with the remaining four members each taking a limb. Fast application is best. While the leader explains the process to the patient and oversees the team, the limbs are immobilized.

The selection of restraint type and position should be individualized; it is not necessary to restrain an agitated elderly patient with dementia in the same manner as an aggressive, muscular patient with cocaine intoxication. Only devices specifically designed for restraining patients should be used. A variety of materials exist including polyurethane, polypropylene, leather, and soft cloth; closure is with Velcro or buckles. The type available is often institution specific. Leathers are sturdy and nearly impossible for patients to remove, but the locked buckles preclude rapid release if needed. For elderly patients, padded mitts prevent disruption of devices, such as intravenous lines, and vest and waist posies anchor the patient and prevent wandering. Firm cervical collars may protect thrashing patients from injuring their necks or biting staff and spit masks limit staff exposure to bodily fluids. Avoid the use of makeshift ties out of bedclothes; they have to be applied extremely tightly to function, may tighten further as the patient writhes, and have associated increased risk of iatrogenic harm.

The recommended position for patient restraint has varied over the years. The supine position is the preferred position in the restraint of agitated patients in the ED. It facilitates access to the patient for medical interventions, such as neurologic assessment, intubation, or central line placement, and is the position of choice when cervical spine precautions must be maintained. Side position is useful if the patient has an aspiration risk; consider administering such patients an antiemetic. Two, three, or all four limbs may be immobilized at the major joints (ie, knees and elbows). If only two limbs are tied down, they should be contralateral arms and legs. Ideally, one arm should be tied upward and the other downward. This decreases the amount of force and momentum struggling can generate.

Respiratory compromise in patients who are restrained has been an ongoing concern. The use of hobble restraints (binding the ankles, binding or handcuffing the wrists behind the back, and then attaching the wrists to the ankles) places the patient in the prone position and is associated in rare cases with unexpected death caused by positional asphyxia.[25] One study measured the effect of restraint position (hobble, prone, and supine) on oxygenation and vital signs after exercise to assess their effects on the mechanics of the chest wall. Whereas mean arterial oxygen tension and carbon dioxide tension were unaffected by position, with hobble restraint there were significant decreases in forced vital capacity, forced expiratory volume, and maximal voluntary ventilation when compared with prone and supine positions. All restraints cause a restrictive pattern in pulmonary function tests; however, this difference did not significantly impact subjects' oxygenation or ventilation.[26] This indicates that it is not primarily the patient's position but their comorbidities and state of agitated delirium that predispose to asphyxia and sudden death while restrained. Still, the position used remains a concern. Hobble restraints, the prone position, and restraints that compress the neck or chest wall should not be used.

Potential complications
Physical restraints may cause several complications. The most common is skin breakdown from the site of the restraint, which may have associated neurovascular damage. This is significantly increased in makeshift restraints. Less commonly, patients who continue to struggle may induce rhabdomyolysis, a condition that has the potential to lead to acute renal failure and death.

Several sudden deaths have been reported in patients who are physically restrained, although this is a rare occurrence.[25,26] A review of coroner's records in Ontario from 1988 to 1995 found 21 cases of unexpected death of people with excited delirium who were in physical restraints.[27] Of these, 18 were prone and 3 had pressure on their neck. Eight who were prone also had compression of their chests and two were in hobble restraints. Eight had cocaine-induced delirium but none had lethal levels of cocaine in their system at the time of death. The Hartford Courant published a five-part series investigating restraint-related deaths: from 1988 there were 142 fatalities of which 23 died in a prone position, and 20 died with inadequate reassessment by the staff.[28] One third of deaths were caused by asphyxia and one quarter from cardiac-related causes. Disturbingly, over one quarter were children. In contrast, one observational, prospective study in an adult ED demonstrated a low complication rate of 20 (7%) of 298 with physical restraints.[29] Half of these events were the patients getting out of the restraints. The rest included vomiting, spitting, and increased agitation. Three patients (approximately 1%) injured themselves or others. Nearly 30% required a combination of chemical and physical restraint but this had no impact on the complication rate.

Constant observation and reassessment of a restrained patient is crucial. Unwatched patients have toppled gurneys, vomited and aspirated, and damaged nerves by fighting the restraints. Training staff in signs of patient distress or positional asphyxia and how to alleviate them may decrease these situations and limit patient harm.

Chemical restraints should supplant physical restraints when safety allows. At the earliest safe time, remove restraints (regardless of the order's scheduled expiration time on the chart). Before freeing the patient, delineate the expectations and criteria for keeping off the restraints. The restraints should be removed completely. Some people advocate a stepwise approach of restraint release (eg, removing one arm, then an opposing limb in 5-minute increments with the last two limbs freed concurrently). Patients must, however, never be left alone with incomplete restraints in place.

Psychotic illness

Psychiatric patients are brought to the ED during psychotic episodes. Historical clues that agitation is from a psychiatric rather than organic etiology include a past psychiatric history, and oriented, logical (even if bizarre) thought content. People with severe mental illness, particularly paranoid schizophrenia, mania, and the personality disorders, are more likely to have a history of violence compared with people without severe mental illness; past behavior increases the risk of violent acts in the ED. It is important to recognize that it is the symptoms of mental illness, not the diagnosis itself, which confer the risk of violence. Although violence is elevated somewhat in patients with mental illness, most of these persons do not commit violent acts and when they do, it is often in association with substance abuse, environmental stressors, or a history of violence.[30] Schizophrenic patients can be violent particularly because of paranoid delusions, in which they believe that others want to harm or have harmed them; their psychosis causes them to misinterpret their social surroundings as a threatening environment, and they respond inappropriately with hostile behavior. They may experience command hallucinations. Manic patients are violent because of psychosis or gross disorganization of behavior or thoughts. Their targets of violence are usually random. Persons with antisocial personality disorder may use violence in a way to seek revenge or bolster their images and are rarely remorseful after the attack. Borderline persons can use violence as a form of manipulation or to lash out when they feel they have been rejected or abandoned.

The management of these patients can be complicated if they are noncompliant with treatment and refusing treatment in the ED.

CLINICAL VIGNETTE 5

A 28-year-old woman with a history of schizophrenia is brought in by her brother for increasing paranoid behavior over the last week after stopping her medications 3 weeks ago. She has responded very well to oral antipsychotic medication in the past. Her psychiatrist is willing to admit her to the hospital, but a bed is not ready. She is becoming more agitated but is refusing medication at this time. Her brother asks for her to be medicated.

Is it appropriate to administer psychiatric medications to this patient against her will? Regardless of family requests, the physician should only give such drugs if it is medically warranted. Specific behaviors that are representative of clinically significant agitation and for which intervention should be seriously considered are listed in **Box 3**. If these conditions are not present, other approaches to patient management, such as verbal de-escalation techniques, should be used while waiting for consultation with a psychiatrist. Removing family members to the waiting room may defuse intensifying situations.

Once the physician has decided a medication is indicated, another question must be addressed: do patients have the right to refuse antipsychotics and other treatments? This volatile question has been extensively studied and debated over the past several decades and centers around the often incongruous goals of preserving patient dignity while meeting treatment needs.[31] It remains without a definitive answer partly because of the lack of consistency between the federal and state judiciaries.[31] The US Supreme Court has declined to hear the handful of such cases put forth for consideration so the legal precedents remain from the varied state judiciaries. More recently, the focus on the right of patients to refuse medications has moved from one that was treatment oriented to one that is danger oriented.[32] In this later stance, medications are administered against the patient's will when they are at risk of causing direct harm to themselves or others, or are gravely disabled and unable to care for themselves.

One common belief is that the competent patient should still have the right to deny medication and control what happens to their bodies; however, competence is a legal, not clinical, construct. Medical professionals, especially in a busy emergency room, do not have the luxury of time to obtain legal consultation and must instead evaluate the patient's capacity, which is a clinical determination of the patient's mental functions. Importantly, individuals are not incompetent merely because they have a psychiatric illness. The woman in the previous vignette could be declared competent if she was able to meet four criteria: (1) understand the relevant information communicated by the physician regarding her medical condition including its nature, the recommended treatments, the consequences of not receiving treatment, and possible

---

Box 3
Behaviors in psychiatric patients representative of clinically significant agitation

Explosive or unpredictable anger

Intimidating behavior

Physical agitation, such as pacing

Physical or verbal abuse to self

Hostile verbal behavior

Resistance to care

Impulsiveness, reaction to pain out of proportion or injury or illness

Data from Allen MH, Currier GW, Carpenter D, et al. The expert consensus guideline series. Treatment of behavioral emergencies. J Psychiatric Pract 2005;11(Suppl 1):405–25.

alternatives; (2) communicate the treatment choices; (3) appreciate the situation or medical condition and its consequences; and (4) reason about the treatment options with rational manipulation of the relevant information (eg, comparing the options and offering reasons why she prefers one treatment option over another).[33] If found incompetent, then a surrogate decision-maker should be obtained (in this case, likely her brother unless other family or guardians are present).

Once the decision is made to medicate psychotic agitation, there are several different chemical restraints available for use.

Chemical Restraints

High risk: the ED physician must tailor pharmacologic treatment to each situation
Chemical restraints are used to decrease anxiety and discomfort, minimize disruptive behavior, prevent escalation of behavior, and aid in reversing the underlying cause of agitation. Thrashing patients in physical restraints may induce hyperthermia and even rhabdomyolysis; they should be sedated before they injure themselves. Medications may act by treating the psychoses and violence directly; however, more frequently they alleviate the symptoms without addressing the underlying cause, often by increasing inhibitory neuron activity and dampening excitatory neurons. The physician should continue to search for causes of agitation even after a medicated patient is calm.

The ideal chemical restraint has efficacy, rapid onset, and titratability. There are several such drugs available for use in the ED. The physician must have a wide arsenal because each medication has specific indications and complications. For example, haloperidol works nicely at calming an agitated schizophrenic, whereas a benzodiazepine can be more appropriate for a trauma patient with amphetamine intoxication. In general, patients should be asked to voluntarily take these medications before forceful institution. For those refusing, as the psychiatric patient in the last vignette, the intramuscular route is preferred when no intravenous access is available and the patient is uncooperative with taking oral medications. Forcing a pill orally may lead to a human bite injury. One last caveat is never to order any of these medications on an "as needed" basis when used for chemical restraint.

Benzodiazepines

Benzodiazepines, in particular lorazepam and midazolam, are the most widely used sedative hypnotics and a preferred first-line choice for the acute management of agitation caused by sedative-hypnotic drug and ethanol withdrawal, cocaine, and sympathomimetic ingestions and muscle hyperactivity. They cross the blood-brain barrier and bind to γ-aminobutyric acid, the major inhibitory neurotransmitter in the central nervous system, and enhance its inhibitory effects at all levels of the central nervous system including the spinal cord, hypothalamus, hippocampus, substantia nigra, cerebellar cortex, and cerebral cortex. This has a calming influence and a depressant effect on psychomotor and cognitive functions. It acts to slow respirations similarly to that during sleep. Patients experience a relief of anxiety, euphoria, disinhibition, and somnolence. These drugs have a high therapeutic window and good safety profile, which has contributed to their prevalence. Prominent side effects are sedation, hypotension, and respiratory depression, which can be synergistic with alcohol use and other depressants. All benzodiazepines cross the placental barrier and are class D medications; they should be avoided in pregnant women. Violent patients who are oversedated and have marked respiratory depression from benzodiazepine use should have supportive care, including supplemental oxygen. Jaw thrusts, bag-valve mask ventilation, and endotracheal intubation are rarely necessary. Avoid the use of flumazenil because of the frequency of epileptogenic coingestions and use of combination therapy with typical antipsychotics.

Lorazepam is the most frequently used benzodiazepine because it has quick onset, short half-life, and a route of elimination with no active metabolites. It is given in 0.5- to 2-mg increments as frequently as every 15 minutes. It is available in oral, intramuscular, and intravenous formulations. Parenteral administration works within 15 to 30 minutes and lasts over 3 hours.

Midazolam should be considered in patients who need rapid sedation, because its mean time to onset is 18 minutes. Initial dose is 5 mg intramuscularly, repeated every 15 minutes as needed. Its use is limited by its shorter duration, lasting approximately 45 minutes compared with 2 hours for other agents, and increased need for rescue doses.[34] For patients who require brief symptom control, however, this is an excellent alternative and part of many prehospital treatment algorithms.

Antipsychotics

Antipsychotics are a broad group of medications that have varying binding affinities to the dopamine and serotonin receptors in the brain. Butyrophenones (haloperidol and droperidol) are a subtype of phenothiazines or typical antipsychotics. They are considered high-potency typical antipsychotic medications because they have a stronger affinity for the dopamine-2 receptor. They are the main class of typical antipsychotics used in the ED for undifferentiated acute agitation. They are efficacious; easy to use and titrate; have a long history of clinical experience; and are readily available in oral, intramuscular, and intravenous routes.[35] These medications should not be given to patients with a history of Parkinson's disease, allergy to this class, or anticholinergic drug intoxication. More relative contraindications include pregnancy and lactation. Refer to **Table 2** for appropriate dosage and pharmacokinetics.

Haloperidol remains the most widely administered antipsychotic medication in the ED because of its high effectiveness and relatively low cost. Two review articles summarized the extensive evidence base for its use in treating agitation.[36,37] For most patients, the initial dose is 5 to 10 mg and may be repeated every 30 minutes. It is quite rare for patients to require more than three doses to achieve sedation. The dose should be decreased in elderly patients. There are oral, intramuscular, and intravenous formulations; the intravenous form is not approved by the Food and Drug Administration (FDA), although it is commonly administered by this route.

Although its use has dramatically decreased since the controversial 2001 FDA "black box" warning (see later), droperidol has a shorter half-life than haloperidol, a more rapid onset of action, absence of long-term side effects, potent sedative properties without long-term cognitive impairments, and is generally as effective for controlling aggressive and disruptive behavior in psychiatric patients.[38] A randomized, double-blind trial with 68 patients requiring chemical adjuncts to physical restraints found that in equal doses intramuscular droperidol has more rapid control of patients than haloperidol.[38] There was no significant difference in the two drugs when given intravenously. The intramuscular dose is 5 to 10 mg and the intravenous dose is 2.5 to 5 mg every 15 minutes as needed. The American College of Emergency Physicians issued a class B recommendation for the use of droperidol over haloperidol in patients requiring rapid sedation.[39]

Atypical antipsychotics include clozapine, olanzapine, ziprasidone, risperidone, aripiprazole, and quetiapine. They have various mechanisms of action to treat schizophrenia's negative symptoms (poverty of thought, withdrawal, and poor motivation) and positive symptoms (psychoses and hallucinations). When compared with the phenothiazines, these newer neuroleptics all have a lower affinity and more selective

Table 2
Medications available for use in chemical restraints[a]

Medication	Dose	Time of Onset	Half-Life	Contraindications
Benzodiazepines				
Diazepam	5–10 mg PO 2–10 mg IM/IV repeat q 3–4 h PRN	1–2 h PO 20–30 min IM	30–60 h	Liver disease Pregnancy
Lorazepam	1–2 mg PO 0.5–2 mg IM <2 mg/min IV	16 h PO 20–30 min IM 5–20 min IV	~14 h PO (end-stage renal disease 30–70 h)	Sleep apnea Severe renal impairment Avoid in pregnancy
Midazolam	5–15 mg IM q 15 min 1–2 mg IV q 2–3 min 1 mg IV (geriatric)	15–20 min IM 1–5 min IV	2–6 h (13 h in renal failure)	Pregnancy
Phenothiazines (typical antipsychotics)				
Haloperidol	5–10 mg PO 5–10 mg IM 1–2 mg IV	2–6 h PO 30–60 min IM/IV	12–18 h	Movement disorder Severe liver disease Breast Feeding
Droperidol	0.625–1.25 mg IM/slow IV q 3–4 h; max of 2.5 mg each dose	30 min IV	2–4 h	Prolonged QTc Caution in alcoholics
Atypical antipsychotics				
Risperidone	1–3 mg PO	30–60 min	20 h	Caution in dementia
Olanzapine	10–20 mg PO 5–10 mg IM q 4 h 5 mg IM (geriatric) Max: 30 mg/24 h	5–8 h PO 15–45 min IM	20–5 h	Prolonged QTc Recent myocardial infarction Diabetes mellitus Elderly (use with caution)
Ziprasidone	10 mg IM q 2 h or 20 mg IM q 4 h Replace with oral as soon as possible	4–5 h PO 60 min IM	14 h PO 4–10 h IM	Prolonged QTc Recent myocardial infarction Diabetes mellitus Elderly (use with caution)
Ketamine	1 mg/kg IV 4–5 mg/kg IM	1 min IV 4–5 min IM	15 min IV 30–60 min IM	Heart disease

Abbreviations: IM, intramuscularly; IV, intravenously.
[a] History of hypersensitivity to a specific agent is a contraindication to use.

antagonism for the dopamine-2–dopaminergic receptors in the mesolimbic rather than nigrostriatal pathways in the brain and block serotonergic $5\text{-}HT_{1A}$ and $5\text{-}HT_{2A}$ receptors. This provides more tranquilization than sedation. Their use is increasing as first-line treatment in the psychiatric setting and ED, and they were given a class B recommendation for such use by the American College of Emergency Physicians.[39] Several medications are available in intramuscular or rapidly absorbable formulations. The use of oral medications facilitates transition to outpatient therapy.

Risperidone is equivalent to haloperidol for the treatment of psychosis, although its use in the acute setting is constrained by its lack of an intramuscular formulation. Olanzapine is approved for the treatment of acute agitation in schizophrenic and bipolar-manic patients. It is available in intramuscular or oral formations at 5 to 10 mg. The oral tablet is rapidly dissolving and an excellent way to medicate cooperative patients. It is strongly sedating, with over 150 times the antihistamine potency of diphenhydramine. Studies on the efficacy of intramuscular olanzapine versus haloperidol found no difference in the requirements for repeat doses or lack of response at 2 hours. Olanzapine has the least effect on the QTc interval of the antipsychotics.[40] There were less extrapyramidal side effects and need for anticholinergic treatment in those given olanzapine. There are several relative contraindications to its use, most notably patients who are elderly (increased risk of death caused by cardiovascular events); predisposed to hypotension; have narrow angle glaucoma (exacerbated by anticholinergic effects); and those with diabetes mellitus. Aripiprazole and ziprasidone stabilize the dopamine system with an agonist-antagonist effect at varied dopamine receptors throughout the brain. Ziprasidone is approved for the treatment of acute agitation in schizophrenic and bipolar-manic patients. It has not been extensively studied in patients with acute undifferentiated agitation in the ED, although it is increasingly given for this indication. It may be administered at 10 mg intramuscularly every 2 hours or 20 mg intramuscularly every 4 hours. The oral formulation has equivalent doses and should replace intramuscular therapy as soon as possible. A double-blind randomized trial that compared ziprasidone with midazolam and droperidol in the treatment for acute undifferentiated agitation found that there was a greater rate of persistent agitation at 15 minutes in patient given ziprasidone, and after effect onset it resulted in deeper sedation.[34] Further research into the use of these atypical antipsychotics for violent and agitated patients is warranted.

Antipsychotic side effects
There are several adverse reactions that may occur after use of antipsychotic agents. See **Table 2** for an overview of reactions and their treatments.

Movement disorders, tardive dyskinesias, and extrapyramidal symptoms are the most common and troubling side effects of the antipsychotics and may limit use. They occur more frequently in people treated with typical rather than atypical medications. These reactions happen in less than 10% of patients within 24 hours of ED care. Even one dose may trigger acute dystonic reactions that include torticollis; jaw, tongue, lip, and throat spasms; laryngeal dystonia; oculogyric crisis; and facial grimacing. Most of these short-term side effects are easily treated with benztropine mesylate, 1 to 2 mg intravenously or intramuscularly, or diphenhydramine, 1 mg/kg intravenously or intramuscularly. Relief is rapid and dramatic in most cases. Importantly, patients should be discharged on several days of the oral formulation of these medications to prevent return of the dystonia. Therapy with high doses of antidote can paradoxically worsen agitation, probably because of worsened akathesias.

More serious reactions include the neuroleptic malignant syndrome of autonomic instability. Signs and symptoms of this potentially fatal disorder include tachycardia, hyperthermia, altered mental status, and muscle rigidity. Death and critical illness may result from ensuing severe hyperthermia. This was observed after a single intramuscular dose of haloperidol in one ED patient.[41] Prompt treatment includes immediate cessation of the neuroleptic along with cooling measures, benzodiazepines, and dantrolene.

Additionally, all antipsychotics can have cardiotoxic actions, including prolongation of the QTc interval, which predisposes to torsades de pointes and other ventricular tachyarrhythmias.[42] Droperidol in particular has received particular attention to the concern of QTc prolongation. The medication was removed from European pharmacies and a controversial black box warning was issued by the FDA addressing this side effect. Anesthesiologists examining whether droperidol prolonged the QTc and caused torsades gave this medication to 16,791 patients; none developed torsades.[43] Another group of 12,000 patients, this time from the ED, received droperidol without any dysrhythmic events.[44] Along with other smaller studies, these reports indicate that this black box warning may be excessive and warrants re-evaluation. The risk of torsades was previously thought to be lower with atypical than typical antipsychotics; however, a retrospective cohort study reported that the risk of sudden cardiac death is essentially identical in users of either type of drug.[45] Both groups had twice the rate of sudden death than nonusers, with a dose-dependent increase in risk. Most of these patients were taking these medications for long-term behavioral treatment. If torsades occurs, the treatment is intravenous magnesium, increase of the heart rate with pacing or chronotropic agents, or defibrillation when unstable.

Some side effects are specific to the atypical antipsychotics. They have a propensity to cause hypotension and hemodynamic instability and should be avoided in patients with severe alcohol intoxication or who received a benzodiazepine less than 1-hour prior. This reaction usually responds with fluid, but vasopressors may be necessary in severe cases. Preferably, a peripheral α-agonist, such as phenylephrine, should be used. They all have the propensity to prolong the QTc and predispose to cardiac arrhythmias. Olanzapine, clozapine, and quetiapine have produced life-threatening hyperglycemia and diabetic ketoacidosis (DKA) in a small subset of patients. This risk is greatly increased in those who have diabetes mellitus.

Combination therapy

There are several studies comparing combination use of benzodiazepines and antipsychotics with either drug alone. Most have supported that dual use achieves more rapid sedation with lower incidence of side effects; this combination therapy is a class B recommendation for the treatment of acutely agitated patients from the American College of Emergency Physicians.[39,46,47] In an inpatient psychiatry unit, the combination of lorazepam, 2 mg, and haloperidol, 5 mg, was more efficacious than solo agent administration.[47] Similar results were published in an ED setting, with better control at 1 hour in patients given a benzodiazepine and haloperidol together.[46] Of note, it is unclear whether the combination is superior to equivalent dosages of the single drug because the researchers were reluctant to give higher doses of a benzodiazepine at once.

CLINICAL VIGNETTE 6

At change of shift, your partner signs out a 58-year-old man with severe schizophrenia and chronic obstructive pulmonary disease brought from a locked psychiatric facility after a mechanical fall with a forehead contusion and nasal fracture. The decision was made to image the patient looking for evidence of TBI. The patient is sedated with haloperidol and lorazepam for a CT scan, which shows no evidence of TBI. It is now

4 hours later and the patient is not waking up. You obtain a arterial blood gases and the P_{CO_2} is 115.

High risk: Agitated Patients with Medical Comorbidities

Patients with medical comorbidities, especially those involving the cardiopulmonary systems, have an increased risk of serious side effects including respiratory depression during procedural sedation. The severe airway complication in the prior vignette was missed because of inappropriate reassessment. An excellent noninvasive monitoring technique increasingly available in EDs is the end-tidal carbon dioxide monitor. This device measures the partial pressure of CO_2 in each expired breath. When displayed in graphical form it is called a "capnograph." Previously used primarily in intubated patients, several reports have supported its role as an aid in evaluating the ventilatory sufficiency of spontaneously breathing patients.[17] It can rapidly identify many complications of procedural sedation including apnea, laryngospasm, bronchospasm, upper airway obstruction, and respiratory depression. Rising values on the capnograph, especially a CO_2 level greater than 50 mm Hg, herald development of airway complications before clinically observed hypoventilation. Furthermore, levels above 70 mm Hg indicate almost complete ventilatory failure. A full discussion of capnography is beyond the scope of this article and has been published previously.[17]

For all these reasons, end-tidal CO_2 monitors should be used in all patients given sedating medications for procedural sedation or analgesia especially if medical comorbidities are present to prevent adverse outcomes.

CLINICAL VIGNETTE 7

A 14-year-old boy is brought in to the ED after threatening his mother with a knife. He has been acting strangely over the last 2 weeks according to his brother. He is starting to pace around the room and knock supplies out of their containers.

The Violent Pediatric Patient

Children and adolescents who are agitated, psychotic, or violent present at significantly lower rates than adults. Nevertheless, the prevalence of these behavioral emergencies in this younger population is increasing with pediatric illicit drug use. It can be highly upsetting for patients, parents, and medical providers. Despite this, agitation must be treated as swiftly in children as in adult counterparts. Physicians must be facile with the indications for and use of restraints in this population and be comfortable with their use. The child and the parents should be informed before the institution of restraints. Chemical restraint may also be needed, but when possible, it is prudent to discuss this possibility with parents.

Studies on the use of chemical restraints in children are sparse, particularly with regard to the newer atypical antipsychotics. Most of the dosages and side effects are extrapolated from adult studies and clinical observation. Thankfully, this need is exceedingly rare in preadolescents because other methods of calming children typically succeed.

As in adults, antipsychotics and benzodiazepines are commonly used. The Phenothiazines remain favored over newer antipsychotics, because the safety of the atypical agents in pediatric patients is unknown. Children who receive droperidol for aggressive behavior are frequently able to re-engage in daily activities within 2 hours with no untoward side effects. One dosing regimen is as follows: the dosing for haloperidol differs from that of adults in children 6 to 12 years old. Patients in this age group may receive an initial intramuscular dose of 0.025 to 0.075 mg/kg/dose (maximum 2.5 mg), with a repeated dose in 1 hour as needed. Children above 12 years of age may receive adult doses. The typical dose of lorazepam is 0.5 to 2 mg, or 0.05 to 0.1 mg/kg/dose.

Risperidone is approved for the treatment of adolescent schizophrenia, manic episodes in children with bipolar disorder in ages 10 to 17, and for irritability in autistic children ages 5 to 16. Risperidone comes in an oral solution and oral disintegrating tablet. Start with a dose of 0.5 mg orally. Note that the oral solution is not compatible with cola or tea.

Recurrent visits to the ED for psychiatric or behavioral problems has been shown to be associated with violence, both as a homicide victim or perpetrator.[48] Intervention and mentoring programs can modify the future behaviors and injury rates of violent individuals, particularly those under age 25, presenting to the ED.[49,50] Tragically, this opportunity is frequently missed. A Toronto-based study noted that most adolescents are discharged directly from EDs without any intervention.[51]

CLINICAL VIGNETTE 8

An 87-year-old man is found wandering in the street unable to give police his address. He is wearing a Medic-Alert bracelet indicating he has Alzheimer's dementia. The social worker has contacted his family, but they will not be in for 2 hours. The patient is becoming increasingly agitated with yelling and attempts to get out of the bed.

The Agitated Geriatric Patient

Elderly patients predisposed to dementia-related agitation may manifest these symptoms on arrival, or the symptoms can be unmasked and exacerbated by the unfamiliar ED environment. The hospital lacks familiar cues and is stimulating. When agitated, these patients may unwittingly harm themselves by pulling intravenous lines or falling from the bed, or may hurt caregivers by lashing out and gripping. Providing a quiet environment and redirecting distressed patients are highly effective, but may not be sufficient. Medicating agitated geriatric patients, who frequently have dementia, is a challenge. These elderly patients have a greater risk of adverse reactions because of their extensive medications, coexistence of chronic illness, different physiologic responses to drugs, and baseline altered pharmacokinetics from drug absorption to metabolism to excretion. Additionally, psychotropic medications are increasingly found to have specific risks in patients with dementia.

Antipsychotics are effective in treating psychotic symptoms of delusions and hallucinations and nonpsychotic agitation (frequently dementia related) in this population. One meta-analysis of randomized trials found a small increased risk of death in elderly patients with dementia-related behavioral disorders given an atypical antipsychotic compared with placebo primarily through an increased risk of sudden cardiac events, rapid cognitive decline, and strokes.[52] Subsequently, the FDA issued a black box warning for atypical psychotics use in geriatric patients, citing this increased risk of mortality.[53] More research has suggested that typical antipsychotics carry equivalent rates of deadly adverse reactions and should not be administered in lieu of the atypical agents in this population.[54] Of note, medications in these trials were given for several months; there are no studies examining the risk of death in elderly patients treated acutely in the ED. Risperidone and olanzapine have the best evidence for efficacy over other psychotropics, but carry the same risk of adverse events.[55] Elderly patients may be chemically restrained with antipsychotics if there is sufficient need, but the practitioner should be aware of these risks and use these agents only when absolutely necessary.

With advancing patient age, the pharmacokinetics and pharmacodynamics of benzodiazepine metabolism changes: brain receptors become more sensitive, and distribution and elimination of these agents is altered. This is particularly true of the benzodiazepines, such as chlordiazepoxide and diazepam, which are metabolized by the hepatic oxidative pathways. The P-450 cytochromes break down these compounds more slowly, leading to their longer accumulation in the body. Lorazepam is not metabolized in this manner, and its pharmacokinetics is less altered by age and is a safer choice in this population. Its shorter half-life offers dosage flexibility. Midazolam has a rapid onset and short half-life; the liquid oral formulation may be used in patients who ingest it willingly and ably. It can facilitate care in demented patients who must undergo diagnostic testing or procedures.

CLINICAL VIGNETTE 9

A 25-year-old man is found minimally arousal on a bus stop bench with an empty alcohol bottle in hand and brought for medical evaluation. The patient has normal vital signs, wakes to sternal rub to give his name, and has no signs of trauma. He is placed in a gown, and after thorough examination is placed in the hallway near the nursing station on monitor for observation. After nearly 2 hours, the patient wakes, is oriented but still obviously intoxicated, and gets up from his gurney. He stumbles upright with his gown falling off his body, requests his belongings, and reports he is ready for discharge.

High Risk: Discharging Intoxicated Patients Prematurely

A significant portion of ED visits are caused by alcohol-related diseases or injuries, comprising almost 8% of visits between 1992 and 2000.[56] That number has only increased in recent years. Alcohol may impair the evaluation, treatment, and disposition of patients. This is not solely caused by increased disinhibition and violence. It may also mask symptoms of underlying medical problems that emerge once the substance metabolizes. It is crucial to observe the intoxicated patient for resolution of any abnormal behaviors once sober and document the reassessment in the chart. Vital signs should be checked frequently and patients should not be released unless these values are within normal limits. Patients in significant alcohol withdrawal (extreme psychomotor agitation, tachycardia, tremors, and hallucinations) need admission.

It may seem easier to discharge patients who vocally demand their release. The emergency physician may be held responsible for events occurring outside the hospital, however, if an intoxicated patient harms another person or himself. Factors that must be evaluated before discharging an intoxicated patient include competency, suicidality, and homicidality. The determination of a patient's decision-making capacity is discussed previously. Alcohol abuse is a significant risk factor for both suicide and homicide. Approximately half of people who commit suicide are intoxicated at the time.[57] Often, such thoughts clear when the intoxication clears. If homicidal or suicidal ideations are expressed and persist, however, a psychologist or psychiatrist should be consulted and the patient held for appropriate evaluation.

If the patient is deemed appropriate for discharge, physicians should briefly offer information about local detoxification programs and further medical care. Although lack of time in a busy department is a hurdle, such interventions are efficacious. As little as 4 minutes of advice has been shown to be valuable to patients. It is hoped that such interventions will work to decrease emergency physicians' perception of lack of time as a barrier to provide information about detoxification programs and further medical care. Healthy people 2010 aims to reduce alcohol-related ED visits and in conjunction with the Society for Academic Emergency Medicine Substance Abuse Task Force recommends that each ED have a referral system for substance abusers. This system should include a list of easily accessed community organizations (ie, Alcoholics Anonymous) and treatment centers.[58]

SUMMARY

The vignettes throughout this article highlight the myriad of patients who can present to the ED with agitated or violent behavior. Providers must be facile at quickly identifying causes of and treating such behavior, and at preventing escalation, while protecting themselves and other ED personnel. Interview techniques, physical restraints, and a variety of chemicals are available for use when necessary. Although there are precedents that endow providers with the legal right to restrain dangerous patients, it is the responsibility of all emergency providers to know the latest regulations and ensure correct documentation.

REFERENCES

1. Larkin GL, Claassen CA, Emond JA, et al. Trends in U.S. emergency department visits for mental health conditions, 1992 to 2001. Psychiatr Serv 2005;56(6): 671–7.
2. Jenkins MG, Rocke LG, McNicholl BP, et al. Violence and verbal abuse against staff in accident and emergency departments: a survey of consultants in the UK and the Republic of Ireland. J Accid Emerg Med 1998;15(4):262–5.
3. Gerberich SG, Church TR, McGovern PM, et al. Risk factors for work-related assaults on nurses. Epidemiology 2005;16:704–9.
4. Lavoie FW, Carter GL, Danzl DF, et al. Emergency department violence in United States teaching hospitals. Ann Emerg Med 1988;17(11):1227–33.
5. Kowalenko T, Walters BL, Khare RK, et al. Workplace violence: a survey of emergency physicians in the state of Michigan. Ann Emerg Med 2005;46(2):142–7.
6. Lavoie FW. Violence in emergency facilities. Acad Emerg Med 1994;1(2):166–8.
7. Casteel C, Peek-Asa C, Nocera M, et al. Hospital employee assault rates before and after enactment of the California hospital safety and security act. Ann Epidemiol 2009;19(2):125–33.
8. Rankins RC, Hendey GW. Effect of a security system on violent incidents and hidden weapons in the emergency departments. Ann Emerg Med 1999;33(6):676–9.
9. Ordog GJ, Wasserberger J, Ordog C, et al. Weapon carriage among major trauma victims in the emergency department. Acad Emerg Med 1995;2(2):109–14.
10. Tintinalli J, Peacock F, Wright M. Emergency medical evaluation of psychiatric patients. Ann Emerg Med 1994;23(4):859–62.
11. Olmedo R. Phencyclidine and ketamine. In: Flomenbaum NE, Goldfrank LR, Hoffman RS, et al, editors. Goldfrank's toxicologic emergencies. New York: McGraw-Hill; 2002. p. 1034–45.
12. Guldner GT, Petinaux B, Clemens P, et al. Ketamine for procedural sedation and analgesia by nonanesthesiologists in the field: a review for military health care providers. Mil Med 2006;1171:484–90.
13. Green S. Ketamine sedation for pediatric procedures: part 2, review and implications. Ann Emerg Med 1990;19:1024–32.
14. Svenson JE, Abernathy MK. Ketamine for prehospital use: new look at an old drug. Am J Emerg Med 2007;25(8):977–80.
15. Melamed E, Oron Y, Ben-Avraham R, et al. The combative multitrauma patient: a protocol for prehospital management. Eur J Emerg Med 2007;14(5):265–86.

16. Miner JR, Heegaard W, Plummer D. End-tidal carbon dioxide monitoring during procedural sedation. Acad Emerg Med 2002;9(4):275–80.
17. Krauss B, Hess DR. Capnography for procedural sedation and analgesia in the emergency department. Ann Emerg Med 2007;50(2):172–81.
18. Cordell WH, Keene KK, Giles BK, et al. The high prevalence of pain in emergency medical care. Am J Emerg Med 2002;20(3):165–9.
19. Wilson J, Pendleton J. Oligoanalgesia in the emergency department. Am J Emerg Med 1989;7(6):620–3.
20. Elbogen EB, Johnson SC. The intricate link between violence and mental disorder: results from the national epidemiologic survey on alcohol and related conditions. Arch Gen Psychiatry 2009;66(2):152–61.
21. Dawe S, Davis P, Lapworth K, et al. Mechanisms underlying aggressive and hostile behavior in amphetamine users. Curr Opin Psychiatry 2009;22(3):269–73.
22. Stretesky PB. National case-control study of homicide offending and methamphetamine use. J Interpers Violence 2008;24(6):911–24.
23. Centers for Medicare & Medicaid Services (CMS), Department of Health and Human Services (DHHS). Medicare and Medicaid programs; hospital conditions of participation: patients' rights. Final rule. Fed Regist 2006;71(236):71377–428.
24. Joint Commission. Available at: http://www.jointcommission.org/Standards/. Accessed April 12, 2009.
25. Annas GJ. The last resort: the use of physical restraints in medical emergencies. N Engl J Med 1999;341(18):1408–12.
26. Stratton SJ, Rogers C, Green K. Sudden death in individuals in hobble restraints during paramedic transport. Ann Emerg Med 1995;25(5):710–2.
27. Chan TC, Vilke GM, Neuman T, et al. Restraint position and positional asphyxia. Ann Emerg Med 1997;30(5):578–86.
28. Pollanen MS, Chiasson DA, Cairns TJ, et al. Unexpected death related to restraint for excited delirium: a retrospective study of deaths in police custody and in the community. CMAJ 1998;158(12):1603–7.
29. Weiss E. Deadly restraint: a Hartford Courant investigative report. Hartford (CT): The Hartford Courant; 1998.
30. Zun LS. A prospective study of the complication rate of use of patient restraint in the emergency department. J Emerg Med 2003;24(2):119–24.
31. Perlin ML. Decoding right to refuse treatment law. Int J Law Psychiatry 1993; 16(1–2):151–77.
32. Appelbaum P. The right to refuse treatment with antipsychotic medications: retrospect and prospect. Am J Psychiatry 1988;145(4):413–9.
33. Appelbaum PS. Assessment of patients' competence to consent to treatment. N Engl J Med 2007;357(18):1834–40.
34. Martel M, Sterzinger Ä, Miner J, et al. Management of acute undifferentiated agitation in the emergency department: a randomized double-blind trial of droperidol, ziprasidone, and midazolam. Acad Emerg Med 2005;12(12):1167–72.
35. Buckley P. The role of typical and atypical antipsychotic medications in the management of agitation and aggression. J Clin Psychiatry 1999;60(Suppl 10): 52–60.
36. Yildiz A, Sachs GS, Turgay A. Pharmacological management of agitation in emergency settings. Emerg Med J 2003;20(4):339–46.
37. Allen M. Managing the agitated psychotic patient: a reappraisal of the evidence. J Clin Psychiatry 2000;61:11–20.
38. Thomas JH, Schwartz E, Petrilli R. Droperidol versus haloperidol for chemical restraint of agitated and combative patients. Ann Emerg Med 1992;21(4):407–13.

39. Lukens TW, Wolf S, Edlow JA, et al. Clinical policy: critical issues in the diagnosis and management of the adult psychiatric patient in the emergency department. Ann Emerg Med 2006;47(1):79–99.
40. Konikoff F, Kuitzky A, Jerushalmi T, et al. Neuroleptic malignant syndrome induced by a single injection of haloperidol [letter]. Br Med J 1984;289:1228–9.
41. Mehta D, Mehta S, Petit J, et al. Cardiac arrhythmia and haloperidol. Am J Psychiatry 1979;136:1468–9.
42. Nuttall GA, Eckerman KM, Jacob KA, et al. Does low-dose droperidol administration increase the risk of drug-induced QT prolongation and torsade de pointes in the general surgical population? Anesthesiology 2007;107(4):531–6.
43. Shale JH, Shale CM, Mastin WD. A review of the safety and efficacy of droperidol for the rapid sedation of severely agitated and violent patients. J Clin Psychiatry 2003;64(5):500–5.
44. Ray WA, Chung CP, Murray KT, et al. Atypical antipsychotic drugs and the risk of sudden cardiac death. N Engl J Med 2009;360(3):225–35.
45. Battaglia J, Moss S, Rush J, et al. Haloperidol, lorazepam, or both for psychotic agitation? A multicenter, prospective, double-blind, emergency department study. Am J Emerg Med 1997;15(4):335–40.
46. Garza-Trevino ES, Hollister LE, Overall JE, et al. Efficacy of combinations of intramuscular antipsychotics and sedative- hypnotics for control of psychotic agitation. Am J Psychiatry 1989;146(12):1598–601.
47. Crandall CS, Jost PF, Broidy LM, et al. Previous emergency department use among homicide victims and offenders: a case-control study. Ann Emerg Med 2004;44(6):646–55.
48. Zun LS, Downey L, Rosen J. The effectiveness of an ED-based violence prevention program. Am J Emerg Med 2006;24(1):8–13.
49. Zun LS, Downey LV, Rosen J. Violence prevention in the ED: linkage of the ED to a social service agency. Am J Emerg Med 2003;21(6):454–7.
50. Snider C, Lee J. Emergency department dispositions among 4100 youth injured by violence: a population-based study. CJEM 2007;9(3):164–9.
51. Schneider LS, Dagerman KS, Insel P. Risk of death with atypical antipsychotic drug treatment for dementia: meta-analysis of randomized placebo-controlled trials. JAMA 2005;294(15):1934–43.
52. Advisory UFaDAPH. Death with antipsychotics in elderly patients with behavioral disturbance. Available at: http://www.fda.gov/cder/drug/advisory/antipsychotics.htm. Accessed April 1, 2009.
53. Wang PS, Schneeweiss S, Avorn J, et al. Risk of death in elderly users of conventional vs. atypical antipsychotic medications. N Engl J Med 2005;353(22):2335–41.
54. Sink K, Holden K, Yaffe K. Pharmacological treatment of neuropsychiatric symptoms of dementia: a review of the evidence. JAMA 2005;293:596–608.
55. McDonald AJ III, Wang N, Camargo CA Jr. US emergency department visits for alcohol-related diseases and injuries between 1992 and 2000. Arch Intern Med 2004;164(5):531–7.
56. Mental health and suicide facts. 2004. Available at: http://www.hentalhealth.org/suicideprevention/suicidefacts.asp. Accessed May 15, 2009.
57. D'Onofrio G, Bernstein E, Bernstein J, et al. Patients with alcohol problems in the emergency department, part 2: intervention and referral. Acad Emerg Med 1998;5(12):1210–7.
58. Haddad PM, Sharma SG. Adverse effects of atypical antipsychotics: differential risk and clinical implications. CNS Drugs 2007;21(11):911–36.

Index

Note: Page numbers of article titles are in **boldface** type.

Emerg Med Clin N Am 28 (2010) 257–263
doi:10.1016/S0733-8627(09)00147-3
0733-8627/09/$ – see front matter © 2010 Elsevier Inc. All rights reserved.

emed.theclinics.com

Moving?

Make sure your subscription moves with you!

To notify us of your new address, find your **Clinics Account Number** (located on your mailing label above your name), and contact customer service at:

Email: journalscustomerservice-usa@elsevier.com

800-654-2452 (subscribers in the U.S. & Canada)
314-447-8871 (subscribers outside of the U.S. & Canada)

Fax number: 314-447-8029

Elsevier Health Sciences Division
Subscription Customer Service
3251 Riverport Lane
Maryland Heights, MO 63043

*To ensure uninterrupted delivery of your subscription, please notify us at least 4 weeks in advance of move.

Printed and bound by CPI Group (UK) Ltd, Croydon, CR0 4YY

03/10/2024

01040450-0008